T0092193

OUR NHS

OUR NHS

A HISTORY OF BRITAIN'S BEST-LOVED INSTITUTION

ANDREW SEATON

YALE UNIVERSITY PRESS
NEW HAVEN AND LONDON

For information about this and other Yale University Press publications, please contact:
U.S. Office: sales.press@yale.edu yalebooks.com
Europe Office: sales@yaleup.co.uk yalebooks.co.uk

Set in Adobe Garamond Pro by IDSUK (DataConnection) Ltd
Printed in Great Britain by TJ Books, Padstow, Cornwall

Library of Congress Control Number: 2023931523

ISBN 978-0-300-26827-0

A catalogue record for this book is available from the British Library.

10 9 8 7 6 5 4 3 2 1

For my parents, Linda Seaton and John Seaton

CONTENTS

ILLUSTRATIONS

IN TEXT

PLATES

ABBREVIATIONS

ABLC	Association of British Launderers and Caterers
AHA	Area Health Authority
AMA	American Medical Association
AMI	American Medical International
BBC	British Broadcasting Corporation
BIPO	British Institute of Public Opinion
BIS	British Information Services
BMA	British Medical Association
BUPA	British United Provident Association
CCG	Clinical Commissioning Group
CHGEM	Community Health Group for Ethic Minorities
CHP	Community Health Partnerships
CNH	Committee for the Nation's Health
COHSE	Confederation of Health Service Employees
CPRS	Central Policy Review Staff
CPS	Centre for Policy Studies
DH	Department of Health
DHSS	Department of Health and Social Security
EMS	Emergency Medical Service
EU	European Union
FFM	Fellowship for Freedom in Medicine
GDP	Gross Domestic Product
GP	General Practitioner

HCA	Hospital Corporation of America
IEA	Institute of Economic Affairs
IMF	International Monetary Fund
ITV	Independent Television
LCC	London County Council
LIFT	Local Improvement Finance Trust
LSE	The London School of Economics
NALGO	National Association for Local Government
NHS	National Health Service
NICE	National Institute of Clinical Excellence
NPM	New Public Management
NUPE	National Union of Public Employees
ODA	Overseas Doctors Association
OHE	Office of Health Economics
OPEC	Organization of the Petroleum Exporting Countries
PEP	Political and Economic Planning
PFI	Private Finance Initiative
PPE	Personal Protective Equipment
PPP	Private Patients Plan
RAWP	Resource Allocation Working Party
RCN	Royal College of Nursing
RHB	Regional Hospital Board
SMA	Socialist Medical Association
TUC	Trades Union Congress
WHO	World Health Organization
WPA	Western Provident Association

PREFACE

Like almost all people born in Britain, I was delivered by someone working for the National Health Service (NHS). Growing up, I had an extensive set of connections to the service that were far from unique. My mother worked as a care assistant in a residential home for the elderly, and then as an NHS hospital cleaner. Two of her sisters were nurses. Later, while at home in Exeter during the vacations from my undergraduate degree, I cleaned the wards of that same hospital. One day, while mopping a chiropody unit, I paused and watched from afar as a large digger demolished the ward I had been born in. The buildings changed, yet this thing I knew as 'The NHS' continued. By training, historians are rarely encouraged to place themselves in their research. The pursuit of pure 'objectivity' – in reality, an impossible task – was baked into the discipline's professionalisation during the nineteenth century. Yet, if you grew up in Britain, it is difficult not to relate oneself with the history of the NHS, which, as my own experiences testify, has touched the lives of nearly everyone in the country since its establishment.

The inspiration for this book came from watching the Opening Ceremony of the London Olympic Games in 2012, where the NHS featured prominently. Why, I wondered, was a medical system so important to projections of British identity? And why had the NHS lasted long enough to take on this significance, when other parts of the postwar welfare state or public industries had fallen away? Answering these questions required undertaking research beyond the official records of the Ministry of Health held in the National Archives at Kew, and prompted me to explore a range of local collections, activist archives and personal papers. I trawled through folders of documents, tracked down episodes of long-cancelled television programmes, and pored over piles of photos. The resulting book interrogates the history of what is frequently described today in Britain as 'Our NHS'. It considers the roots of the service, how it modernised and resisted opposition and why it came to take on such prominence. I also discuss the costs of these historical developments. This book is not a mawkish account, driven by 'loving' the NHS. The service was not always supported; it could do harm, and its nationalist framing sometimes excluded people. Nor do I offer a declinist interpretation driven by the latest newspaper headlines. This book is a work of history, not a policy study of the contemporary NHS. The media's focus on 'NHS crisis' – which, of course, stems from real concerns – often obscures the historical picture recounted in these pages, full of surprising continuities or different ruptures than we might expect. I hope I have written a book that does some justice to the significance of this totemic postwar health service and the politics it represents, the people who worked in it and the patients it treated.

ACKNOWLEDGEMENTS

The research for this book began while I completed my doctorate within the Department of History at New York University (NYU). The Remarque Institute, NYU London, NYU Madrid, New York Academy of Medicine, Rockefeller Archive Center and American Philosophical Society (APS) provided much-needed funding or a place to write while I finished my PhD. I am also appreciative of funding provided by the North Atlantic Conference on British Studies (NACBS), Britain and the World, the Society for the Social History of Medicine (SSHM), the 'Cultural History of the NHS' project at the University of Warwick, the 'Waiting Times' project at the University of Exeter and the 'Surgery & Emotion' project at the University of Roehampton to present my work, as well as audiences at the events held by these organisations – among several others – for their feedback. I have been assisted by the archivists, librarians and fellowship coordinators in the many sites I visited, with particular mention to Arlene Shaner at the New York Academy of Medicine and Adrianna Link at the APS. I completed *Our NHS* while a Junior Research Fellow at St Anne's College, University of Oxford. I enjoyed working with many wonderful colleagues at St Anne's, but I particularly want to thank Suzanne Jones, Patrick McGuinness, Tinashe Mushakavanhu, Portia Roelofs, Matthew Leigh, Peter Ghosh and Uta Balbier for their conversation and encouragement. While I was a Junior Research Fellow, the History & Political Economy Project – founded by Christy Thornton and Quinn Slobodian – also provided generous funds to help me finish archival research.

As these names suggest, I would not have completed this book without other people. Perhaps the most important person to thank is Guy Ortolano for his boundless advice and support as my doctoral advisor and beyond. David Edgerton helped me begin my research on the NHS a decade ago at King's College London and he has aided me in thinking through its claims in conversations since. I am grateful to the following people for reading book chapters (or prior versions of them): Peter Baldwin, Olof Bortz, Hilary Buxton, Lila O'Leary Chambers, David Cowan, Jennifer Crane, Aled Davies, Daniel M. Fox, Martin Gorsky, Beatrix Hoffman, Laura King, Julie Livingston, Peter Mandler, Gareth Millward, Martin Moore, Colm Murphy, Susan Pedersen, Sally Sheard, Kyle Shybunko and Rosemary Taylor. As an alumnus of the New York–Cambridge Training Collaboration in Twentieth-Century British History (NYCTC), my research has been enriched by the following colleagues: Alex Campsie, Laura Carter, Sam Coggeshall, David Cowan, Anna K. Danziger Halperin, Lucy Delap, Roslyn Dubler, Freddy Foks, Alice Gorton, Lottie Hoare, Alma Igra, Emily Jones, Jon Lawrence, Lynton Lees, Nicole Longpré, Ellie Lowe, Harry Mace, Peter Mandler, Sarah Mass, Helen McCarthy, Katrina Moseley, Laura Quinton, Emily Rutherford, Abigail Sage, George Severs, Divya Subramanian, Chika Tonooka, Sam Wetherell and Hannah Rose Woods. I am thankful for Aled Davies's thoughts and responses to many annoying email requests for obscure data sets or quotes. The book would not have taken the shape it did without the input and support of Lila O'Leary Chambers. I record my appreciation to Ossie Fernando, Jack Pizzey, June Rosen and Yvette Vanson for speaking with me about their lives and the NHS. Thanks to my editor, Joanna Godfrey, for her enthusiasm for the book and help in shaping it, the rest of the team at Yale University Press, and the anonymous scholars that the press arranged to review the manuscript.

I want to thank the following people for their friendship while writing this book: Jack Allen, Sara Barila, Shilpa Bisaria, Tom Bristow, Hilary Buxton, Lila O'Leary Chambers, Michelle Donnelly, Stephanie Donnelly, Emily Feltham, Orlando Goodall, Matthew L. Jones, Catherine Mas, Jessica Quiason, Daniel Rey, Parijat Samant, Elliot Short,

Kyle Shybunko, Carmen Talbot, Katherine Travers and Tony Wood. Aled Davies and Kate Davies provided laughter during many stays at their home while completing research. Special thanks to Ashish Ravinran and Sam Thypin-Bermeo for their friendship. The memories of the time we spent together in New York will always be with me. Cheers to my brain surgeons – Jafar J. Jafar and James Palmer – for sorting that sticky issue out. I express my love to my family, Jack Seaton, Helen Whitton, Stephen Whitton, Adam Whitton and Nadia Whitton, for all their support. My parents, Linda Seaton and John Seaton, have always believed in me. I dedicate this book to them both.

INTRODUCTION

When June Rosen first met Aneurin Bevan, he was wearing his pyjamas.[1] Just eight years of age, Rosen could not fully grasp her parents' conviction that this man was about to change the lives of 45 million people. All the same, with the Minister of Health staying as a guest in her home, Rosen helped to bring him breakfast in bed. Suffering from a cold, she was instructed to keep her distance. But even from the doorway, Bevan – the Welsh ex-miner and socialist firebrand – impressed with his shock of silver hair. Later that day, Rosen's father – a local Labour councillor – drove their visitor to Park Hospital on the outskirts of Manchester for a special ceremony. It was 5 July 1948, and Bevan had made the trip to inaugurate a new institution, the 'National Health Service', which promised comprehensive medical care to all citizens, without direct charge.

Seventy-five years later, anyone looking to fill a rainy afternoon can purchase a jigsaw puzzle that memorialises the events of that day.[2] The puzzle's thousand pieces form a colour painting of Bevan in front of Park Hospital, holding hands with a girl similar in age to Rosen. The Welshman stares imperiously into the distance, flanked by enough doctors, nurses and patients to raise the question of whether anyone is actually left in the hospital. Released in the 'Nostalgia' series of the company Falcon Deluxe, the picture offers a harmonious scene of the 1940s, full of smiles, sunshine and racial diversity. This jigsaw is just one instance of the esteem that surrounds the NHS in the early twenty-first century. In 2012, the NHS featured centrally in the Opening Ceremony of the London Olympic Games. With professional dancers dressed as nurses and children jumping on beds, Britain projected to the world that a system of medical provision lay at the heart of its identity.[3] Over and over again, people across the UK tell pollsters that the service is the thing that makes them 'most proud to be British'.[4] In an increasingly secular society, the institution is discussed as something akin to a religion.[5]

Our NHS explains why the service came to assume such significance in British life. In doing so, it argues that the social democratic politics that the NHS represents endured well beyond the moment of their supposed demise. This book is a story about how a welfare institution first emerged, modernised, engaged with the world and survived the rise of neoliberalism. These pages differ in tone from both celebratory histories that present the NHS as destined for greatness and dour obituaries charting a terminal descent into 'privatisation'. Instead, I look at the NHS from the inside out, shifting from the doctor's consulting room, to the aspiring surgeon travelling across formerly imperial borders, to critics hatching plans for the institution's replacement, to members of the public baking cakes decorated with the service's initials. *Our NHS* reveals the surprising resilience of a health service that is perpetually in 'crisis', yet perennially lasting, offering an account that incorporates those who wanted to tear it down and those who kept it afloat.

MAKING 'OUR NHS'

Founded in 1948 by Clement Attlee's Labour government, the NHS is a taxpayer-funded, universal and free-at-the-point-of-use health system coordinated by central government. In contrast to the citizens of many other industrialised nations, Britons do not rely on third-party providers or direct patient payments. Instead, the government dominates the medical sphere and no personal health insurance is required, although roughly 10 per cent of the population have insured themselves privately over the past thirty years.[6] The service's operation has been reconfigured by internal reforms over the decades, but throughout this restructuring it has retained its state-centred and universalist principles.[7] Despite its distinctive administrative scaffolding, Britain's NHS fits within the broader pattern of changes to medical care in most industrialised nations during the twentieth century.[8] Like other health systems, the NHS provided widening access to – and occasionally pioneered – developments in pharmaceutical, surgical and technological medical science that included the contraceptive pill, hip replacements and magnetic resonance imaging (MRI). Hospitals concentrated medical expertise and swallowed the lion's share of budgets, while their colleagues in general practice became grouped together in shared facilities like health centres, reflective of an international shift towards 'primary care'. And, as elsewhere, health goals remained unfulfilled, hierarchies between practitioners and patients persisted and new challenges appeared on the horizon, underlining the longstanding arguments made by medical historians that health care rarely moves in a straight line towards progress.[9]

Yet, for all that it shared with overseas counterparts, the NHS came to be seen by Britons as unique, as this book will show. Rather than a natural or inevitable process, the growth of the public's affection towards the NHS was a historical process that required work. In short, 'Our NHS' had to be *made*, both as an institutional reality and as a cultural icon. The service's guarantee of health care to all citizens undoubtedly earned it a great deal of goodwill, but the lack of doctors' bills alone did not make the service the prominent component of national life that it is today. Previous history books about the NHS have largely overlooked this point because they tend to focus on elite politicians, civil servants and prominent doctors, mapping the sequence of the service's internal reorganisation without also considering its relationship to the outside world.[10] Similarly, economists have concentrated on administration out of a purportedly value-neutral pursuit of 'efficiency' or 'cost-effectiveness'. Instead, *Our NHS* attends to a much wider cast of activists, campaigners, medical experts, patients, academics, architects, trade unionists, film-makers, novelists and musicians, among many other figures and organisations.[11] I discuss the service's practical development alongside many of the principal cultural, social and ideological currents of the twentieth and twenty-first centuries. The result is a history of the service that attempts to uncover the importance of this pivotal institution at home and on the world stage.

Although the NHS is now praised by all sides of the political spectrum as a shared national inheritance, historically it represents an achievement of the left. Many hands made the service, but socialist medical reformers, left-wing intellectuals and cultural figures, trade unionists and Labour Party politicians played the leading role in its survival and swelling reputation. They deliberately furnished the NHS with a caring and egalitarian image, embedded communal modes of care in the lives of Britons, countered the hostile denunciations of 'state medicine' advanced by their political opponents, linked the service to 'Britishness' and founded national traditions to celebrate its history. The NHS emerged from a moment where figures across the political spectrum put forward proposals to coordinate medical services, but these plans would not have led to the NHS as it is known today, either in organisational or cultural terms. The nationalised and state-centred structure of the NHS is the legacy of the medical left. In the decades after 1948, the service's supporters made key contributions to extending the state's reach and embedding communal principles in medical care, as well as bolstering its stature against free-market critique. Indeed, the extensive links between the Conservative Party and free-market intellectuals and organisations who wanted to marginalise or even replace nationalised medicine – some given serious consideration for the first time in this book – further undermine the suggestion that the NHS always enjoyed consensus.

Our NHS begins with the service's inception, showing how it did not, at first, claim any of its later esteem among the wider population. Many historians endorse the widespread assumption and commonsense assertion that the British people embraced the service with open arms.[12] In fact, when reformers first presented their plans for a state-coordinated health system during the mid-1940s, large sections of the public greeted their proposals with ambivalence, trepidation, or even hostility.[13] It took a wide-ranging effort by the advocates of such a scheme to shift apprehensions about 'state medicine' towards a more humanistic idea of a 'National Health Service'. Amidst interwar concerns about Britain's dwindling birth rate, the care promised to mothers and children formed an important dimension of these attitudinal changes. The NHS, its proponents also suggested, would boost industrial production by safeguarding the health of working-class families. Some historians' later acceptance of the notion that the service enjoyed immediate popularity stems from the success – and lasting power – of the cultural arguments made by its supporters from the moment of its inception.

After a difficult beginning, and in the context of a postwar 'baby boom', the NHS needed to make its hospitals and doctors' surgeries fit for the future. This book illustrates how governments modernised the service over the next three decades. Concrete hospital wings and steel-framed health centres made this transformation visible to the Britons who entered such facilities.[14] The process of modernisation entrenched communal modes of care, bringing patients from different backgrounds together in large, shared hospital wards or open-plan waiting rooms.[15] Modernisation also displayed an attentiveness to the 'popular individualism' that gained purchase in Britain during the postwar period, precipitated by rising living standards, softening class divides and changing attitudes towards gender and sexual relations.[16] On the back of efforts by the service's supporters, community-oriented social services could be reconciled with the individual needs amplified by these social changes. By the 1970s, the health service had largely responded to these trends and enmeshed itself in villages, towns and cities across the UK. Though far from perfect in execution, this modernisation started to bear fruit in a decade defined by economic crisis that undermined other social services and state-owned industries. If comparable public institutions became dogged by a reputation as bureaucratic and rigid, the health service's degree of adaptability helped ensure that it escaped such a fate.[17]

Britain's relationship with the world also shaped the NHS's operation and reputation. *Our NHS*'s consideration of these global dimensions illuminates the emergence of what I call *welfare nationalism*. Welfare nationalism refers to a belief that welfare services express something essential about the nation.[18] This sentiment can encourage feelings of superiority over other nations and marginalised social groups, such as immigrants. Whereas a heightened conviction in social services is usually associated with the left, and boasts about the nation with the right, welfare nationalism fused the two together and helped endear the NHS to both ends of the political spectrum. At first, it was the NHS's founders and supporters who considered how the institution related to other countries. Bevan believed Britain's health service would serve as a beacon of inspiration, famously describing it as 'the envy of all other nations of the world'.[19] To his delight, hundreds of foreign commentators and experts – principally from the US – quickly flocked to the UK and studied the first nationalised universal health system in a major democracy.[20]

As Britain's empire began to collapse and the nation's international standing became uncertain, American opinion about the NHS mattered. Indeed, US policymakers sometimes used the service as confirmation of Britain's diminished stature in the postwar era. When the Labour government decided that it would withdraw troops from the Persian Gulf and Southeast Asia in order to reallocate money to domestic priorities in 1968, US Secretary of State Dean Rusk seethed that he 'could not believe that free aspirins and false teeth were more important than Britain's role in the world'.[21] Rusk had missed the point – the NHS was important to Britain's role in the world. However, as the NHS suffered persistent critique by conservatives across the Atlantic, and when US attempts to enact its own system of national health insurance failed, the British service's supporters retreated from their earlier faith that the institution would inspire others and came to embrace welfare nationalism instead. Rather than emphasising the institution's international promise, they now stressed its exceptional – and 'British' – qualities. By the 1970s, the differences with care found in other nations, especially the US, became more prominently discussed by the service's defenders. Thereafter, significant parts of the public seemed to agree with the sharp lines drawn between the NHS and foreign health systems. Put another way, this quintessentially 'British' institution began as part of an international movement, and it was only when this internationalism collapsed that the NHS became recoded as a uniquely British achievement.

The increasing emphasis on the service's 'Britishness' sat uneasily with its workers and patients who were born overseas. Like most other industrialised nations expanding access to health care in the postwar period, the UK relied on foreign doctors, nurses, technicians and ancillary workers.[22] While many British commentators, politicians and patients voiced appreciation for their contributions, some did not welcome Black or Brown faces at the local health centre or hospital. Opponents of the NHS weaponised the welfare nationalism around the service to make xenophobic and racialised claims about the 'replacement' of British-born medical practitioners with overseas professionals who, they suggested, possessed inferior qualifications and linguistic capacities. Moreover, the hostility directed at Commonwealth immigrants during the 1960s by figures such as the politician Enoch Powell also involved the NHS.[23] Powell and his supporters refused to acknowledge that migrants possessed any 'right' to access NHS care. To them, the service was an institution that should exclusively serve those born within Britain's national borders, regardless of immigrants' contributions to the economy or the NHS itself. By the 1970s, then, welfare nationalism was starting to command support for the service from both left and right. A Labour Party policy had become recast as a national endowment, enabling its continued viability – but at a cost to the service's staff and patients who arrived in Britain in the wake of decolonisation.[24]

During the 1980s, as so much of Britain's welfare state endured sustained hostility, the postwar modernisation programme combined with welfare nationalism to ensure the NHS's unlikely survival. The decade began with the election of a Conservative government led by Margaret Thatcher, which sought to enact proposals to marginalise or even abolish the NHS, spurred on by the economic turbulence of the 1970s.[25] Many historians downplay the scale of Conservative ambitions, coming close to accepting Thatcher's famous reassurance that the service was 'safe with us'.[26] Instead, *Our NHS* shows how the Conservatives, at first, embraced the longstanding neoliberal argument that replacing universal, public provision with private health insurance would boost overall spending on medical care and encourage self-reliance among the population. This position represented a challenge to the welfare nationalism that had been building elsewhere on the political right. However, these alternatives to the NHS failed to attract sufficient public enthusiasm. In fact, their reputation actually went backwards in the 1980s, as supporters of the NHS promoted the view that private health insurance was inequitable and, given its deliberate association with US care, 'foreign'. Some Britons might have insured themselves privately for elective procedures to escape waiting lists, but few wanted public provision replaced wholescale. As a result of campaigning by its supporters, Britain's health service became popularly understood as the antithesis of the unequal medical system found across the Atlantic. Shedding its postwar association with families and manufacturing, and now fortified by powerful nationalist convictions, the NHS survived a decade that other forms of welfare, such as mass council housing, or public industries, like British Telecom, did not.[27]

Prior scholars have attributed the persistence of institutions like the NHS in the 1980s to 'path dependence', a concept borrowed from economics.[28] They suggest that the difficulties and expense of taking a new direction in policy explain the continuation of older arrangements. In other words, the decisions of the past constrain those that might be made in the present. Though not without its merits, path dependence has limits as an explanation. *Our NHS* demonstrates how the continuation of nationalised medicine was not an inevitable outcome but required, as in the moment of its foundation and early years, active effort. Political argument, social attitudes, cultural representation and international links mattered. Neither the supporters nor the detractors of the NHS thought the service's structures enjoyed any special immunity from being replaced. I demonstrate how the actions they took prevented that outcome.

Our NHS closes by reflecting on the consequences and aftermath of the marketisation that reshaped the institution as a new millennium dawned.[29] Inspired by the view that the private sector could help the state deliver social services more efficiently, both Conservative and Labour governments introduced reforms which enmeshed the NHS with markets. External contractors took on work in the health service, like cleaning, as part of moves towards 'outsourcing' in the 1980s. Two decades later, consulting firms, private equity interests and construction companies formed international consortia that funded and built British medical facilities, such as hospitals, under the 'Private Finance Initiative' (PFI). For many contemporaries, and scholars since, this development amounted to the demise of the NHS's founding principles.[30] In contrast, this book argues that marketisation did not equate to the 'privatisation' of the institution. The introduction of markets into the service never went as far as their proponents hoped, private companies frequently found themselves retreating, and the state not only continued to provide the vast majority of care, but even expanded into new areas. Though altered in structure, operation and feel from its beginnings, the NHS was not overwhelmed by market forces. Given the dizzying array of legislation passed by governments, and the many declarations of the service's actual or imminent 'death' from the 1980s onwards, it demonstrated a surprising degree of continuity.

In these same years, the anxieties felt by activists, campaigners and trade unions regarding marketisation encouraged them to identify with 'Our NHS' more explicitly and rally public support like never before.[31] They invented new traditions such as celebrating the service's 'birthday' on 5 July – a commonplace today that dates not from the Attlee 1940s but from the Thatcherite 1980s. Beginning as a trade union response to budget cuts and outsourcing, the institution's anniversaries grew into national, government-backed occasions featuring street parties, fun-runs and baked goods. NHS anniversaries involved a process of history making, presenting the service's past as a story of immediate public celebration in 1948 and linear progress wrought by the state in medical care since. This social democratic interpretation of the service's past was so influential that some professional historians joined the Olympic organisers in replicating it. Yet this reading of the NHS's history obscures the contradictions, oppositions and struggles evident in these pages. The smoothing out of the service's past as a matter of consensus required erasing the distinctive strategies that supporters had marshalled to ensure the institution's survival. As a result, the NHS's cultural meaning could be more easily appropriated for different ends, even by politicians who subjected the institution to unprecedented and sustained financial pressure after 2010. For all these unexpected outcomes, NHS birthdays reflected a degree of popular approbation that its founders could never have imagined. The health service staked a claim as the best-loved institution in Britain.

The NHS's past is widely understood in the UK as a story of inevitable success and a distinctively 'British' tradition. It is also lamented as the tale of a once-great institution that slipped inexorably into the hands of all-powerful market forces. *Our NHS* offers a different interpretation by emphasising the service's survival, the shortcomings of its opponents and the fostering of popular support. I uncover the contests, successes and unexpected social exclusions that have taken place over the last seven and a half decades. Combining the practical realities of the NHS's development with its changing social and cultural reputation, this book carries implications for how we think about political change in the twentieth and twenty-first centuries.

THE ENDURANCE OF SOCIAL DEMOCRACY

The NHS embodies the politics of social democracy, an ideology which first emerged during the late nineteenth century.[32] In broad terms, social democrats use the state to mitigate the inequality and fracturing of community bonds caused by industrial capitalism. Whereas conservatives and liberals championed markets as the best instrument for human improvement, social democrats looked to the state. The principal advocates of social democratic goals in Western industrialised nations were left-wing intellectuals, political parties and trade unions. As opposed to revolutionary socialists, these figures and organisations sought to win power through the ballot box. Though it encompassed many movements and traditions after its foundation in 1900, the Labour Party became the leading proponent of social democratic policies in Britain.[33] Alongside economic strategies to reduce unemployment, the party embraced public welfare services as a means of supporting the primarily working-class Britons harmed by unequal access to essentials such as food, housing and medical care. Indeed, Bevan presented the NHS as testament to the value of social democratic politics, hailing the institution as 'a triumphant example of the superiority of collective action and public initiative applied to a segment of society where commercial principles are seen at their worst'.[34]

Beyond social democracy's significance as an approach to statecraft, economics and intellectual life, *Our NHS* also calls attention to how people experienced this form of politics.[35] The commitment among social democrats to strengthening community bonds entailed the pursuit of a future in which people from different backgrounds would live and work among one another on more equal terms. This faith in 'communalism', as it is described in these pages, could take different guises, such as the aspiration for working-class and middle-class tenants to live on the same council estate or for their children to attend the same schools.[36] Bevan placed the NHS 'alongside the rest of the communal agencies, by means of which the New Society is being gradually articulated'.[37] In the health service, communalism expressed itself through shared medical spaces, such as combined, public wards or open-plan waiting rooms. While other health systems could also possess these features, the figures and groups involved with the NHS's development favoured communal designs over individualised alternatives and used the state to make them a reality, sometimes to a higher degree than their counterparts overseas.[38] The aspirations to create a more egalitarian society through communal environments, and the lived experiences of what followed from these convictions, make the concept of 'social democracy' preferable to alternative framings of this period's politics. For instance, the 'developmental state' provides significant explanatory power as a framework, but focuses upon government structures, economic theory and technocrats over and above culture and lived experience.[39] I seek to combine both ends of the scale, showing how even seemingly mundane facets of everyday life, such as a trip to the doctor, can reveal the priorities and legacies of a larger postwar project. I am inspired by historians who, despite other interpretative differences, are united by a desire to challenge prior work which cast the post-1945 decades within a supposed political 'consensus'.[40] By looking for the sources and endurance of social democratic politics, *Our NHS* provides a different approach to the shared problem of how best to rethink these years.

The NHS's foundation in 1948 signals the importance of the postwar Labour governments to social democratic politics in Britain. On the back of a landslide election victory in 1945, Labour under Attlee sought to remodel the nation through policies ranging from full employment to the nationalisation of key industries and infrastructure like coal mines and railways.[41] The government also expanded the pre-existing framework of local and national social services into something that contemporaries were describing as a 'welfare state' by the end of the 1940s.[42] These strategies, Labour believed, would not only rebuild the nation after the devastation of total war but offer a path away from the economic depression and unemployment that defined what many British people bitterly remembered as the 'hungry thirties'.[43] The appropriate balance between the government and markets remained hotly debated as the country ended its wartime mobilisation. Moreover, the state did not become wholly 'welfarist' from this point onwards, underlined by the fact that the postwar Labour government spent almost as much money on military commitments as social services.[44] But the NHS – as a state institution, funded by taxation, boasting a workforce overwhelmingly employed in the public sector and providing a universal service organised around communal modes of care – reflected principles best understood as social democratic.[45] Buoyed by sustained levels of GDP growth averaging just over 3 per cent per annum, the historian Eric Hobsbawm joined many other scholars by describing the period between 1945 and the mid-1970s as a 'Golden Age' underpinned by 'a sort of marriage between economic liberalism and social democracy'.[46]

Yet, every purported golden age is destined to close, and historians have pinpointed the 1970s as the moment when social democracy seemingly collapsed.[47] The economic crisis that followed the 1973 OPEC oil embargo, soaring inflation, rising unemployment and labour unrest undermined its capacities and confidence. These structural shocks encouraged critics in think tanks, businesses and political parties on the right to advance a different political ideology: 'neoliberalism'.[48] Although a contested term, neoliberalism in this book refers to a political ideology premised on free markets and competitive individualism.[49] This brand of politics did not necessarily 'roll back the state', but instead deployed the state to secure markets from outside interference.[50] While it is important to guard against conceptual simplifications, historians rightly seek categories and chronologies to make sense of an endlessly complicated human experience. To that end, neoliberalism and social democracy offer an essential means of thinking in broad terms about politics, economy and society since the Second World War.

Thatcher's election victories and international influence as a champion of free markets affords Britain a prominent role in histories of neoliberalism's ascent.[51] During the 1980s, Conservative governments deregulated financial markets, privatised publicly owned industries and reshaped parts of the welfare state by transforming universal services into residual ones that only served the poor.[52] In Britain, as in the US under Ronald Reagan, the former USSR after the collapse of the Berlin Wall or China under Deng Xiaoping, the power of capital surged, creating a political and economic regime that seemed unassailable.[53] The triumph of neoliberalism, historians suggest, even seemed to win over the earlier critics of capitalism, like the Labour Party – reborn in the 1990s as 'New Labour' – who now warmed to markets as a force for good and extended their reach in social services like health care.[54] Exhausted and betrayed, social democracy can appear to have little more than a 'brief life' in historical accounts of the post-1945 era.[55]

I upend these narratives by focusing instead on the *endurance* of social democracy. *Our NHS* shows how a social democratic institution acquired resilience in the postwar decades, resisted crisis and neoliberal assault, and indeed expanded its stature and reach beyond the point of its much-heralded demise. Scholars have begun to question the absolute dominance of neoliberalism, highlighting its inability to translate ideological priorities into policies.[56] Despite narratives of the welfare state's collapse during the 1970s, these historians have pointed to the ways that it became better funded and more egalitarian.[57] Other scholars have shown how social democrats did not simply roll over when economic crisis arrived but advanced strategies to preserve – and even renew – its forms and values.[58] In these accounts, the defenders of social democracy are restored as dynamic historical actors, capable of missteps, but also successes, no less than their opponents. However, even the revised picture presented by recent scholarship still places British social democracy's expiration date somewhere around 1979, when Thatcher walked through the door of No. 10 Downing Street.[59]

Our NHS explores the limits of neoliberalism but also the strengths of what came before. I highlight how proponents of free markets struggled to overcome the earlier work and counter-movements of their opponents, even at the point when histories of the rise of neoliberalism suggest that the latter collapsed into irrelevance. Such a position requires affording social democracy the same capacities that historians provide other ideologies, like liberalism, which are allowed afterlives in a manner not typically extended to ideologies on the left.[60] The foundation of massive state structures, and the embedding of communal values that millions of people experienced after 1945, carried long-term significance. This argument means recognising that the successes and failures of an ideology amount to more than just the performance of an associated political party at elections.[61] The electoral record of the Labour Party – in power on its own or in coalition during just thirty-three years of the twentieth century – is patchy, but the political success of the health service that they founded is remarkable. This book casts light on political change that cuts across the party in government, blending policy and medical expertise with the cultural and lived dimensions of social democracy.

Neither social democratic or neoliberal approaches to the NHS remained static. In broad terms, the former retained its core commitment to use the state to mitigate inequality and bring people of different backgrounds together in communal environments, and the latter preserved its faith in markets and competitive individualism. Nonetheless, both shifted in emphasis over time. During the mid-twentieth century, social democrats associated the NHS with supporting families and an industrial economy. By the end of the century, in the wake of social change and deindustrialisation, they shed these priorities and adopted a position combining a recast programme of 'modernisation' – which provided a greater role for markets – with a heavier emphasis on welfare nationalism. The neoliberal approach to the health service began by calling for its outright replacement with free-market alternatives like private health insurance. When this strategy failed, its proponents insisted on the NHS's internal marketisation, albeit as something of a consolation prize compared to initial neoliberal aspirations.

Attending to the endurance of social democracy highlights the NHS's place within the fate of a much broader ideological project, as well as the potential for that project to adapt and even flourish. Whereas other parts of the welfare state or public industries fell away in Britain after the 1970s, such as the New Towns programme or the National Coal Board, the NHS – even as it changed – largely grew stronger. This fractured survival means that Britain cannot be considered a wholly social democratic country today. The UK did not experience the same twentieth century as Scandinavian countries like Sweden, which possessed – despite undertaking its own neoliberal reforms – stronger collective wage bargaining, subsidised childcare and lower levels of inequality.[62] Calling attention to how social democratic politics might endure does not mean ignoring the expanded power and reach of free-market capitalism across the world, nor does it entail denying the shortcomings or inequities found within institutions like the NHS. This book amply shows how social divisions – along the lines of class, gender, race and others besides – permeated a purportedly 'universal' health service, and how its popular support drew upon nationalist sentiment that sometimes fostered, and still fosters, racial exclusions. *Our NHS* critically interrogates the phrase that inspires its title, seeking to understand where such sentiment came from, how it was deployed and what costs it carried. Even if it is not a feel-good 'people's history', this book remains a *peopled* history seeking to conjoin multiple perspectives to explain both the standing and survival of a service that is often taken for granted.[63]

UNDERSTANDING THE NHS

The NHS is a suitable candidate to reveal the endurance of social democracy. Although forming a single wing of the welfare state, it reached the start of the twenty-first century with an annual budget larger than the total GDP of Hungary, standing as the world's fifth largest employer behind only the likes of the Chinese People's Liberation Army and McDonald's, and attracted broad public celebration rivalled by few other institutions.[64] Some might question whether the history of the welfare state or social democratic politics should be told through the example of health care, considering that the money allocated to it by governments expanded in all industrialised nations during the late twentieth century, regardless of those nations' broader welfare arrangements or political culture.[65] In this reading, health care is presented as a 'special' area of social policy that should be treated separately. However, the focus on rising public subsidy does not tell the whole story. After all, the state's financial outlay for health care could expand, but then so could private spending. Taxpayers' money might have been channelled to private companies. New barriers to accessing medical care could also emerge. For example, even in a country that enjoyed generous welfare provision like Finland, total government spending on health care increased, but patients still faced direct payments in hospitals and health centres after the 1990s.[66]

Moreover, the opponents of the NHS who feature in this book rarely saw health care as a special or untouchable dimension of state welfare. Instead, they railed against what one critic scorned as 'the almost pathological obsession on the part of the British public, in the face of all fact and logic, with the indestructible virtues of a comprehensive and free National Health Service'.[67] To the advocates of neoliberalism, the NHS posed as much of a problem – and sometimes even more of a problem – as social housing, state pensions or unemployment benefits. Given the success that free-market policies enjoyed in reshaping other areas of British life, it is essential to consider their reach, and lack of reach, into health care arrangements.

This book is not a total history of the NHS. It does not encompass every medical development, administrative reform or type of patient. These pages acknowledge – and frequently evidence – the heterogeneous nature of the NHS. However, I maintain focus on the service's overall development, and the shifts in its reputation, to cast light on the broader question of the relationship between social democracy and neoliberalism. As a result, the book follows a different path from earlier histories, which placed greater emphasis on mapping the institution's internal reforms. *Our NHS* begins by focusing on the service's foundation and postwar modernisation, then examines its changing place on the world stage and the rise of welfare nationalism, and concludes with its survival against free-market opposition. Throughout, I weave in the stories of individual hospitals, health centres, trade unions, think tanks, activists, medical professionals and patients. I recognise the variation between the forms that the NHS took in the constituent nations of the UK but proceed with the view that the overwhelming commonalities between these systems and the public experiences of them allow for joint consideration. The principal parts of the NHS referenced in the book are hospital services and general practice, alongside – to a lesser extent – public health. No more important than other forms of care such as mental health or sexual health services, these areas have been chosen because they were the most heavily relied on by the majority of the population, and the most widely discussed, throughout the NHS's history.[68]

Our NHS offers a new historical interpretation of an internationally famous health system, questioning both its uncritical celebration and predictions of its demise. In doing so, it challenges the predominant account of political change across the twentieth and twenty-first centuries. This history should serve as a counterpoint to the media-driven narratives of 'crisis' that surround both the institution and the politics that it represents. While not diminishing the seriousness of the problems confronting the NHS and social democracy, taking a longer view reveals how both have long faced challenges and yet endured. *Our NHS* begins with the struggle to found a new health service, a battle still unfolding on that Monday morning in 1948 when June Rosen brought Bevan his breakfast.

PART I

FOUNDATION AND MODERNISATION

1

THE NATIONAL HEALTH

During the spring of 1948, the doctor-turned-politician Edith Summerskill (1901–1980) delivered an evening BBC radio broadcast to promote the new 'National Health Service' due to start in three months' time.[1] A feminist campaigner recognisable on newsreels by her trademark black hat, Summerskill had become the Labour MP for West Fulham ten years earlier and now served as the Parliamentary Secretary for the Ministry of Food (Figure 1). She used her transmission to share how 'the suffering of a woman' first drew her into the political arena. In 1923, full of nerves as a young and newly qualified doctor, Summerskill went to a downtrodden working-class area on a cold, wet night to help a woman give birth. The husband answered the door, 'pallid and shabby with the familiar signs of long unemployment'. Summerskill entered the house and soon faced a woman her own age laying on a mattress, protected from the chill by only a tattered blanket. Next to the bed stood an infant's crib. The couple's first child gripped its bars, forehead swollen and legs crooked – 'the classic picture of rickets', diagnosed the doctor. Years later, Summerskill vividly recalled how the young woman 'clutched my hand, with her own moist, bony fingers'. The patient wore a brass wedding ring, pitifully twisted with a piece of cotton to stop it falling off a hand emaciated by hunger. Like any good orator, Summerskill used this harrowing episode to drive home the point of her radio message. The National Health scheme, she promised, would – alongside other welfare measures introduced by the postwar Labour

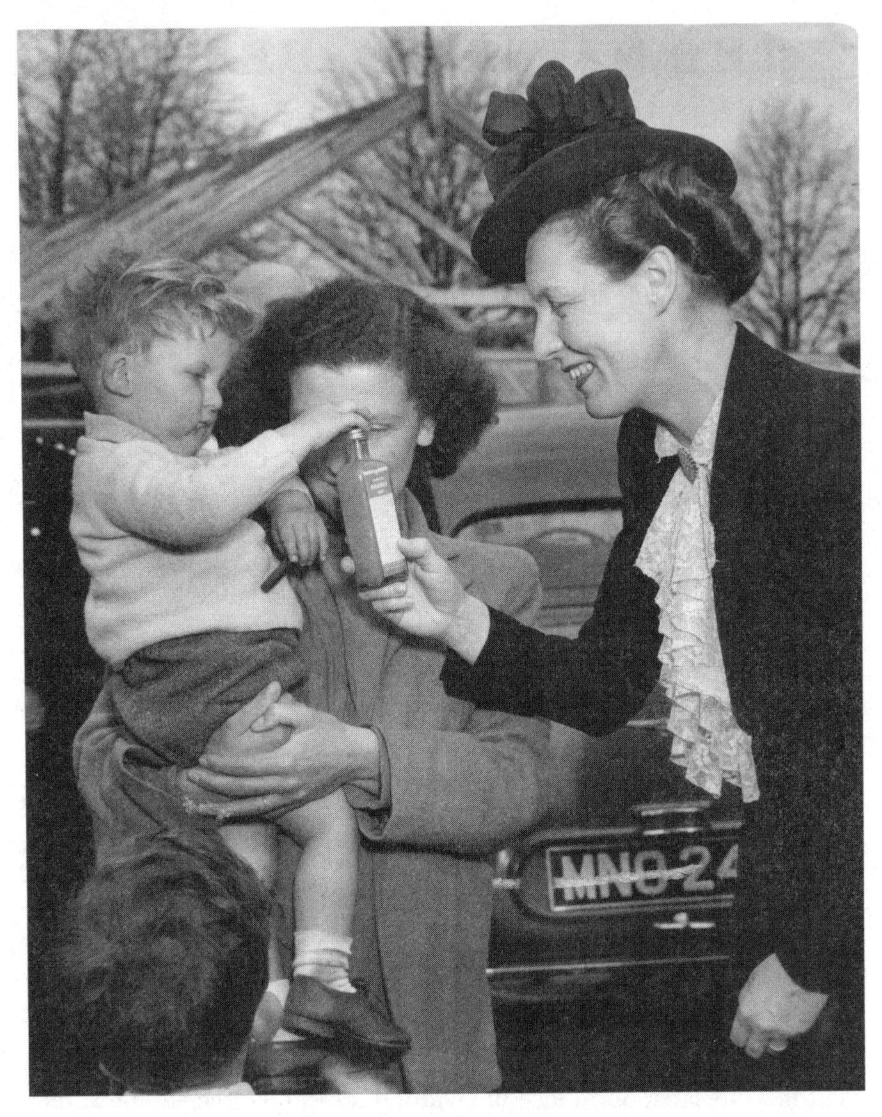

1. The Labour politician Edith Summerskill campaigned during the interwar years for a national system of 'state medicine', which she believed would support the health of women and children, reverse Britain's declining birth rate and boost economic production.

government – make such a bleak scene impossible by guaranteeing support from the cradle to the grave. But where did the idea to use the state to coordinate, provide and fund the majority of medical care come from? And what did the public think about these plans?

As might be expected with an institution that later took on such prominence, scholars disagree on the nature of the NHS's inception. Writing just after the Second World War, the social policy expert Richard Titmuss argued that the service stemmed in large part from the heightened expectations and political radicalism engendered among the population by total war.[2] People having come together in air-raid shelters or sharing the experience of rationing, he suggested, led them to look favourably on wartime proposals for a future health system based on equality of access.[3] Much later, the historian Daniel M. Fox argued that a different form of consensus, between experts, mattered the most.[4] The support among medical professionals and policymakers for the principle of 'hierarchical regionalism' – meaning, planning health services with research centres at the top to serve defined geographical areas – explained why these elite circles embraced something like the NHS. The historian Charles Webster rebutted Fox's claims and presented the creation of the service as a matter of conflict, not agreement, with the Labour Party playing a special role in longer-term discussions over its organisation and abolishing payment in medical care.[5]

Despite their differences in opinion about the impetus for the NHS, these scholars all rightly agree that the service did not appear in 1948 out of a vacuum. Indeed, the NHS arrived on the back of a half-century of proposals for a coordinated, universal 'state medical service'. Summerskill, for instance, advanced such a cause by helping found the Socialist Medical Association (SMA) in 1930.[6] Yet this organisation – and many other associations, activists and intellectuals in the interwar years – did not believe that the application of state planning to medical care mattered merely in terms of improving health care's efficiency. Nor did such an approach just boil down to an ethical imperative, though breaking down the barriers to accessing medical treatment was undoubtedly seen as important. What is sometimes missed in histories of the NHS's inception is how reformers consistently maintained that the service would help address the most pressing challenges facing Britain at the time, including reversing a declining birth rate and, relatedly, securing economic growth. 'The National Health', as Britons often called the NHS after its foundation, was an institution designed to address these problems. The service therefore reflected the core principles of social democracy in its reliance on the state to mitigate inequality and its ambition to bring people together in communal facilities. These goals fused with a mid-century priority to support traditionally gendered families in an economy primarily based on industry and manufacturing.

However, Britons did not automatically or unanimously welcome the service. For all the ink spilled on historical accounts of the NHS's origins, public opinion is usually overlooked. If wider attitudes are mentioned, they are usually depicted in abstracted terms as – following Titmuss – a reflection of the 'Spirit of '45', where an ethos of 'fair shares for all' led the public to unquestioningly welcome the state as the best solution to the nation's problems.[7] In fact, when asked during the war, sizeable numbers of people expressed misgivings about a government-coordinated system of medical care.[8] At the heart of these apprehensions, and sometimes hostility, lay a view that the state restricted choice and enforced regimentation. This scepticism followed older trends. As the historians Jose Harris and Pat Thane have made clear, since the Victorian period, many Britons expressed a desire for independence in relation to state welfare services.[9] Some people continued to voice confidence in a liberal style of governance, where the state ostensibly ruled at a distance and did not get involved in the private lives of citizens.[10] Moreover, the public did not completely condemn the health services that these older political traditions had brought into being. The *New Statesman* may well have hailed the coming of the NHS as 'one of the great advances in social history', but as Summerskill's presence in the BBC studios testified, the public needed to be persuaded.[11]

HEALTH CARE BEFORE THE NHS

As the world's first industrial nation, Britain was long acquainted with the ill health and inequality that accompanied coal mines, factories and slums. The interwar years marked a period of improvement in the nation's health from the Victorian era, but stubborn challenges persisted.[12] Tuberculosis continued to haunt both the older smoke-filled towns and the newer suburbs. Instances of childhood afflictions such as diphtheria and whooping cough were reduced but still shortened lives. Though levels of mortality caused by such infectious diseases fell across the interwar period – largely due to improved housing and nutrition – they began to be overshadowed by diseases caused by people living longer, such as cancer and heart afflictions. The medical services that patients relied on to treat all these conditions were based on municipal, voluntary and private initiative.[13] These services interlocked with a welfare state that had emerged during the first half of the twentieth century.[14] Although many members of the public fell through gaps in this provision, interwar health services displayed signs of innovation that made its replacement in 1948 far from inevitable.

The general practitioner (GP) formed the front line of medical care in most communities during the interwar years, typically working alone or with one or two other colleagues in a partnership.[15] Patients visited GPs in surgeries based out of their homes or in converted premises like a shop front. Some doctors mixed their own medicines on site. The Northern Irish GP Tom McQuay claimed that many patients would almost demand a bottle of ointment or tonic at the end of a consultation to make them feel as if they had got their money's worth (usually about three shillings per visit).[16] Most practitioners undertook extensive rounds of home visits, swooping into a patient's home to deliver a diagnosis – or sometimes even a spot of minor surgery – during the day or night. In an environment where local doctors competed for patients, McQuay sometimes performed up to ninety visits a day to top up his earnings.

Millions of Britons gained access to GP services through what was colloquially known as the 'panel' system, established under the terms of the 1911 National Insurance Act.[17] If a worker earned less than £250 a year, their visit to the GP was free of charge, underwritten by a fund based on contributions from individuals, employers and the state.

Introduced by the Liberal Chancellor of the Exchequer, David Lloyd George, health insurance sat among other earlier welfare measures – such as old age pensions – that used state intervention to mitigate poverty among the working classes. This 'New Liberalism' had marked a departure from the more *laissez-faire* approach of Victorian Liberals like William Gladstone, and responded to the electoral threat of the new Labour Party, who promised a far greater role for the state in the economy and society.[18] The Liberals' ideological manoeuvres did not meet their intended goals, and Labour became the Official Opposition after the First World War, forming its first governments under Ramsay MacDonald in 1924 and between 1929 and 1931. Despite the electoral decline of the Liberal Party, by 1938, 20 million insured workers – approximate to 54 per cent of the British population – were entitled to treatment as a panel patient under their 1911 Act.[19]

National health insurance did not provide universal care or access. Reliance on a panel doctor, while a lifeline to many, carried stigma compared to paying privately. In GP surgeries, panel patients sometimes waited in separate rooms to private patients.[20] Many working-class panel patients felt that the care they received was inferior to the attention given to their private counterparts.[21] The existing state assistance for medical care also excluded people slightly higher up the income ladder. Middle-class professionals earning a salary above the income limit, such as the growing number of administrators and those employed in the scientific and technical sectors during the interwar years, found themselves without coverage under the 1911 Act. This omission led to a high degree of middle-class spending on private insurance premiums and personal anxiety during times of severe illness or unemployment.

In general, national health insurance did not apply to women, and it excluded all children. Many younger women who had gained access to a panel doctor while employed in the expanding interwar retail, clerical and light industry sectors regularly lost coverage when they married or had children. Expected to stay home, married women often relied on a man's wages and his willingness to spend money on the family over his own leisure. All too often, though, a husband's session in the pub left little money for his wife's trip to the doctor. In its lack of provision for these women, national health insurance reflected what the social policy expert Jane Lewis describes as a 'breadwinner' model of welfare, premised on an idealised vision of patriarchal gender relations with men in the workplace and women in the home.[22] As a result of policymakers' unwillingness to undermine a man's responsibility to care for his family, married women stood in a much more disadvantaged position when accessing medical care than their husbands.

The lack of coverage in national health insurance for a man's 'dependents' created hardship during the interwar period, for both working-class people and professionals on unstable incomes. Decades later, Summerskill's patients still remembered the feelings of insecurity that these gaps caused among poorer communities during the 'Slump' that followed the 1929 financial crash. Before entering politics, Summerskill maintained different GP surgeries in London. These practices served a predominantly female and working-class body of patients, with many women seeking Summerskill out as a rare woman doctor also willing to provide birth control. Patients from large and poor families referred to her as the 'sixpenny doctor' as she often charged less than other practitioners and made reductions for women and children who did not enjoy the benefits of a man's insurance.[23] One woman recalled how 'every day was a battle for survival not only for us; but for the majority of families living in poverty'. Doctors like Summerskill were respected for charging low prices, and the support she gained among local women contributed to her election to Parliament. 'You can imagine the impact when a doctor offered treatment at *6d*', another patient who did not possess health coverage later enthused.

The rationing of health care by individual means exacerbated wider standards of ill health. During the Great Depression, maternal mortality rose, peaking at 5.9 deaths per 1,000 births in 1933, representing an increase on the 3.9 per 1,000 between 1921 and 1925.[24] Near the end of the 1930s, the nutritionist Sir John Boyd Orr found that undernourishment afflicted roughly half the British population, and fell hardest on women and children.[25] Though difficult to attribute to a single cause, lack of access to medical services worsened these key health metrics, particularly during high unemployment when many working families faced the stark choice of eating or seeing the doctor. Social investigators of various political persuasions found that government inaction harmed the health of the vulnerable.[26] The encounter with malnourishment and rickets that Summerskill described on her radio broadcast confirmed the realities of these grim statistics.

The most popular novel of 1930s Britain, *The Citadel* (1937), exposed a fiction-reading public to the harms that gaps in existing general practice provision caused.[27] Written by the Scottish GP and author A.J. Cronin, the book forcefully critiqued private medicine. The events of the novel, told from the perspective of the fictional Dr Andrew Manson, loosely mirrored Cronin's own career as a doctor and medical inspector of coal mines in South Wales during the early 1920s. Manson undertakes a journey from medical assistant in the deprived Welsh mining community of Drineffy to a private physician for the rich in London's salubrious Harley Street. However, when serving the West End's elite clientele, Manson realises how money corrupts the medical profession. After one of his colleagues kills a working-class patient through malpractice, Manson leaves Harley Street and forms a group practice with doctor friends made earlier in his career. The novel presented cooperation and the pooling of expertise as a superior means of organising health services, compared to an existing disaggregated system structured around charity and money.

Distinct from general practice, hospitals formed the second line of medical care.[28] Many institutions dated back to the eighteenth or nineteenth centuries, their Georgian or neo-Gothic façades looming over communities across the UK. Two types existed during the interwar period: municipal hospitals and voluntary hospitals. The municipal hospitals were managed and funded by local government and provided about two-thirds of all non-psychiatric hospital beds.[29] Many municipal hospitals began as infirmaries attached to workhouses under the 1834 Poor Law Act. By the end of the nineteenth century, they also cared for non-paupers. The 1929 Local Government Act empowered county boroughs and county councils to take over and improve these older Poor Law institutions. On the one hand, trailblazers such as the London County Council (LCC) achieved notable success, showcasing the confidence of municipal medicine in the 1930s. Indeed, public health fell within the remit of local government, with individual Medical Officers of Health (MOsH) overseeing a range of initiatives, from sanitary inspectors to tuberculosis sanatoria. On the other hand, many councils struggled to match the likes of the LCC, and the social stigma of attending the old Poor Law institutions endured. As in general practice, then, hospital care proved uneven in quality across the UK.

The voluntary hospitals ranged from prestigious teaching institutions in major cities, such as Guy's in London or the Edinburgh Royal, to medium-sized institutions in towns, to small cottage hospitals that might be found outside of crowded urban areas. Independent from central or local government, they provided the remaining third of hospital beds in the UK and funded their activities through patients' payments, historic endowments and charitable fundraising. The role of charity in their finances created unevenness in provision, as affluent areas usually possessed more money to fund their local hospital. The requirement that poorer patients prove their financial need through a means test to access care in voluntary hospitals also fostered resentment. Nonetheless, these institutions possessed longstanding roots in communities. Local dignitaries, aristocrats and minor royals populated their fundraising committees that organised a range of activities such as dances, galas, whist-drives and university rag weeks.[30] 'Flag days' were a common fundraising technique during the first half of the twentieth century. Introduced during the First World War, these occasions saw nurses, hospital administrators and volunteers taking to the streets to sell miniature Union Flags. Although some people may have crossed the street when they heard the rattle of a collection tin, few denied the value of the work that the voluntary hospitals performed.

The early twentieth century witnessed an expansion in both the total number of hospitals and the number of beds that they provided. In England and Wales alone, hospital bed numbers swelled from 112,750 in 1891 to 225,556 in 1921, and reached 263,103 in 1938.[31] These increases resulted from changes in expert and lay opinion. Hospitals came to be seen not as places where the poor died – as in the eighteenth and nineteenth centuries – but instead as safe locations to access treatment and novel technologies such as X-rays. As the historian George Gosling demonstrates, middle-class patients now entered institutions that their forebears might have avoided.[32] Contributory schemes – where workers paid weekly deductions of *2d* or *3d* from their wages in return for admission to a hospital without charge – provided greater access for the working class.[33] At their peak, these schemes covered some 20 million people as their benefits extended to 'dependents'. These insurance arrangements could evolve into sizeable enterprises. In Aneurin Bevan's (1897–1960) hometown of Tredegar in South Wales, the Workmen's Medical Aid Society became the most famous example of this brand of working-class mutualism, providing five doctors, a surgeon, two pharmacists, a physiotherapist, a dentist and district nurse to approximately 95 per cent of the mining town's population during the 1920s.[34]

As the expansion of hospitals and novel insurance mechanisms suggest, the interwar period was far from a stagnant era in health provision, even if all regions did not enjoy an equal degree of quantity or quality in service. Other new developments included the foundation of pioneering 'health centres' that combined curative and preventative medicine by bringing together GPs, public health officials, nurses, dentists and other professionals under one roof. In 1920, the Dawson Report had called for an extensive network of such centres, and notable experiments with the model in Finsbury and Peckham demonstrated their possibilities.[35] The modernist architecture of the Finsbury Park Health Centre – given glass bricks and an open-plan reception area by its Russian architect, Berthold Lubetkin – offered glimpses of a different future for medicine.[36] The question of how to secure this future occupied reformers across the interwar years.

THE REFORMERS

Against this tapestry of services, a body of medical reformers – of various political backgrounds – challenged the status quo. The government had established the Ministry of Health in 1919 and it oversaw initiatives ranging from administering national health insurance to council house construction. However, the ministry's formation did not lead to the government coordination of health services, leaving reformers frustrated with a medical system plagued, in their view, by confusion and inconsistencies. Questions of efficiency, differences between regions and issues of economic injustice all came up for debate. But beyond the administrative technicalities of what a new health system might look like, these reformers considered much wider national problems, including economic productivity and a perilously dwindling birth rate. The solution, more and more figures and organisations believed, lay in the state.

The phrase 'National Health Service' had appeared for the first time in 1911. Dr Benjamin Moore deployed the term – alongside others like 'National Medical Service' – in his book *The Dawn of the Health Age* (1911), which called for a centralised system of medical care coordinated by the state.[37] Rising from a working-class background to become the first chair of biochemistry in the UK at the University of Liverpool, Moore's tract reflected his socialist beliefs. As disease did not respect class boundaries, he asserted that his proposals were 'best for both the millionaire and the pauper'. He reserved particular scorn for voluntary hospitals, and presented them as a 'public sore and festering spot' due to their apparent disorganisation, underfunding and paternalistic attitudes to the working class. In an attack on voluntarism that came to exemplify many left-wing arguments for medical reform, Moore wanted to end 'feeble sentimental tears over the sufferings of the poor and doling out charity to them', and called for 'a system which will end these sufferings'. 'We require a Cosmos evolved out of this Chaos', Moore declared. He predicted that state medicine could save at least 300,000 lives a year 'without costing the nation a single penny', because protected individuals would then become, or continue to be, productive workers.

Moore's interventions overlapped with other early calls during the Edwardian period to widen the scope of the state's involvement in medical care. Forceful demands for some form of national health system had arrived in the influential 1909 Minority Report of the Poor Law Commission, authored by the leading economists and social reformers Beatrice Webb and Sidney Webb. This husband-and-wife team were foundational members of the Fabian Society, a socialist intellectual group committed to building a future that escaped the inequalities of industrial capitalism through non-revolutionary means.[38] They expressed no love for the Poor Law, which was premised on a harsh regime of moral judgement and means testing. Like Moore, the Webbs attacked the existing provision of health care that had emerged from such Victorian legislation on ethical and economic grounds.[39] The requirement that individuals prove their destitution, in their view, deterred patients from seeking treatment and caused 'an untold amount of aggravation of disease, personal suffering and reduction in the wealth-producing power of the manual working class'. They posited that expenditure on treating disease among the sick poor by local authorities would be 'more suited to a State Medical Service than that of the Poor Law'. The former, suggested the Webbs, would mark a more caring and rational future for medicine. Although the Webbs' recommendations in the Minority Report did not become government policy, their calls for a 'State Medical Service' marked the beginning of a swelling clamour for reform.

Proposals for a state medical system grew in popularity during the interwar years, a period of disruption after the First World War, the 'Slump' following the 1929 financial crash and – despite Britain's more conservative mainstream electoral politics than its European neighbours – swelling political radicalism.[40] An organisation dedicated to convincing the Labour Party of the necessity of a state medical system emerged in this atmosphere: the Socialist Medical Association (SMA). Helmed by its first president, the surgeon and Labour MP Dr Somerville Hastings, the SMA stressed the advantages of utilising the state to provide a truly 'public' medical service in meetings, pamphlets and medical journals.[41] They believed that such a system would end the blight of inequality. The SMA also extended the economic logic of their Edwardian forebears. In a typical 1931 article titled 'Can We Afford to

Leave the Nation's Health to Private Enterprise?', Hastings argued that sickness cost Britain £300 million per year, partly due to the loss of any child as a 'productive unit' to disease.[42] Though not communist, the organisation drew inspiration from the young USSR. In 1932, a delegation that included Summerskill explored the possibilities of state medicine by visiting 'polyclinics' – the Soviet equivalent of a health centre – in Leningrad and Moscow.[43]

The SMA differed from their predecessors in a number of respects. For one, they believed that the state should take on a greater role in the provision of medical care. Setting alarm bells ringing among the medical profession, they thought doctors should be full-time salaried government employees and coordinated in health centres, similar to the model facilities in Finsbury and Peckham. Second, compared to figures like Moore who thought workers should still pay contributions for their health care, the SMA argued that a future scheme should be free at the point of access. Any direct monetary involvement in medicine, they argued, created an 'economic barrier' between doctor and patient that deflated attendance at the local surgery and made medical experts 'more concerned with mere externals than an intimate knowledge of the science of his profession'.[44] Removing money from medicine, they reasoned, would help mothers and children in their shared status as non-wage-earners, advance medical science, and improve care by bringing doctors and patients into a closer relationship with one another.

The SMA maintained that their plans would not just create better care and economic efficiency but also avert a potential disaster: namely, Britain's declining birth rate. As in many industrialised nations during the first half of the twentieth century, Britain's birth rate – which fell from nearly six live births for the average married woman in 1860, to just over two by 1940 – provoked anxiety across the political spectrum.[45] Though varying between social classes and regions, couples controlled their fertility as the emotional and financial costs of raising children increased. These everyday decisions about children caused widespread political apprehension. In the interwar period, the foremost intellectuals writing on the birth rate, including the sociologists

Alexander Carr-Saunders and D.V. Glass, clustered around the London School of Economics (LSE), which had been founded by the Webbs.[46] Both men formed the Population Investigation Committee in 1936, a body that undertook statistical research and reported to the government on the 'population problem'.[47] Applying novel techniques in demography, they warned of a loss of British prestige on the world stage and a fall in standards of living as 'large-scale methods of production' would have to be 'abandoned'.[48] These claims about population dovetailed with a widespread interest in eugenics during the interwar years, where figures from across the political spectrum used contemporary theories of heredity to advance proposals that they felt would improve health and social welfare.[49] Although eugenics later went underground after the Second World War due to its association with Nazism, it had long proved influential in British discussions of the quantity – and quality – of the population.

Other figures echoed these dire warnings about the birth rate but went further in recommending solutions. Enid Charles's *The Twilight of Parenthood* (1934) foretold that the current rate of decline might even lead to 'extinction in some of the leading civilized communities of the modern world'.[50] Identifying the cause of this phenomenon through statistical methods, this Welsh socialist claimed that children had become an onerous 'expense' for families, and summed up this burden by stating that 'the choice between a Ford and a baby is usually made in favour of the Ford'. Painting the '*laissez faire* economy' as 'biologically self-destructive', Charles demanded greater government support for the cost of raising children, including comprehensive maternal and medical services. For her, health services should feature within a broader 'social-democratic plan of recognizing motherhood as a profession safeguarded by State endowment of the family'.

These arguments – and especially the influence of the SMA – persuaded the Labour Party to commit to a 'State Medical Service' in 1934.[51] Though some of the details remained vague, the party pledged to establish a unified medical system that provided universal care, free at the point of use. Given the successes of Labour-run councils like the

LCC, they believed local government should provide these services. This stance promised national coordination and funding while protecting on-the-ground knowledge of local health needs. The party had taken a programmatic step forward from its earlier belief that full employment and better pay stood as the best way to improve health outcomes. To be sure, left-wing voices did not monopolise the groundswell of proposals for medical reform during the interwar years that led Labour to adopt such a stance.[52] The conservative think tank Political and Economic Planning (PEP), for instance, drew its funding from private companies and expressed a more conservative bent than the likes of the SMA.[53] Yet, in an important 1937 report, PEP similarly recommended coordinating hospitals in a national network. By the outbreak of the Second World War, then, systematic reform was well discussed among activists, medical experts and intellectuals. After armed conflict broke out in September 1939, it became a subject of public interest.

THE SECOND WORLD WAR AND THE MEDICAL FUTURE

For nearly six years, Britain fought a difficult war.[54] But after 1942, with the UK claiming victory in the Battle of Britain and the US entering the conflict, thoughts turned to peace. Amidst the whine of air raid sirens and the rubble of the Blitz, plans began to be laid for a brighter future.[55] Proposals for medical care lay among the many transformative schemes put forward. Beyond mere recovery to a pre-war standard, reformers spanning the political spectrum sought to leave behind the insecurity that had blighted the interwar years and harness the power of the state to build a healthier Britain. While an agent of destruction, the war also presented a window of possibility to advance some of the radical ideas advanced earlier by the Fabians and the SMA. However, the social solidarities forged in wartime did not immediately translate into public acceptance for systemic change in medical care.

The publication of a report in 1942, *Social Insurance and Allied Services*, electrified the reconstruction debates. Authored by the Liberal social reformer and economist Sir William Beveridge (1879–1963), the report gained popularity far beyond what its dull title might suggest. During the Edwardian period, Beveridge had abandoned a promising legal career to work among the working-class inhabitants of London's East End, driven by a belief that applied social science could help end poverty. He was a somewhat awkward man in his personal relationships, but even if he could annoy with his brusqueness, few doubted his intellectual capacities or commitment to tackling social inequality. After building a formidable reputation in policy circles, Beveridge was asked by the government during the Second World War to research the future of welfare services, primarily in an attempt to keep him busy. What became known as the 'Beveridge Report', though, caused the wartime government more headaches by proposing a full-scale universalist welfare state, without the need for a means test, in order to defeat the 'five giants' of want, disease, ignorance, squalor and idleness.[56] Beveridge recommended a flat rate of national insurance tax to be paid by every wage-earner into a fund managed by the government that would, in return, offer a flat rate benefit for sickness, unemployment and old age. Although radical in many ways, his ideas entrenched a 'breadwinner' model of welfare by assuming that paid employment was the sole preserve of men and that women, upon marriage, should be supported by the government but stay in the home.[57] All the same, the ambition of Beveridge's report made him an international celebrity, with copies translated into multiple languages and even eventually found in Hitler's bunker.[58]

Among the problems that Beveridge aimed to address lay the 'limitation of medical service, both in the range of treatment which is provided as of right and in respect of the classes of persons for whom it provided', which represented, to him, the area where 'Britain's achievement' fell 'seriously short of what has been achieved elsewhere'.[59] 'Assumption B' of his report accordingly called for a 'national health service' to ensure that the restoration of an individual to good health become 'a duty of the State'. Though a Liberal, Beveridge drew on the existing direction of travel in socialist circles – including his old friends, the Webbs – in his health service proposals. His report provided a powerful, and popular, message that health care should be organised by the state in a rationalised system to facilitate industrial productivity. Moreover, he asserted that health care represented a 'right' for all citizens, even if he also insisted that citizens had a responsibility to protect and improve their own health. Thousands of people purchased copies of Beveridge's plan, and conversations about its merits could be overheard during factory lunchbreaks as well as around the dinner table.[60]

SMA goals became more achievable in the wake of the Beveridge Report's positive reception. Discussions over adopting their full platform at Labour Party conferences began to swing in their favour. While the Labour Party had committed to a 'State Medical Service' in 1934, eight years later delegates pressed for a more thorough and explicit 'Right to all forms of medical attention and treatment through a National Health Service'.[61] In 1943, the party vowed to introduce such measures in natalist terms. When comparing the health of the working classes to the health of those sitting on the benches of the House of Lords, the ex-suffragist and Labour politician Barbara Ayrton-Gould argued that, 'If the entire population were certain that all their children could have the same opportunities of health from the cradle to the grave as the children of the peers you would go a great way towards solving your birth rate problem'. Some delegates more readily attacked voluntary hospitals and 'all their horrible charitable associations'. These assertions underlined how health care was now becoming couched in a social democratic language of 'rights' to be guaranteed by the state – something too important to leave to charity, mutualism or the market.

The Labour Party committed to establishing a free and comprehensive 'National Service for Health' in 1943, stating in strident terms that 'full health is the greatest asset of an individual, and a healthy population is the greatest asset of a nation', albeit coupled with a somewhat anxious hope that 'the population, instead of diminishing sharply and progressively, will be kept replenished by a sufficiency of children, well-born and well-nurtured'.[62] In a pamphlet released in the same year titled *Wanted – Babies: A Trenchant Examination of a Grave National Problem* (1943), Summerskill explained the declining birth rate as a 'silent revolt' by housewives when presented with the choice between having children, or education and full-time paid employment.[63] In her view, women toiled just as much as men in raising children, yet received no recognition. The solution lay in paying family allowances directly to women and a state medical service. Summerskill justified public money spent on the 'embryo worker' by claiming that they would 'eventually produce the real wealth of the country' and therefore provided a 'magnificent return at a very high rate of interest for the investment made in his childhood'.

As in earlier years, the left did not monopolise discussion of the medical future, but it did do more during the Second World War to popularise what a state service might look like. New philanthropic organisations like the Nuffield Provincial Hospitals Trust and venerable professional groups such as the Society of Medical Officers of Health may have also beaten the drum for a more coordinated service.[64] But left-wing advocates, such as later SMA president Dr David Stark Murray, confidently promoted the possibilities of the state for a wider audience in accessible forms like his Penguin paperback *The Future of Medicine* (1942).[65] Murray emphasised improved curative and preventative measures, including support for maternal and child health, as an issue 'of primary importance in the health of the nation'.

With proposals for a 'national health service' entering the mainstream, pollsters sought to gauge the average Briton's view of the idea. The public did not unanimously agree that the state should take the lead in distributing the promise of medical science. An April 1941 Gallup opinion poll found only a narrow majority – 55 per cent – in favour of 'all doctors and hospitals under state control with their services free as education is now'.[66] Two years later, the social research organisation Mass Observation took to the streets to further probe public attitudes towards the proposals touted by the Beveridge Report.[67] The 1943 Mass Observation report 'Feelings about Hospitals' sent Mass Observers scurrying across five London boroughs to collect a hundred interviews about the future of Britain's health services. They found that 42 per cent of people were in favour of 'State Hospitals', whereas only

13 per cent were in favour of voluntary hospitals, 8 per cent preferred municipal hospitals, 11 per cent wanted to retain 'all sorts of hospitals; as at present', and 21 per cent expressed 'no opinion'. If respondents claimed to prefer state control overall, a mix of preferences existed among the populace. For all the faults that reformers laid at the feet of the interwar health system, the public did not completely condemn it.

This split in opinion remained relatively stable throughout the war. In 1944, the photojournalism magazine *Picture Post* followed the British Institute of Public Opinion (BIPO) as they interviewed a cross-section of Britons about health care proposals.[68] Asking 'On the whole, would you like the idea of a publicly run National Health Service, or would you prefer Hospitals and doctors to be left as they are?', BIPO found that only 55 per cent of the public opted for the former. As the photos of housewives and shipbuilders that accompanied the *Picture Post* article made visible, individuals stood behind these aggregated polling numbers (Figure 2). The replies to Mass Observation studies, scribbled on scraps of recycled paper by the organisation's investigators, provided insight into individual beliefs.[69] These responses showed that for all the wartime debate about reconstruction, and the popular interest that key documents like the Beveridge Report attracted, most people tended to think about the future through their prewar experiences. For instance, few remarked on the Emergency Medical Service (EMS) – a centralised, state-run hospital network which had been set up at the start of the conflict for the thousands of casualties expected by aerial bombing.[70] This absence was notable given Londoners' higher exposure to the EMS compared to people in other parts of the country. Reformers faced difficulty in generating enthusiasm about a nationalised health system by pointing to the more rationalised measures introduced during the war, or straightforwardly building on the ethos of 'fair shares for all' shaped by experiences like the Blitz. Widespread participation in evacuation, rationing, air raids and civil defence organisations did not immediately translate into a broad acceptance of government coordination in health care.

Instead of wartime measures like the EMS colouring opinions, many people continued to invoke memories of the 1920s and 1930s. The

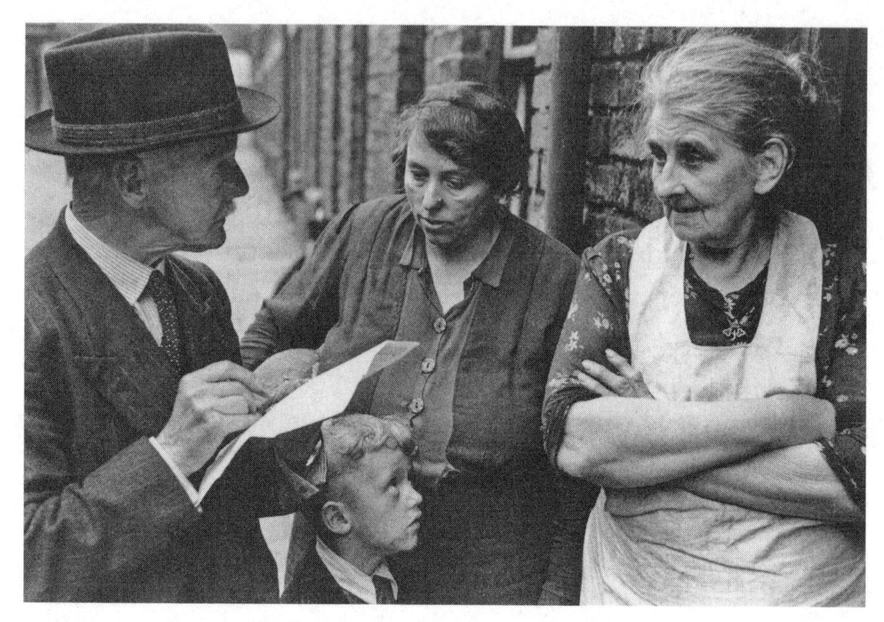

2. When polled during the Second World War, Britons expressed a range of opinions about proposals for a new 'State Medical Service'. The opposition voiced against such plans often centred on a belief that greater government involvement would make health care bureaucratic and impersonal.

anti-socialism of the interwar period crept into the reasoning of those who opposed any future state control of hospitals. Before the war, the press and Conservative Party regularly marshalled 'the public' as a respectable sphere of politics that excluded trade unions and the labour movement, particularly during moments such as the 1926 General Strike.[71] This powerful construction carried longer-term implications for popular reactions to the idea that the state should take the central role in health care. 'Well England is a capitalist country, thank God, and I think all this talk of State control is bunk', declaimed one middle-aged man in a typical oppositional response.[72] Another woman asserted, 'I hate anything which is controlled by the government'. Others thought that state oversight would make health care 'mechanical'. Mass Observation commented on 'expressions of really deep-seated fear' about the impersonal nature of nationalisation, alongside anxieties that 'the State-paid doctor would stiffen into an automaton, a civil servant for whom every patient meant simply one more form to fill in'.[73] Although these responses bore the hallmarks of interwar anti-socialism, they also reflected wartime frustrations with government intrusions into everyday life. If members of the public sometimes voiced irritation about being told to put gas masks on their babies, pull their curtains during blackouts or volunteer themselves to the army or civil defence organisations, then many did not welcome the possibility of increased state involvement in their medical affairs either.[74]

To some, state medicine heralded the death of choice. 'Well, people want to have a choice, not be forced into a hospital like a prison', one woman argued in an evocative example.[75] Her response tracked with other observations collected in 'Public Attitudes to State Medicine', a 1943 Mass Observation survey based on 2,000 interviews and 200 contributions from the organisation's network of panellists, which showed respondents fretting over an 'end' to the local GP and their replacement by an unknown government employee.[76] Despite the inability of the poor to exercise much practical selectivity in their doctor, 66 per cent of those surveyed thought it a 'bad idea' that the state should choose a person's doctor, as opposed to only 11 per cent in favour.[77] Letters to local newspapers from readers sometimes presented 'state medicine' as a 'deadly threat to personal liberty', or, in their most extreme, a form of dictatorship or slavery.[78]

Such views did not prevent Clement Attlee's Labour Party from winning the 1945 General Election in a landslide victory over Winston Churchill's Conservatives. Health care did not sit at the top of the new government's agenda. Labour's manifesto, *Let Us Face the Future* (1945), prioritised the nationalisation of key industries, full employment and council house construction above the establishment of a 'National Health Service'.[79] However, the party's promise to 'work specially for the care of Britain's mothers and their children', as 'healthy family life must be fully ensured and parenthood must not be penalised if the population of Britain is to be prevented from dwindling', illustrated how far the earlier combination of optimism with cautioning about the economy and the birth rate had travelled. In Labour's view, a state medical system would help rebuild the war-ravaged country by boosting production and supporting families.[80] Now they had to breathe life into the longstanding aspirations for a national health service. Convincing Britons of its merits proved to be its own sort of battle.

FOUNDING THE 'NATIONAL HEALTH SERVICE'

As the new Minister of Health and Housing under Attlee, Aneurin Bevan had responsibility for legislating the new service, as well as securing the participation of medical professionals and the public. With the years-long campaign for a state medical service to draw on, Bevan was not totally adrift. He knew it needed to be coordinated by the government, free from direct payment and universal in scope. However, an important question still had to be answered: namely, just how far should the state control the organisation and provision of medical care? Although Bevan believed government planning would pave the way to a New Jerusalem, this issue provoked open divisions within his own party, with health practitioners and among the public.

The decision about whether to nationalise the municipal and voluntary hospitals formed the first point of contention.[81] Bevan's desire to bring these facilities under state control reversed the earlier position – held by almost all medical reformers, the SMA and the Labour Party – that local councils should take responsibility for both. The problem lay in the fact that many members of the public did not want 'state medicine' to envelop the familiarity of their local voluntary hospital. During the war, responses to Mass Observation had revealed apprehension about the implications of the potential banishment of charity from health care. The 'Feelings about Hospitals' survey found 'a definite association between people's feelings about how hospitals should be run, and whether or not they had ever been patients at any hospital', especially among ex-patients of voluntary hospitals.[82] Their supporters among the public invoked tradition in voicing support for their continued existence, with one 'firm believer in the Voluntary System' justifying her stance by stating that 'it has stood the test of time'.[83] Some thought that voluntary hospitals should only lose their independence to local councils, rather than central government. 'I think they're best run locally, where local conditions are understood', claimed one man, adding that 'State interference would ruin them'. Others believed that voluntary hospitals should receive financial grants from central government but manage themselves, with one man expanding on the point: 'The Beveridge Report is all right, provided it isn't put into the hands of a lot of damned bureaucrats: only people who understand the running of hospitals should be allowed to have any say in it'. The Mayor of Bournemouth stressed community ownership of such institutions in his opening address to the 1946 Labour Party conference, and described his local voluntary hospital as 'very dear to the hearts of the people'.[84] 'They have worked unsparingly for it down the years' he continued, alluding to a 'great fear that they will be deprived in the future from giving that service which has been for them an expression of their sympathy and Christian charity'.

Municipal hospitals possessed a prominent defender in Herbert Morrison, Leader of the House of Commons and Attlee's deputy. In Cabinet discussions, Morrison drew on his experiences as the former Labour leader of the LCC in the 1930s, where he had overseen an authority that supplied the most municipal hospital beds in the world by 1939.[85] He maintained that the proven successes of this model could be replicated across the country, with councils given financial support from the government but otherwise pursuing their own agendas that best suited local conditions.

Despite these pleas for both voluntary and municipal hospitals, Bevan remained convinced that the best course of action lay in their nationalisation. Government control, he believed, would end the confusion and inefficiencies of a hospital system that had developed piecemeal since the eighteenth century. It would distribute health care more evenly across the nation, particularly in industrial and rural areas. Echoing the logic of earlier reformers on the left, Bevan also imagined the NHS as a key support for the 'planned' economy of the future. It followed that hospitals should be integrated within this vision of the postwar era, not left to their own devices. While Bevan acknowledged the contributions made by voluntary hospitals, he asserted that they had been 'established often by the caprice of private charity' and therefore paid no heed to providing equality across services, especially in specialisms like cancer treatment or cardiology.[86] He derided prioritising the purported 'localism and intimacy' of the 'very small hospital' above other considerations. 'I would rather be kept alive in the efficient if cold altruism of a large hospital than expire in a gush of warm sympathy in a small one', he remarked. Bevan also pulled no punches when it came to hospitals run by local authorities. 'If we are to carry out our obligation and to provide the people of Great Britain, no matter where they may be, with the same level of service', he declared, 'then the nation itself will have to carry the expenditure, and cannot put it upon the shoulders of any other authority'. He admitted that the battle to build a new and comprehensive service would be long, but stated that it represented a cause that would 'lift the shadow from millions of homes'.

Attlee ultimately sided with Bevan, deciding to trust his Minister of Health over Morrison. With this internal disagreement out of the way, in 1946 Labour passed the National Health Service Act, enshrining the Minister of Health with a 'duty' to promote a comprehensive health service in England and Wales. The government would become the central instrument of medical coordination and provision.[87] All voluntary and local authority hospitals were transferred to the Minister, managed through Regional Hospital Boards (RHBs). If local councils lost control of their municipal hospitals to the RHBs, then the NHS Act still charged them with establishing health centres that would bring together curative and preventative services. In a nod to their prior successes, local government also retained its responsibility for public health, although questions would soon arise regarding preventative medicine's formal separation from hospitals and general practice in the tripartite structure of the NHS. Dental, pharmaceutical and ophthalmic care also fell within the remit of the state. The totality of these services would be available to all citizens without direct cost, replacing the pre-existing plurality of private, mutualist or charitable models of health care with a social democratic 'right' to treatment, guaranteed by the state. In 1947 and 1948, the government introduced largely identical NHS Acts in Scotland and Northern Ireland, respectively.

Although this legislation emerged from a political debate about the future of health care that ranged across the political spectrum, its state-centredness and nationalised structure represented the particular legacy of the political left, and especially Bevan. On the one hand, figures from the Liberal Party and the Conservative Party had also called for the government coordination of medical care. After all, Beveridge endorsed such an approach in his 1942 report. At the end of the war, the Conservative Minister of Health, Henry Willink issued a White Paper which proposed, as its title suggested, *A National Health Service* (1944).[88] On the other hand, although this White Paper also called for a free and comprehensive health service, it would not have created the 'NHS' in either structural or cultural terms. For instance, the 'Willink Plan' did not suggest the nationalisation of the hospitals, nor did it compel local authorities to construct health centres. The proposals did not express anywhere near as much faith in the central state as Bevan or the medical left. Willink's scheme would have created a more disaggregated system that would have been difficult to translate into a cohesive cultural idea of 'the NHS'. For his part, Beveridge insisted upon not being seen as the institution's architect. 'As I go about the country I find myself continually being hailed as the inventor of the Health Service', he later complained.[89] Beveridge believed that charity should have been given more of a role in the NHS Acts and refuted the idea that his report and the medical service that followed it were synonymous. 'Let me emphatically deny any such claim on my part', he maintained, 'I am not the inventor'.

Regardless of Labour's distinctive contributions, the medical profession had long been wary of government intervention in their work and were primed to oppose the NHS. Their primary professional organisation, the British Medical Association (BMA), had campaigned against the 1911 National Insurance Act.[90] During the interwar years, the BMA fretted over the growing interest in 'state medicine' spearheaded by socialists and other reformers. The SMA's suggestion that doctors become salaried workers horrified the BMA. Beyond their own professional status, they felt that an increased role for the state in medicine would erode standards of care. In a 1939 speech, the organisation's former Secretary Dr Alfred Cox insisted that in a world becoming 'more and more machine made and mechanized' where 'the individual tends to become more and more swamped in the mass', it was 'an imperative duty . . . to keep our profession, and the rights and privileges and welfare of the individual, free from the shackles of standardization – a condition which is the inevitable result of government control'.[91]

As soon as Labour took office, the BMA sallied forth from their headquarters in Bloomsbury to do battle with Bevan. Between 1945 and 1948, the organisation negotiated in tense meetings, balloted their members to rally feeling against the service and sought to win the backing of patients.[92] In their campaign against the NHS, they presented the longstanding left-wing demands for 'state medicine' as a less personal alternative to existing measures. During a 1945 public debate on the question of 'Is State Medicine Desirable?', one critical doctor depicted Labour's proposals as restricting choice and insisted that while the party might nationalise other industries, like coal, 'they could not nationalise something which was on a higher moral and ethical plane'.[93] When an interviewer asked the GP Margaret Teuter Samuel what she first thought about the NHS proposals, she simply replied: 'Disgraceful, disgraceful'.[94] A former Chairman of the BMA compared the scheme to Nazi Germany and suggested it would make Bevan a 'Medical Fuehrer'.[95] When the NHS Acts passed, the BMA balloted its members, returning a 54 per cent vote against joining the service. Bevan – not a man to be outdone in a war of words – described the BMA as a 'small body of politically poisoned people'.[96]

The doctors did not lack wider support. Among the Britons who had heard of the dispute between the BMA and Bevan, 30 per cent stated that their 'sympathies are with the doctors', as opposed to 28 per cent 'against' them.[97] The BBC received angry complaints about its 'prejudiced and utterly one-sided' reporting of the disagreement that seemingly favoured the Labour government.[98] These affinities between the public and the medical profession sometimes followed directly from their everyday interactions. Doctors, nurses, dentists and opticians were respected members of a local community. Their thoughts on what the NHS would look like mattered. Diaries revealed how patients asked searching questions of these professionals about the new system. Most of the professional opinions they received were critical. After a woman from Gateshead asked her GP for his thoughts in May 1946, she wrote 'My doctor says it will be good for doctors but not for patients'.[99] Critical views from medical practitioners changed patients' minds. A pottery worker from Stoke-on-Trent recorded in his diary days before the service's introduction that 'The nation's health should – indeed must – be the nation's first charge'. But after a consultation with his own GP later in the month, he rearticulated his doctor's pessimism that the service 'is foredoomed, if not to utter failure, it will be quite incapable of coping with the public needs and thereby inefficient'.[100]

Nonetheless, concessions made by Bevan to the medical profession eventually helped turn the tide against the BMA. Enid Russell-Smith, a career civil servant at the top of the Ministry of Health, accompanied Bevan to the exhausting negotiations with the medical profession's representatives. As the first British woman to gain a black belt in karate, she might have been tempted to deploy her skills in martial arts against the 'bloody-minded doctors' and 'revolting dentists' that they spoke with.[101] Yet, come the 'appointed day' of the NHS's inception, Bevan eventually won the support of enough doctors through a series of concessions. GPs were allowed to continue to take private patients. Consultants could do the same in the hospitals. Bevan ruled out doctors becoming salaried professionals, as the SMA had long called for. Instead, GPs would become 'independent contractors' to the NHS, employed by the service's Executive Councils, rather than by local or central government. In some ways, this concession extended the pre-1948 circumstances of GPs under national health insurance, bringing them closer to the priorities of the state but allowing them to stand at a distance. The prestigious teaching hospitals continued with a degree of independence by maintaining their own governing boards. In the final BMA plebiscite (which balloted the whole medical profession), 54 per cent voted to cease negotiations with Bevan. As the minister later quipped, he had 'stuffed their mouths with gold'.[102]

The displeasure that many health professionals directed at the NHS did not end. On 5 July 1948, medical students at St Thomas's Hospital, London, scrawled 'BOOT OUT BEVAN' in white paint on the wall opposite the Houses of Parliament.[103] Embarrassed hospital officials quickly covered the graffiti with a tarpaulin. Nevertheless, on the same day, the vast majority of English, Welsh, Scottish and Northern Irish doctors continued with their work, now under the state's stewardship. Nationalising hospitals proceeded efficiently – a remarkable feat considering the 1,143 voluntary hospitals and 1,545 municipal hospitals in England and Wales alone. Yet forging some of the bureaucratic dimensions of the NHS proved difficult. As late as the spring of 1948, Russell-Smith at the Ministry of Health privately wrote how she was 'almost frightened by the vast mass of stuff there is to get through before July'.[104] When reports arrived from post offices that they had not received enough sign-up forms for prospective patients, she hurriedly sent her 'valiant staff' to train stations to place emergency supplies on passenger trains. Such efforts ensured that the NHS could begin at all.

Nonetheless, another key part of Bevan's victory over the doctors involved marshalling public opinion in favour of the service. Given the misgivings about 'state medicine' expressed by many people across the first half of the twentieth century, shifting popular attitudes about the coming NHS required an active effort.

PROMOTING THE NHS

The ability to access health care free at the point of use immediately transformed lives. Britons who had long put off seeing a doctor, dentist or optician cold now do so without direct charge. This expanded provision, though, was not enough to unseat long-held misgivings about 'state medicine' alone. As the wartime Mass Observation surveys showed, large sections of the public needed to be convinced. Labour addressed this problem in two ways. First, they attuned the structure of the NHS to specific needs and safeguarded values like choice. Second, they launched a public relations campaign that successfully reworked popular understandings of their ambitions. Instead of an impersonal, bureaucratic machine, the public began to see 'the National Health' as a caring, family-centred institution that marked a clear break with the past.

Structurally, the NHS's emphasis on family care quickly won accolades across social classes. All women and children could now access family doctor and hospital services without financial barriers or the indignity of means testing. Mass Observation documented the feelings of appreciation for the security now guaranteed by the state. 'A Report on the National Health Service' (1949), based on 110 interviews across Britain, found that the 'attention to maternity cases and to children's ailments is usually the most highly praised of all'.[105] In a typical example, one working-class woman, who 'didn't used to go much to the doctors', gladly took advantage of the new NHS when she broke her arm.[106] While she thought the deductions in National Insurance were 'a lot of money to pay out every week', she noted that her husband's insurance payments before 1948 'was just for himself and now we're all covered by it'. Another working-class woman widowed from the war with three children similarly observed, 'It's very good for people that have children, because some people used to have to have children in degrading conditions because they couldn't afford to pay the hospital bills'. Middle-class families also acknowledged the benefits of medical universalism. One woman with three daughters claimed, 'Each time I used to go up, it used to cost me 3/s or 3/6s for each visit for myself and the children, and now we don't pay anything'. Another middle-class respondent described the NHS as 'excellent' because 'I have two children and for anybody with children it is a very good thing'. When Mass Observation asked her what she liked best, she replied that though before 1948 'anyone who worked could be covered by Health Insurance . . . for the children there was no such scheme'. Despite the many improvements in health provision during the interwar years, the previous system had not gone far enough to earn the undivided loyalty of the public.

Men, and particularly fathers, expressed their appreciation for the new NHS, reflecting the gradual embrace of a mid-century masculine identity as the 'family man' who seemed more comfortable at home than men of earlier generations.[107] 'I like it because my wife and children are covered', said one thirty-five-year-old father from Paddington, previously the only one in his family covered by a panel doctor.[108] The NHS, he enthused, meant he could now 'bring them up healthy'. Similarly, a young agricultural worker thought 'insuring the whole family on the man's contribution is a tremendous benefit', because 'it was quite unreasonable for a working man to have to pay out a lot of money if his wife or children was ill, and the result was that they were often neglected'. During the war, Mass Observation detected a higher degree of support among men than women for the principle of the state's involvement in medical care, perhaps reflecting their greater familiarity with government assistance in accessing GPs through national health insurance.[109] Their responses once the NHS arrived also suggested how the provision of health care to whole families dovetailed with changing expectations about parental roles and a swelling belief that a child's total wellbeing should be supported.

The NHS's approach to charity provided another point of connection between the service's structural dimensions and the public. Labour did not banish voluntarism from British health care in 1948, but they did curtail it. Bevan's orders to remove collection boxes from hospital waiting rooms symbolically demonstrated that people would no longer have to rely on charity for their medical needs. Despite some voices of support for voluntary hospitals during the interwar and wartime period, Mass Observation had uncovered a vein of anger about the role of charity in medicine. Responding to a question about 'hospitals collecting subscriptions, and having flag days', a striking eighty-three out of eighty-four answers focused on flag days alone. Among respondents, 55 per cent saw this fundraising method in a negative light, 25 per cent were positive and 18 per cent offered a more balanced comment.[110] People with a critical opinion of flag days lambasted them as a 'public annoyance', 'degrading' and 'all wrong'.[111] 'Finish with all that hypocrisy', charged one person, adding that hospitals 'shouldn't have to beg in a country of plenty'. Respondents described flag days as a relic of the past, finding them 'archaic' or 'out of date'. In a 1947 survey, contributors may have thought of giving to hospitals and funds for disabled people as among 'the most praiseworthy causes', but a sizeable body also took this opportunity to lambast flag days.[112] Even if flag days had provided only a small amount of the total funding of voluntary hospitals compared to insurance schemes in the interwar period, they attracted an outsized degree of vitriol. Clearly, most of the public shared Bevan's view that an overreliance on charity in health care was unfair and outdated.

The government also facilitated support for the NHS by protecting choice in medicine, described by Bevan as 'one of the most important safeguards for the public'.[113] Patients continued to choose their own doctors within the service. Labour resisted calls to shepherd patients towards particular doctors. This decision went against the views of some reformers – including members of the SMA – who believed that such direction might secure a more even distribution of GPs across Britain.[114] Bevan's concessions to the doctors in allowing them to continue with private patients also ensured that choice under the NHS included the option to pay for medical care outside of the system, if the individual so desired.

However, the institutional framework of the NHS alone could not address the obstacles nationalised medicine faced in securing public acceptance, even if it demonstrated a responsiveness to their concerns. Persuasion played a central role in generating support for Labour's economic and welfare policies after 1945, no less true with the new NHS.[115] Films, radio broadcasts, press advertisements, an informational display for factories and women's organisations, speeches, posters and leaflets all promoted the NHS, both in terms of the services it offered and what it symbolised.[116] Central government cooperated with local councils to aid their communications about the service. This promotion played a key role in shaping early opinion, particularly for those who did not use it immediately after July 1948. In fact, only 38 per cent of people had any contact with the NHS in its first three months, and publicity efforts filled the gap.[117]

Labour took their messaging directly to homes. The government sent a four-page 'House-to-House' leaflet – which described the NHS and how to join – to every household in England and Wales between late April and May 1948, with Scotland producing its own version. Bevan personally stewarded its production, eagerly 'trying it out' on his media friends and working closely with Thomas Fife Clarke, founding member of the British Institute of Public Relations and head of the government's Central Office of Information (COI).[118] Both men ensured that the leaflet was released separately from another pamphlet on National Insurance and secured Treasury funding for higher quality paper, a not insignificant victory given continued paper rationing (Figure 3).[119] The effort put into the publication extended to a Welsh-language translation and lengthy discussions over font and italics. With a print run of over 13 million, this leaflet represented, in the view of one civil servant, 'the most powerful instrument in the armoury of publicity at the launching of the National Health Service'.[120]

The 'House-to-House' leaflet prioritised the notion of choice, reflecting the Ministry of Health's desire to further alleviate the fears about government-organised health care stoked by doctors in their conflict with Bevan. Its first heading, 'Choose Your Doctor Now', preceded a paragraph repeating the word 'choice' and a reassurance that 'Your dealings with the doctor will remain the same as they are now: *personal and confidential*'. Under 'WHAT TO DO NOW', the leaflet encouraged Britons to 'Choose your doctor' by procuring an application form at the Post Office. Primarily aimed at ensuring as wide a sign-up to the NHS as possible, the government strategically highlighted choice of doctor as the entry point to the service. The film *Doctor's Dilemma* (1948) similarly asked millions of cinemagoers, 'Have YOU chosen your family doctor?'[121]

Film proved crucial for the government, as they repeatedly used the popular medium to distinguish the 'National Health Service' from

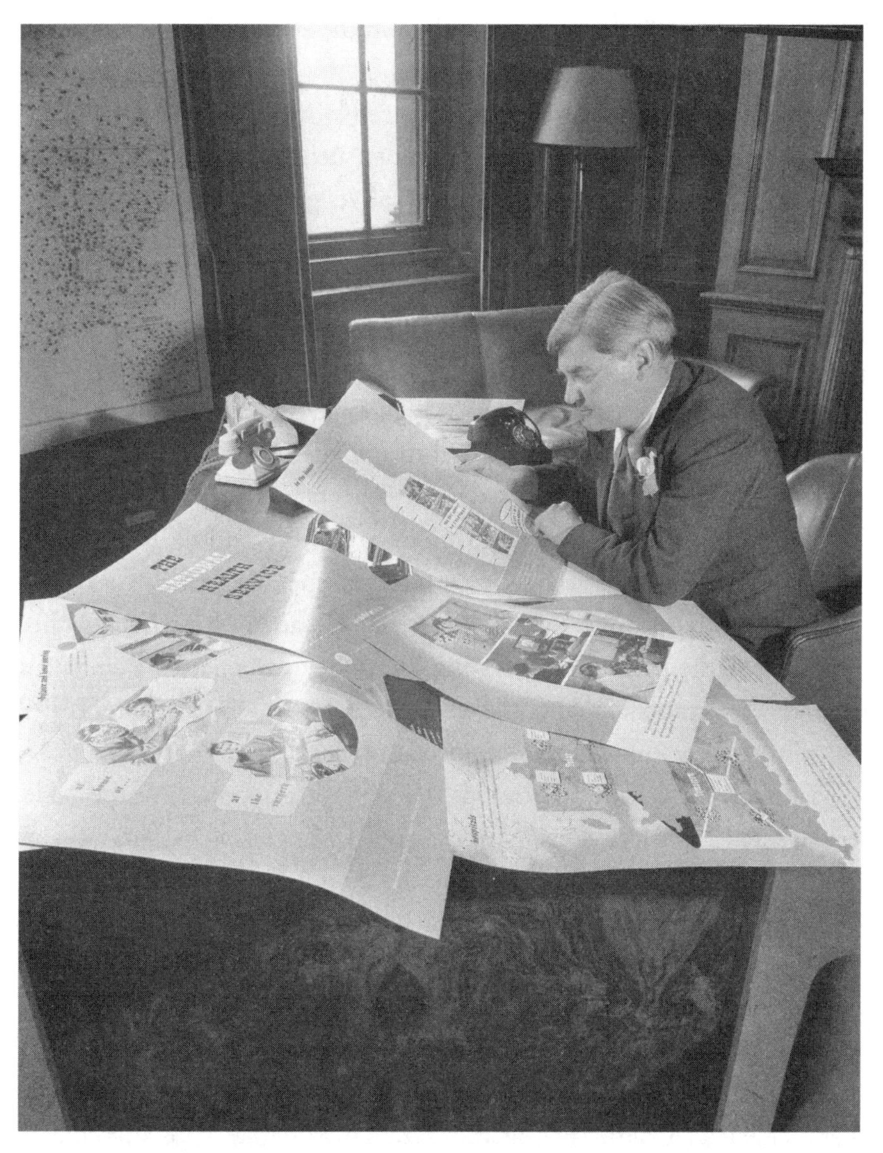

3. Minister of Health and Housing Aneurin Bevan took a keen interest in promoting the NHS through film, posters and radio. This extensive output helped alleviate some of the public anxieties about 'state medicine' by branding the 'National Health Service' as a caring guardian of the family unit, fit for the future.

older understandings of 'state medicine'. *Here's Health* (1948) – a twenty-five minute drama – took place in the months before the NHS and followed the fictional Dr Collins's efforts to assist the Carters, a poor rural family.[122] Written and produced by Budge Cooper, this film followed her other wartime productions, such as *Children of the City* (1944), in emphasising the transformative potential of the state in working-class lives. Directed by her husband, Donald Alexander, *Here's Health* stressed the advantages of the NHS to previously uninsured groups. When Mrs Carter breaks her ankle and Dr Collins is called, he does his best to help but laments the timing as, he explains, 'under the new Health Act . . . you would have been relieved of all the worry about money'. The film then moves to a 'future' under the NHS. Depicted as an improved time for all, it showed the Carters now having their health needs met, free of charge. *Here's Health*'s sombre ending back in the pre-NHS present – with the Carter children spending Christmas apart from their parents due to Mr Carter having to care for his wife – further emphasised the inequities of relying on money and charity. References to 'the new Health Act' and 'the new scheme' presented a different, and more humanised, understanding of nationalised health care.

Through these communications, Labour and supporters of the NHS constructed sharp divisions between a pre-1948 and post-1948 Britain. Narratives of progress flattened out the complexities of the past. The Ministry of Information cartoon *Your Very Good Health* (1948) deployed themes of historical advancement to persuade the public to use the new NHS.[123] This film formed part of the *Charley* series, created by the film-makers Halas and Batchelor to promote different aspects of postwar reconstruction, such as New Towns.[124] In this edition of the series, the main character Charley – a working-class man with a wife and child – comes to see the NHS as an advantage for his family. His initial scepticism is partly overcome by being reminded of the shortcomings of the pre-existing panel system. The film also targeted middle-class opinion. Charley's more affluent neighbour, George, does not think the NHS is designed for people of his means. But, after falling from a tree and needing hospital care, he comes to appreciate the service. With such productions, the Labour government packaged many of the earlier political arguments for a government-run service in a digestible cultural medium, including the social and economic benefits of medical universalism, the advantages of the state's rationalisation of services and its significance to families and children. 'The younger generation will stand to gain the biggest benefits of all', concluded *Your Very Good Health* in another reassertion of the service's futurity through the symbol of the child.

The government and its supporters hoped to minimise worries about choice and regimentation and move popular opinion towards appreciation of a mid-century social democratic ethos where the government was seen as a guardian of the family unit. The poster 'Labour's Health Service Covers Everyone' (1950) offered a visual reminder of the state's role in safeguarding families.[125] On a striking yellow and red background, a man, a woman, an older boy and his grandparents all gaze up at a small girl: a healthy and multi-generational family covered by the NHS. After reading an article in *News Review* magazine about the service in January 1949, a man from Fareham, Hampshire, thought it a 'clear and convincing picture of the advantages of the new National Health Scheme'.[126] His diary recorded recognition of the imagery of historical progress, futurity and the family prevalent across early NHS promotional material. 'It takes an imaginary family and shows how much better off it is today with the benefits now available,' the man observed. Reflecting on having to pay for the service through National Insurance contributions, he maintained, 'But isn't anything so comprehensive worth paying for? Yes, I say, yes indeed'. A July 1949 opinion poll found the NHS ranked highest by all sections of the public as 'the best thing the Labour Government has done'.[127] Among respondents, 30 per-cent placed the institution at the top, above children's welfare measures at 17 per cent. The NHS was clearly becoming popular as part of a broader appreciation for welfare measures that supported families and children, even if the level of support was not overwhelming.

By the end of the Labour government's time in office in 1951, the terms through which the public discussed nationalised medicine exhibited signs of change. While people sometimes continued to invoke the term 'state medicine', this particular formulation declined among the general public and thereafter largely became the language of the NHS's free-market critics. Diaries after 1948 usually referred to the NHS as 'the service', 'health scheme' or just 'the scheme'. Letters to newspapers from the early 1950s onwards showed 'the National Health', 'National Health Scheme' or the 'National Health Service' becoming the predominant descriptors.[128] The gradual replacement of 'state medicine' with these softer phrases further protected the service against the charge that the government would make health care bureaucratic or mechanical.

The cultural embedding of Britain's new health system with caring and forward-looking qualities created the space for more people to associate themselves with the institution. If the public had struggled to express attachment towards the interwar health system because of its disaggregated and uneven nature, then the creation of 'the National Health' as a single, bounded service – free from direct payment – allowed for such feeling. People began to 'thank' the NHS after its establishment.[129] In 1949 one woman expressed 'my thanks to the National Health Service' for a new hearing aid that was, to her, 'a wonderful gift'.[130] Writing to the *New Statesman* in the same year, another man credited the service with curing his daughter of mumps.[131] Articulating a direct connection with the institution itself, he thought her survival was 'a tribute to the doctors and nurses of the National Health Service'. Though he noted that his old private doctor – a 'family friend' who refused to join the NHS – would have acted the same way, this man used his experience to challenge the view that the service made doctors bureaucratic. Clearly signalling his attachment to the NHS, he concluded that 'as for "family friends", the greatest friends of my family are those who saved my baby's life'. This man's description of the NHS as not just a protector of children but also a 'friend' resonated with the ideas that the service's advocates had worked to foster.

***

The making of the NHS was not instant or automatic, but achieved over time. Aspirations for a 'State Medical Service', as it was first described, began in the Edwardian period and gathered pace across the interwar years. Universal, government-provided medicine, various reformers emphasised, would end the blight of poverty, recover the dwindling birth rate and boost industrial production. These aspirations reflected wider social democratic priorities during the mid-twentieth century. Debates over reconstruction during the Second World War, and the publication of the Beveridge Report, provided further stimulus. After 1945, the Labour government ensured that the radicalism of these longer-term ambitions remained more-or-less intact, even if Bevan made concessions to the medical profession. Labour recognised that the success of such a scheme could never be taken for granted and required active promotion. The creation of a gargantuan institution that touched the lives of everyone in the country would always be about more than legislation, hospital budgets and doctors' salaries. Attlee's Labour governments jettisoned their forebears' focus on 'state medicine' in favour of a more humanistic and futuristic notion of a 'National Health Service'. This cultural category opened the space for the public to begin to forge their own connections with the institution. After the NHS's first year, 95 per cent of the UK's 45 million people had signed up to the service. With expectations high, they now entered its hospitals and doctors' surgeries.

2

ON THE WARD

Three weeks after the NHS launched, a pregnant woman named Sarah Campion (1906–2002) booked a bed at Queen Charlotte's Hospital, London. She published an account of her subsequent journey from antenatal clinic to the birth of a boy, Philip, as a book titled *National Baby* (1950).[1] Written in the style of a diary, it documented how 'the National Health' treated mothers. Campion penned *National Baby* in an entertaining style and, reflecting her socialist beliefs, generally spoke in support of the NHS. Yet her book also featured criticisms of the care that she received from 'St. Albion's Hospital', a pseudonym for Queen Charlotte's chosen to shield the identity of the staff and patients that she had encountered.[2] Antiquated buildings, worn-out medical customs and condescending attitudes numbered among the critiques levelled at the hospital and, in turn, the new nationalised health system. Worryingly for the service's supporters, Campion did not stand alone in holding such views. How, then, did the NHS move on from its Victorian and interwar inheritance? And what role did patients and the public play in the process of modernisation that unfolded across the postwar decades?

As Campion recognised, the distinctions either side of 5 July 1948 were not as firm as the NHS's founders claimed. To be sure, the postwar Labour government had begun to rationalise health care through the mechanisms of state planning guided by the NHS Acts. Across the UK, 3,100 hospitals now provided 550,000 beds, overseen by RHBs that coordinated services and allocated government funds.[3] An army of half a million workers ensured that the NHS fell behind only the British Transport Commission and the National Coal Board as the largest employer in the nation. But the quality and feel of Britain's hospitals clashed with the futuristic vision of the service that had been presented to the public in promotional materials like films or posters during its turbulent inception. Most hospitals dated from the nineteenth century: approximately 45 per cent were built before 1891, and 21 per cent before 1861.[4] No new hospitals opened with the inauguration of the service. The funds for renovating or constructing buildings stood at one fifth of the prewar rate.[5] Moreover, some of the unevenness in the quality of care across the UK persisted, and the medical cultures that the patient encountered at their bedside appeared to be largely unchanged.

Out of these uncertain beginnings, and through persistent controversy, the NHS modernised. Between the 1940s and 1970s, a system took shape that provided free-at-the-point-of-use medical care in changed health care spaces organised on communal lines. Both Conservative and Labour governments refurbished older facilities and constructed a number of new ones, while introducing reforms to the everyday provision of medicine. This process of modernisation conjoined with trends elsewhere around the world during the mid-twentieth century. Most industrialised countries built larger hospitals that concentrated developments in high-technology medicine such as radiology, cardiology and oncology.[6] As in other nations, the hospital formed the keystone of the postwar health system. By the early 1960s, they absorbed about 60 per cent of all NHS expenditure.[7] Yet in Britain, the state led the process of modernisation, even if charitable organisations, medical activists, community groups and researchers helped bring the NHS closer to its founding principles. Though the health service experienced instability in its budgets during the 1970s, this decade marked the point of its maturity.[8] The NHS did not succumb to the financial cuts that fatally undermined other parts of the welfare state, despite its persistent underfunding compared to areas like education (a position that would not be consistently reversed until 1984).[9] Nor did it acquire a popular reputation as a failed exercise in public ownership. Even though the immediate postwar years were far from an era of plenty for the health service in terms of funding, the determined efforts of its supporters ensured that it could embed itself in British life.

The process of modernisation did not just boil down to bureaucracy or the grand designs of experts. It was also a social process that attempted to reshape human relationships in accordance with political objectives. In the case of the NHS, these priorities were the advancement of a social democratic communalism that was flexible enough to attend to personal preferences or local needs.[10] Planners and reformers believed that patients of different backgrounds could be brought together on public wards, while still being treated as individuals. This balance between the communal and the personal proved essential in accommodating a flowering 'popular individualism' by the 1960s, as consumerism, feminism and a decline in deference to older social hierarchies took hold.[11] If the historian Tony Judt presented this rising tide of postwar individualism as integral to the eventual undoing of social democracy across Europe, then the NHS questions this interpretation.[12] Rather than build or refurbish NHS hospitals with single rooms that ensconced patients away from one another, patients were encouraged to experience – and in many cases came to prefer – the shared life of the ward. The everyday life of social democracy, with all the possibilities and tensions of its communalism, could be felt in these spaces of care. While historians have given valuable attention to shifting administrative structures or the construction of new buildings, these social dynamics proved equally important.[13] Away from the newspaper headlines about NHS bureaucracy or the hospital designs that fronted glossy architectural journals took place the hidden work of reformulating the associations between patients, the state and medical experts. More mundane – and therefore easily missed – reforms that altered the life of hospitals, such as extending visiting hours or redesigning patients' beds, cemented communal relationships and placed the service on a firm foundation.

HOSPITALS OF THE PAST, FOR THE FUTURE

The social democratic principles that shaped the NHS as an idea and a piece of legislation were poured into a nineteenth-century vessel. Half of the hospitals that the service inherited dated from Queen Victoria's reign.[14] The practices and routines of the service's wards also possessed roots in this earlier era. However, despite these continuities with the past, different groups of patients now entered these facilities in greater numbers. The middle class became attracted to NHS care through both a desire to save money and a mid-century faith in the modern hospital as the best way to access medical expertise. Maternity care reflected these changes in attitudes, with Britons increasingly viewing hospitals as safe places to deliver babies given the care and technologies available.[15] Only 15 per cent of all live births in Britain took place in a hospital in 1927 but this figure grew to 24 per cent by 1933, 35 per cent by 1937, and 54 per cent by 1946.[16] By 1970, government and medical experts were recommending 100 per cent hospital births – a figure never achieved, but testament to the expanded belief in the virtues of these facilities. The prior concerns about the dwindling birth rate – which had given impetus to the interwar and wartime arguments in favour of establishing the NHS – quickly subsided in the face of a 'baby boom' after 1945, as Britain experienced a significant increase in fertility rates. While British women had an average of 1.8 children in 1940, this number rose to 2.8 in 1965.[17] The NHS's initial proponents might have taken heart from such increases, but these new mothers, infants and children still needed to be cared for. Accordingly, the service's early years proceeded with a family-oriented and maternalist emphasis.

Queen Charlotte's Maternity Hospital, London, exhibited the medical past, the medical future and changing patient views at the start of the NHS. The institution began in the eighteenth century as one of Britain's first 'lying-in' hospitals for pregnant women.[18] It moved to a site in Marylebone in the nineteenth century. Between 1929 and 1930, a new hospital structure was built on Goldhawk Road, Shepherd's Bush, which opened under the threat of bombing during the Second World War.[19] The state nationalised Queen Charlotte's in 1948, and, under the NHS, it became linked with the Chelsea Hospital for Women, another venerable institution with origins in the 1870s. Though Queen Charlotte's administrators did not oppose the new state system, some grumbled about the end of the hospital's glamourous charity balls, where the presentation of aristocratic debutantes had once helped finance its activities. The government would now foot the bills that had been covered in the interwar period by charity, insurance or patients' direct payments.

The architecture and design of Queen Charlotte's reflected many Victorian conventions, despite its recent relocation and reorganisation. Its main buildings stood six stories tall, split into wings in the 'pavilion' style. Iron railings surrounded the site and a porters' lodge guarded the premises. The onset of the NHS heralded few signs of structural improvement. Bevan informed the hospital's chairman that although 'a big building programme was called for when materials and labour were available', his institution should make do and 'paint and furnish and generally overhaul'.[20] Even if the main structure of Queen Charlotte's was relatively new, the scattered network of institutions attached to the hospital remained monuments to nineteenth-century medicine. One of its main convalescent facilities, the All Saints Hospital, 60 miles away in the seaside town of Eastbourne, had opened in 1869.

Sarah Campion based *National Baby* on her experiences with this mixture of medical facilities. Born Mary Rose Coulton in 1906, Campion grew up in an affluent Cambridge household (Figure 4).[21] Daughter of the medieval historian G.G. Coulton, she discovered an early love of writing and changed her name to mirror her favourite poet, Thomas Campion. Her novels brought her moderate success, particularly the 'Queensland Trilogy', which had been informed by living in Australia during the late 1930s.[22] She led an unusual life. A staunch socialist, Campion taught Jewish children English in Nazi Germany before being expelled by the government, and lived and travelled in the USA, Canada, South Africa, Australia and New Zealand. Campion resided in Britain during the Second World War and its aftermath, before settling in New Zealand in 1952, where she remained until her death some fifty years later.

Campion's first interactions with the NHS attested to the initial high demand for its services. When attending antenatal clinics at the

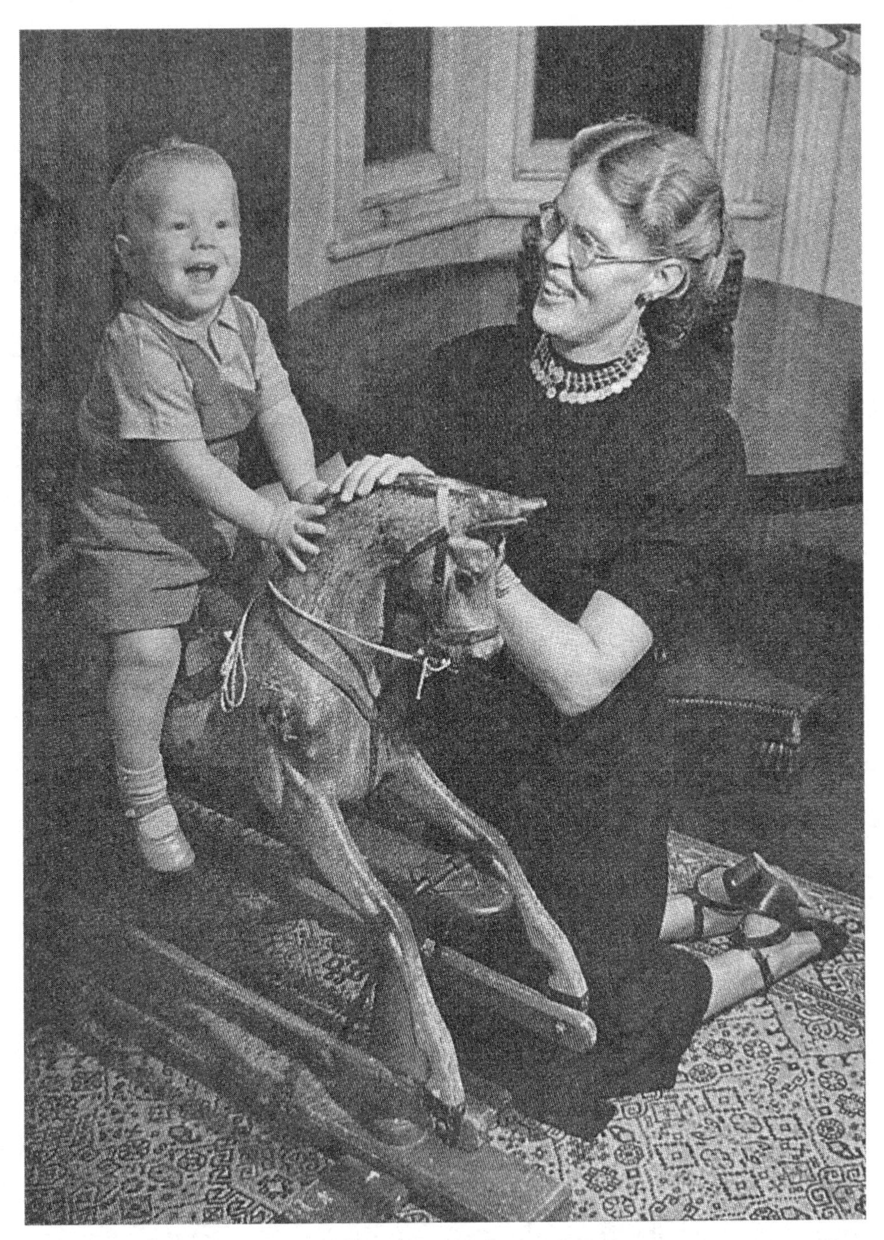

4. The author Sarah Campion expressed support for the new NHS in her published account of giving birth at Queen Charlotte's Maternity Hospital, London. However, she also identified sources of tension on hospital wards related to privacy and patients from different social classes mixing together.

Chelsea Hospital for Women, she joined large numbers of women waiting on long wooden benches to see a doctor. This scene was not uncommon after health care became free at the point of access. In 1947, Queen Charlotte's admitted just over 3,000 in-patients, a figure that rose by 17 per cent during 1950–51 alone.[23] Administrators fretted over how 'the cramped facilities' were 'being strained to the utmost'. But, for Campion, queuing became an important illustration of the NHS's sense of equity. 'Each lays some piece of property in the seat when she leaves it, to stake a claim', she noted, 'and while she is up there the head of the queue moves, we all move, ostentatiously pushing this jetsam before us, as if to demonstrate that we, too, know that fair's fair'.

For all this egalitarianism, Campion encountered resentment among women regarding infractions on their bodily privacy during medical investigations. Queen Charlotte's – like other teaching hospitals – frequently used patients in training medical students. Sometimes these exercises took place without forewarning. One woman at the antenatal clinic told Campion of her surprise at being suddenly in front of 'a whole lot of grinning students'.[24] Gender shaped such concerns, as predominantly male instructors and medical trainees observed and commented on women's bodies in exposed settings. Campion resented 'having my body made the arena for a medical free-for-all', but patients possessed few means of recourse if they objected. During one appointment with a male doctor, Campion felt like she was being 'done like an object on an assembly belt'. After she asked for more information and was dismissed by the doctor, Campion confessed that she felt like 'a nitwit'.

When Campion arrived at Queen Charlotte's to give birth weeks later, she expressed concerns about privacy.[25] After a difficult labour that involved the use of forceps, she spent nine days recovering in a 'blue and spacious ward', with 'acres of parquet' separating the beds.[26] This lengthy period of confinement fell just under the ten days customary for various hospital treatments at the time.[27] In many NHS hospitals, including Queen Charlotte's, wards followed the 'Nightingale' pattern.[28] Named after the Victorian medical reformer and nursing pioneer Florence

Nightingale (1820–1920), these large wards typically housed twenty to thirty beds arranged along two walls, with no firm sub-divisions between patients. The high ceilings and large windows of the 'pavilion' hospital style reduced infection in accordance with a nineteenth-century understanding of disease transmission, where sickness spread through 'bad airs' that Victorians managed through cross-ventilation.

In these open environments, Queen Charlotte's used bedside curtains to provide a degree of privacy. Patients could pull curtains around their bed when they undressed, felt ill or desired a moment of relative solitude. These amenities, though, did not always fulfil their intended purpose. On one occasion, shortly after giving birth, nurses wanted to clean the area around Campion's bed. While the curtains were open, she vomited, which left her feeling 'wholly and nakedly exposed'. 'I feel, rather than see', she recounted, 'the immediate tactful looking-away of every eye in the ward'.[29]

The founders of the NHS were not blind to the apprehensions about privacy that large public wards engendered among patients. Somerville Hastings – President of the SMA – commented on the problem during a wartime lecture on the future of hospitals.[30] While he agreed with others on the left like Bevan that there should be 'no place in the ideal system for the small cottage hospital', he supported a number of practical solutions to make patients feel comfortable in large institutions. 'It would not be very expensive to change all hospital wards into curtained cubicles', Hastings offered. 'The provision of curtains, together with the occasional change of the position of patients in the wards', added the surgeon, 'should go far to satisfy the wishes of most'. Sectioning patients off from sight, if not entirely from sound, offered a potential means of alleviating concerns over privacy while retaining the communal nature of the ward that many figures such as Hastings prioritised as a means of bringing together Britons from different backgrounds.

Despite Hastings's optimism, many NHS hospitals struggled to afford the curtains that Campion encountered. Even moveable screens – which represented a louder, less individualised alternative – were not always present. Their absence confirmed how the uneven provision that had marred the interwar medical system could still exist in the new nationalised service. The government may well have concurred that a 'good means of securing patients' privacy is the use of curtains', but it still relied on voluntary organisations to fill the gaps that the low postwar health budget left behind.[31] Local women's groups regularly highlighted the affronts to patients' privacy that stemmed from financial shortcomings. Organisations such as the Mothers' Union or the Townswomen's Guild remained popular in the postwar years – particularly among the middle class – by offering a variety of educational and leisure activities.[32] They also sometimes became involved in the operation of welfare services, despite the centrality of the state after the Second World War. In 1952, a business and professional women's club in Arbroath, Scotland, demanded more privacy for women in their community's hospital.[33] A local newspaper expressed the gendered standards of decency often at the heart of these controversies by warning that four women were on 'full view' to those passing up nearby stairs. This issue was far from particular to Scotland, as five years later the Somerset Federation of Women's Institutes passed a resolution that curtains and screens should be made mandatory for all patients.

In a testament to the continuing importance of charity in the NHS, women's groups regularly fundraised to buy amenities that helped safeguard privacy. Women Helpers Leagues or Leagues of Friends spearheaded these endeavours within individual hospitals. These groups adapted to the new status of charity in medical care, moving away from supporting hospitals' overall income and towards raising money to fund minor structural improvements or comforts for patients.[34] By 1956, Leagues of Friends or similar organisations supported 2,100 out of 2,600 NHS hospitals.[35] The League of Friends shop became a common sight, generating funds by selling refreshments, as well as books, board games and craft kits to keep patients occupied. Largely staffed by women volunteers, such fundraising mechanisms also made it possible for many hospitals to purchase medical equipment and amenities that included curtains and screens. The League of Friends at Selly Oak Hospital, Birmingham, spent the considerable sum of £1,000 in the late 1950s to provide curtains to a ward with sixty-seven beds.[36]

The existence of amenity rooms, or 'pay-beds', in NHS hospitals provided options to the small minority of predominantly middle-class patients who felt that curtains or screens could never ensure enough privacy. For a fee, individuals could have their own solitary room within a public, NHS hospital. At the point of Campion's arrival at Queen Charlotte's, the hospital possessed six private single bedrooms, costing seventeen guineas a week, and six two-bed rooms, costing twelve guineas a week.[37] Pay-beds were a marginal taste and comprised only 1.2 per cent of all NHS hospital beds between 1948 and the early 1970s.[38] As fees for pay-beds rose in the new nationalised service, Campion encountered affluent patients complaining about 'the sudden leap in the price of privacy'.[39] Nonetheless, letters of appreciation to Queen Charlotte's from occupants of these beds expressed gratitude for the solitude of a single room and relative isolation from other hospital attendees.[40] The use of money to pay for a bed would continue to be seen as a distasteful compromise of the service's values to figures on the medical left. Yet the presence of these patients within the NHS carried advantages by preventing funds moving outside the nationalised system to private hospitals. Instead, they continued to support their local, public hospital.

All the same, the vast majority of patients from professional backgrounds like Campion did not choose to pay for a bed in the NHS and instead entered its public wards. The inclusion of middle-class patients in universal welfare services was key to their success and survival, as they encouraged cross-class support.[41] Indeed, their participation also formed an essential element of the communalism behind the service. However, the presence of middle-class patients brought tensions. The historian Florence Sutcliffe-Braithwaite has shown how, in the immediate postwar years, many middle-class Britons felt that rising working-class incomes and living standards threatened their own status.[42] These professionals felt that popular access to cars, holidays or household amenities eroded the distinctiveness of being middle class. Campion understood how increased mixing between patients of different financial means generated friction, even if she expressed little sympathy for any 'upkeeping of caste'.[43] As one of the 'only members of the professional classes in our ward', she claimed that women of her means were 'resented by our wardmates'. 'We were thought to be getting something for nothing, at the expense of those who deserved it more', she explained.

Although Campion focused on the animosity sometimes directed at middle-class patients in the early NHS, their less well-off counterparts experienced their own difficulties as they entered Queen Charlotte's in expanded numbers. The hospital's concerns about meeting a 'very great increase in the number of patients needing and asking for free transport since 5 July, 1948', suggested the expanded ranks of working-class women now accessing its care.[44] Administrators regularly commented on the marital status of these poorer women. In their contributions to annual reports, the hospital's almoners – who performed a function akin to that of social workers in the early NHS – fretted over the increased numbers of illegitimate births due to wartime disruption.[45] Almoners usually referred to such women as 'girls' – no matter their age – and directed them to hostels and organisations such as the National Council for the Unmarried Mother and Her Child.[46] Moral codes that emphasised respectable marriage saturated the new health service. Some local councils, for instance, continued the practice of loaning unmarried women wedding rings to help avoid stigma when they accessed medical services.[47]

Campion's primary critique of the NHS took aim at its rigidity. Her complaints about what she termed the 'Hospital Mind' revealed how the determined efforts by the service's founders to minimise critical understandings of 'state medicine' did not meet total success.[48] When Campion wanted to pick Philip up from his cot – located at the end of her bed – and hold him, the nurses scolded her with a reminder that contact was only permitted at allotted times. 'I long to pick Philip out of his cot and hand him round for inspection', Campion confessed, 'but the Hospital Mind has now begun to get at me . . . and, being merely the mother of the child, I dare not'. In such passages, *National Baby* frequently placed the individual 'I' in conflict with the collective 'they'. Explaining this distinction, Campion wrote: '*They* are powerful, terrible, unknown. *They* are National Health, Government, a Thou-God-Seest-Me sort of eye, and Don't Do That'. The positioning of individual autonomy in opposition to the regulations of the hospital carried wider implications – for Campion, this paternalism extended beyond the gates of Queen Charlotte's and blemished the NHS as a whole.

However, Campion struck a positive note in the concluding remarks of *National Baby* with her insistence that Britons should 'congratulate ourselves on having the new Health Service to aid us in this enterprise of child-rearing'.[49] The quality of treatment that she received and the financial savings that the service offered, compared to the expense of private care, ranked foremost in her assessment. Campion recognised that issues around privacy and class divides posed challenges to the service's potential success. She pinpointed the middle-class prioritisation of 'a privacy which their ancestors fought their way upwards to gain' as an obstacle to their participation. While she knew 'the new Health Scheme is for all of us: as a middle-class mother I have grave doubts about its free use by the higher income groups as well as by the lower (who use it out of stark necessity, and make no bones about it)'. Campion ended her account with a plea for the professional classes to use the NHS, alongside a demand that the service start 'taking more account of the individual'. Many NHS supporters worked towards this objective when they helped to modernise hospitals in the subsequent decades.

MAKING HOSPITALS HUMAN

By the 1960s, various activists, social scientists and medical experts across the world stressed the need to make hospitals 'human'.[50] These reformers targeted institutions unleashing a seemingly inexhaustible wave of medical advancement. As in other health systems, the NHS had brought in more effective anaesthetic agents like lidocaine, minimally invasive surgery on the ear, nose and throat and new tools for seeing inside the body, such as the fibre optic endoscope, alongside life-saving operations that included the first successful kidney transplant in 1960. However, as the historian Ayesha Nathoo argues, novel forms of media like television sometimes questioned this high-tech world of medicine, dragging controversies such as the uneven success of the first heart transplants into the public domain.[51] The reformers invested in humanising hospitals similarly challenged medical hierarchies by arguing that hospitals needed to take more account of a patient's social background and personal preferences. Although the authority commanded by figures such as matrons on wards would later be romanticised, postwar reformers – and many patients – believed that such excessive deference to medical practitioners caused more harm than good. These arguments infused the NHS's modernisation as it gathered pace. Stemming from national, local and voluntary sources, a wave of reforms sought to better accommodate changing cultural norms, as well as patients' networks of family and friends. Not all of these efforts translated perfectly into practice, and some reiterated existing social divisions. Nevertheless, the modernising NHS came to exhibit an increased willingness to consider patients' social position and their individual needs.

To foster continued support, the NHS needed to accommodate changing gender norms. In the mid-twentieth century, it became more acceptable for men to prioritise father–child relationships and openly participate in intimate family moments.[52] As a result, whereas men once preferred to wait in the pub than attend the birth of their child, now many wanted to be present. Few NHS hospitals allowed such access in the service's early years. The historian Laura King has demonstrated how institutions refused entry to fathers on the grounds of hygiene, disruption to staff, or by claiming that men were unprepared for the realities of birth.[53] This exclusion of fathers could exacerbate feelings of frustration and loneliness among mothers. Campion gave birth without the presence of loved ones, her only company throughout labour being the sounds of other women in pain and the nurses that attended her. 'If ever a child came into the world on a hot tide of sheer bad temper, mine will be that child', Campion had rued.[54] Loneliness shaped her experience of childbirth.

Hospitals increasingly allowed fathers to attend deliveries from the 1960s.[55] This expanded access, though, carried conditions. Like many other institutions, Queen Charlotte's permitted fathers to attend births if they signed a permission form in advance. One father in 1969 objected to this requirement by dismissing the supposed 'risks' involved, insisting that he paid income tax and so had a right to be present, and promising that he would 'behave as a reasonable mature father'.[56] While this man believed that emotional control and his status as a taxpayer justified his presence, the hospital insisted that he complete the paperwork, adding that 'it is not unknown for fathers to keel over in these unaccustomed surroundings and injure themselves in so doing'.[57] Though such negotiations between individuals and hospitals persisted, by the early 1970s approximately 70 per cent of deliveries were now attended by the father.[58] The service had responded to these shifting understandings of masculinity and family life.

The NHS reacted more slowly to other evolving views around gender and sexuality. Unmarried motherhood remained contentious. Increases in extra-marital births across the period – from 5.44 per cent of all births in England and Wales in 1960, to 11.79 in 1980 – did not translate into immediate acceptance.[59] After one woman made a complaint about the condition of her ward at the Chelsea Hospital for Women in 1966, for instance, the hospital's internal discussion of the matter included comment on how the patient 'has been married and divorced twice and has had two miscarriages, one of which was a therapeutic abortion for psychiatric reasons'.[60]

Margaret Drabble's novel *The Millstone* (1965) spoke to the continued maligning of unmarried mothers in the NHS.[61] The book's protagonist, Rosamund Stacey, is a young academic from a middle-class background who becomes pregnant after her first sexual encounter. Her subsequent experience with the NHS in London served as a commentary on contemporary attitudes to illegitimacy in the service. Stacey finds that the fictional 'St Andrew's Hospital' highlights her marital status on the ward with 'a label at the end of my bed with the initial U, which stood, I was told, for Unmarried'.[62] Drabble drew on her own experiences when writing *The Millstone*. In a 1965 interview discussing the book's publication on the popular BBC radio programme *Woman's Hour*, she described it as 'autobiographical' and noted that 'some of the experiences . . . must be my own'.[63] Drabble was married during the births of her first three children, but her exposure to maternity care 'on the National Health' left her feeling that such services were 'very confusing and bewildering'. She recounted being 'parcelled around from doctor to hospital and from clinic to clinic' and criticised the regimented attitudes of staff as well as the lack of information they gave their patients. Drabble confessed a 'love-hate relationship' with the NHS, even though she 'couldn't be more grateful for it, because I don't know what people would do without it and I thoroughly approve of it in principle'. While she reflected its early maternalist claims by presenting the institution as 'a great comfort especially when one has children who are forever being ill', the everyday practice of the service frustrated her.

As *The Millstone* suggested, the NHS embodied many of the contradictions inherent to what the morality campaigner Mary Whitehouse lambasted as the 'permissive society' during the late 1960s and 1970s.[64] The ten years after 1959 witnessed a raft of legislation that modified or overturned the regulation of social issues that included divorce, obscenity, capital punishment, prostitution and same-sex relations. These reforms were not without inconsistencies and often conflicted with public opinion. The NHS, too, sometimes sat at odds with this liberalising agenda. On the one hand, women were given more reproductive options in these years. In 1961, the pill became available on the NHS. Though it could not be gained without charge at first, by the mid-1970s the NHS offered the pill and contraceptive appliances without payment. The National Health Service (Family Planning) Act in 1967 also empowered local authority-funded family health clinics to provide contraceptive advice to unmarried women. In this same year, the Abortion Act permitted the termination of pregnancies within the service. On the other hand, limitations applied. Two doctors still had to agree that certain conditions were met for an abortion, such as the pregnancy risking the mother's life, or harming her or her family's physical and mental health.[65] Doctors made these decisions, rather than women themselves. Citizens in Northern Ireland had more limited access to these NHS services, due to local religious opposition. While the service might have symbolised the ills of 'permissiveness' to some commentators, for others it did not go far enough.

For all these ambivalences, the health service underwent other adjustments in the 1960s that took greater account of patients' social relationships. Extended visiting hours in hospitals marked an important step in this direction. The drive for reform arrived from organisations and figures outside of the NHS. Indeed, this period witnessed the emergence of a greater number of activist organisations campaigning on medical issues, with sixty-six founded between 1960 and 1979.[66] An important figure in explaining the social dimensions of modern medicine was the statistician Ann Cartwright. As one of the few women associated with the Institute of Communities Studies (ICS), she pioneered many techniques in sourcing patients' opinions.[67] After gaining her first experiences in research helping the Attlee Labour government monitor public attitudes to new welfare services, Cartwright developed her expertise in medical care. The work for what became *Human Relations and Hospital Care* (1964) required undertaking over 700 interviews in patients' homes, where Cartwright and her team sourced opinions about recent NHS treatment and medical environments.[68] Cartwright collected evidence that showed a widespread expansion in hospital visitation, among other trends. Family and friends were now able to make a patient's hospital stay more enjoyable, as 88 per cent of the patients interviewed said they could have daily visitors. While the study found that some patients desired even longer visiting hours, improvements had been made since Campion's experience at Queen Charlotte's, when visitors were allowed access for only one hour in the evening. The rigidity of the 'Hospital Mind' that *National Baby* had documented in the 1940s seemed to be thawing.

Children's hospitals also transformed their attitudes to visiting. At the beginning of the NHS, children requiring hospital treatment generally entered institutions alone and parents had limited chances to visit them.[69] Critics of this practice deployed psychological understandings of 'attachment theory' to call for change. Prominent psychologists including John Bowlby and Donald Winnicott drew attention to the emotional damage that children underwent when they were physically separated from parental, and particularly maternal, love.[70] By drawing on the postwar emphasis on the family in Britain, these experts reflected a wider sense that a woman's place was to look after her child in the home rather than take paid employment.[71] They proved effective, and the 1959 Platt Report translated these demands into official policy, recommending improvements for children's hospitals that including unrestricted visiting hours to ensure 'continuity with the home during the time the child is in hospital'.[72] The NHS's acknowledgment of social relationships refracted wider views on gender and family life.

As a sprawling arm of the welfare state, the NHS could only proceed slowly in altering customs across its many branches and facilities. *The Millstone*'s dramatic climax centred on the hospitalisation of Rosamund's child, Octavia, for a complication with her pulmonary artery. In one scene, Rosamund is told by the Ward Sister that 'visiting is quite out of the question'.[73] She only gains access to her child by using her class position and appealing to the surgeon himself, leaving her with a sense of guilt about 'Those that don't even get in. Those without money. Those without influence. Those who would not dare to have hysterics'. This sense of anguish would not have been lost on many readers of the novel, even after the Platt Report. 'My Child in Hospital', a series of *Woman's Hour* radio programmes in 1964, featured women's accounts of being prevented access to their children.[74] It would take beyond the next decade for these exclusions to disappear. Nevertheless, levels of access increased dramatically across the 1970s and 1980s, and became near universal thereafter.[75]

The reforms that drew more family members and friends into hospitals created unexpected results. Efforts to address noise on hospital wards offered a striking example.[76] As patients at Queen Charlotte's network of institutions testified, open, public wards could be loud. The King Edward's Fund for London took special interest in this problem, and published a 1958 report, *Noise Control in Hospitals* (1958).[77] The dominance of the state in the field of medicine did not prevent philanthropic bodies like the King's Fund from working to promote best practice in the nationalised system and suggesting reforms.[78] The organisation detailed a series of recommendations to prevent noise, such as fitting small rubber strips to door frames or stacking items on trollies in a certain way.[79] The King's Fund also produced colour notices to promote the report. Illustrated by Fougasse, the creator of the famous Second World War propaganda posters 'Careless Talk Costs Lives', they reminded staff about the impact of noise on patient care.[80]

However, for all the work of the King's Fund, patients still experienced noise as a problem. The organisation produced a report in 1974 that compared patient attitudes on this issue to their findings at the same hospitals in 1958.[81] In the earlier survey, nearly 50 per cent of patients said they were not bothered by noise. By the early 1970s, this figure had fallen to 20 per cent. Either hospitals had become louder or patients held stricter standards about the acceptable levels of sound. The report identified decreases in complaints about 'squeaking doors and floor boards, noisy chairs and bedpans and sluice room equipment'. Identifying these problems had paid dividends. However, patients voiced increasing annoyance about noise generated from other patients' visitors. Unrestricted visiting, and the admittance of new guests like children, created a louder atmosphere. The reforms in this area therefore had a knock-on impact for other facets of care. 'Now that there are such long visiting hours', one patient lamented, 'I find this very trying'.

The NHS faced difficulties more serious than noisy wards. Nonetheless, the very exposure of these problems could lead to important change, as the case of psychiatric patients made clear. The position of mental health patients in the service had shifted on the back of the Mental Health Act (1959), which spurred a move away from asylums towards what became known as 'care in the community'.[82] But this legislation did not produce immediate results. Barbara Robb, a psychotherapist and health activist, identified widespread neglect towards elderly patients in long-stay mental institutions during the mid-1960s.[83] Robb exposed the conditions that her previous patient, Amy Gibbs, had endured in Friern Hospital, Middlesex, including poor hygiene and emotional abuse. She sent a report – titled 'Diary of a Nobody' – to the government, only to have her findings dismissed by the Labour Minister of Health, Kenneth Robinson. Undeterred, Robb founded a campaigning organisation, Aid for the Elderly in Government Institutions (AEGIS), and published an exposé, *Sans Everything* (1967).[84] Change arrived when Robinson's successor at the Ministry, Richard Crossman, appointed a leading member of AEGIS, Brian Abel-Smith, as his chief advisor on health and welfare.[85] Scandals involving psychiatric institutions continued to emerge after this point, such as in Ely Hospital, Cardiff, in 1969, where nurses claimed that patients were mistreated and that their own complaints had been supressed. On the back of such controversies and the efforts of campaigners like Robb, by the 1970s meaningful reforms led to the establishment of an inspectorate and an ombudsman, as well as greater support for the field of psychogeriatrics.[86] Such scandals did not disappear in the NHS. Yet they demonstrated how external pressure brought attention to patients' social circumstances and, in some cases, forced transformations across the service.

THE HOSPITAL PLAN AND COMMUNALISM

By the 1960s, criticism of the service's largely Victorian hospital stock had become impossible to tune out. The journalist Gerda L. Cohen went so far as to claim that 'no country in Europe can rival our finely-embalmed collection of antiques, some suitable for an 18th-century folk museum and others a monument to skinflint pauper relief'.[87] Amidst this mounting pressure, the Conservative government announced a 'Hospital Plan' in 1962, comprising a ten-year building programme to construct ninety hospitals throughout England and Wales at a cost of £500 million.[88] This outlay would enable, in the words of the government, 'modernizing the whole pattern and content of the hospital service'.[89] The near doubling of NHS expenditure since 1948 – if still not enough to overtake the money allotted to education – allowed for greater spending on new buildings, renovation and ward amenities such as curtains.[90] Rather than separate patients from one another as resources became available to construct individual rooms, hospitals committed to communal dynamics and reflected the values of social democracy. In fact, by the 1970s, a cross-class body of opinion stated their preference for shared medical spaces over the alternatives that isolated them to a higher degree.

When Minister of Health Enoch Powell (1912–1998) first announced the Hospital Plan, the prospect of brand-new hospitals excited architects and commentators. The promise of expanding the number of District General Hospitals where, in the words of the *Architectural Review*, 'the National Health Service mobilizes all its skills and equipment in the service of the public' attracted significant attention.[91] In a reflection of the rationalising impulses of state planning that swelled further during the 1960s, these facilities coordinated the beds and expertise that might hitherto have been provided by multiple smaller hospitals onto a single site. From the outside, the average British hospital built in these years fitted international trends, with a concrete, modernist aesthetic that projected a sense of the forward march of medicine.[92] One favoured approach was known in expert circles as the 'match box on a muffin', so-called because it placed a vertical tower on top of a flat entrance building. The Victoria Hospital, Fife – which opened in 1967 – sported such a design. However, it would be wrong to assume that these concrete hospitals were automatically seen as imposing or rolled out by central planners without care for the communities that they served. As the historian Ed DeVane reveals, planners regularly attuned hospitals to local landscapes through strategies such as limiting their height, which ensured more low-rise designs in the NHS than in the US.[93] These temples to the medical future fit the broader pattern of public sector and welfare state architecture, placing the health service next to council housing tower blocks or shopping centres as instantly recognisable signs of Britain's postwar development.[94]

Yet renovation proved an equally important part of the Hospital Plan. The programme reserved a portion of its funding for the remodelling of 134 older institutions. Sheffield's RHB, for instance, spent over half of their government allocation on upgrading existing facilities.[95]

In many cases, administrators spent money on constructing a single ward block or medical department, rather than a totally new hospital. Throughout the UK, RHBs erected fresh concrete structures that stood next to their interwar or Victorian forebears, offering a kaleidoscope of the past and future of medicine. Even this smaller-scale construction generated enthusiasm in a service previously starved of capital expenditure. Newsreels had descended on St James' Hospital in South London when it merely opened a new waiting area for patients during the mid-1950s, lavishing praise on its 'ultra-modern design'.[96] This degree of excitement for what might have seemed like minor adjustments persisted as the Hospital Plan gathered pace.

Other changes also reshaped the physical infrastructure of hospitals that, in turn, helped balance the NHS's communalism with the increased desire for autonomy expressed by patients. As the service received more money in the 1960s through initiatives like the Hospital Plan, curtains became a regular fixture and alleviated some of the earlier apprehensions around privacy on hospital wards. By the middle of the decade, 57 per cent of patients occupied wards with curtains, 40 per cent wards with a moveable screen, 1 per cent wards with cubicles, and only 2 per cent wards with no possibility of separation from other patients.[97] Although charity continued to play an important role across the NHS, its hospitals relied less on women's groups and voluntary organisations to fundraise for these protections than in the 1940s. In her study, Cartwright showed that some patients felt embarrassed to ask for a screen or complained that nurses did not let them pull curtains while they had visitors, but most now benefitted from options that offered a break from the shared dynamics of the ward.

These increased protections complemented an expanded willingness among hospitals to listen to their patients about personal privacy. Organisations external to the NHS again helped change the public system. At the King's Fund, the occupational psychologist Winifred Raphael led efforts from the mid-1960s to encourage NHS hospitals to adopt patient surveys. Raphael's *Patients and Their Hospitals* (1969) involved ten district general hospitals and over 1,300 patients.[98] Five years later, she reported that seventy-two hospital groups had since started asking patients for their opinions directly, with over half using the survey devised by the King's Fund.[99] These patients seemed happy to participate and generally appreciated the increased attention given to their comfort. The expanded use of surveys allowed hospitals to chart an uptick in satisfaction on the issue of privacy. Of the respondents to Raphael's 1969 study, 94 per cent said they had enough privacy during their stay.[100] While those claiming that they did not have sufficient privacy mentioned problems with curtains not being pulled properly or being able to hear doctors' conversations with other patients, this headline figure suggested significant difference from the 1940s.[101]

The introduction of cubicles numbered among the improvements to patient privacy. Many hospitals took advantage of healthier NHS finances to retrofit their wards with partial separation between beds. These medical spaces began to look different to their counterparts at the start of the service. From the 1960s, sound-resistant panels brought groups of patients together in smaller clusters. In the 1940s, wards in the Mill Road Maternity Hospital, Liverpool, for example, would have appeared familiar to Campion: beds in a row along each wall, and no separation between patients.[102] By the late 1970s, the hospital had parted these same wards into smaller cubicles which provided increased, if not total, separation.[103] Over the beds, curtains – on noise-reducing runners – could be pulled whenever the patient wanted, and personal lights were also available. Taken together, these amenities represented a marked shift from the point of *National Baby*'s publication.

However, the increased attention to personal needs on NHS wards did not come at the expense of the service's commitment to communalism. After all, cubicles were not brick walls, and patients could wander between these sub-divisions to socialise with one another, if they were in good enough health. As the 1960s came into view, the photographer Freddie Mudditt captured these social interactions while staying as a patient at the Ingham Infirmary, South Shields, in the north of England.[104] Bringing his camera with him, he captured not just the everyday routines of nurses in starched white caps fitting sheets and serving meals, but also patients leaning across beds to share a joke with each other (Figure 5). As Mudditt's pictures showed, patients desired a retreat from others at times, but they also wanted to talk and interact. In her research, Cartwright remarked that patients 'sounded as if they were describing a holiday camp rather than a hospital'.[105] Of respondents to her survey, 61 per cent found the company of other patients 'very enjoyable', 34 per cent 'fairly enjoyable' and only 5 per cent 'not very enjoyable'. The communal dynamics of a ward could also bring comfort during serious illness. 'At one time I would have thought it dreadful to have a breast off', confided one woman in Cartwright's study, 'but one lady there had and she got on fine'.

Of course, social divisions sometimes splintered this communalism, particularly for people of colour using the NHS who had recently

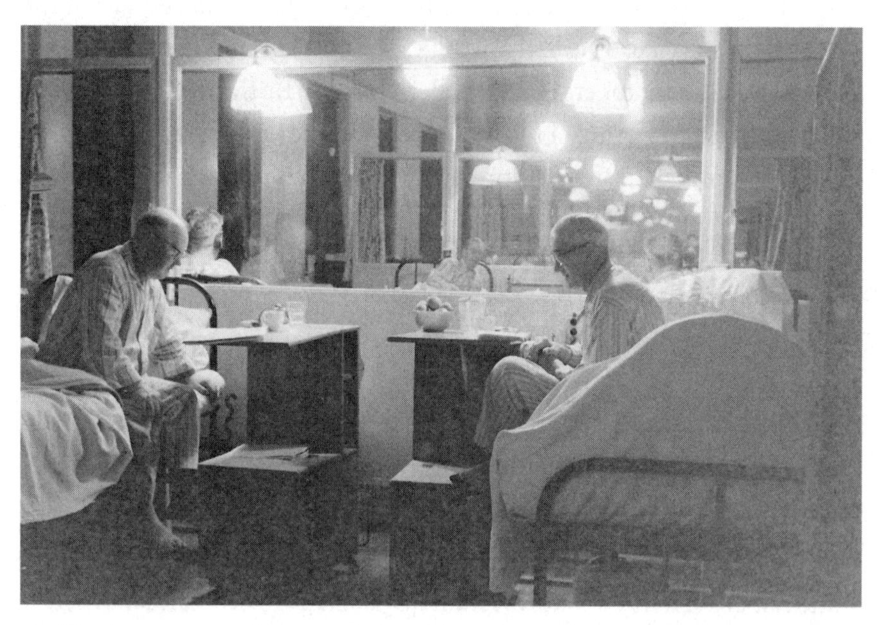

5. The large size and open-plan nature of British hospital wards reflected the communalism of the modernising NHS. As the 1960s came into view, the Ingham Infirmary, South Shields, demonstrated how these spaces facilitated social interaction while safeguarding privacy through small-scale touches like curtains or cubicles.

arrived from countries in the former British Empire. The period between the 1948 British Nationality Act – which provided open access to Britain for every person in the Commonwealth – and the 1962 Commonwealth Immigrants Act – which marked the beginning of restricting such access – witnessed thousands of migrants journey to the UK, where they worked, made new lives and used welfare services like the NHS.[106] In hospitals, they sometimes encountered hostility from their white wardmates. 'Asian visitors by the dozen talking loudly', complained one respondent to the King's Fund survey on sound in hospitals, 'walking noisily and dropping things'.[107] Another patient groaned that 'The whole Asian family seems to come *en bloc*'. These views provided a medical equivalent to the wider stereotype that immigrant families were always large, loud and crammed into overcrowded homes.[108]

Buchi Emecheta's novel *Second-Class Citizen* (1974) spoke to the persistent class and racial tensions that patients might experience in the NHS.[109] Based loosely on Emecheta's own life, the book follows a young Nigerian woman, Adah, as she immigrates to Britain to join her husband, Francis. The NHS forms part of a culture shock on her arrival, and she wonders, for example, when first encountering a lack of payment for treatment, whether it was a 'second-class hospital, a free one, just because they were blacks?' Adah eventually welcomes the care provided by the NHS. Nonetheless, when she gives birth at University College Hospital she feels marginalised due to her poverty and race. As the only Black patient, Adah becomes the subject of gossip among her fellow convalescents. Throughout her hospital stay, she feels embarrassed at her inability to afford a new dressing gown or clothes for her infant. This loosely autobiographical novel illustrated how the communal aspects of a ward exacerbated feelings of insecurity about poverty and race, as talk spread easily between hospital beds.

Yet, overall, *Second-Class Citizen* made a case for the social life of NHS hospitals. As the historian Mathew Thomson argues, by the 1960s, such representations of the service in popular culture could accommodate both criticism of the treatment received and praise for the NHS's values.[110] Emecheta's novel shows how Adah appreciates the convivial atmosphere of a ward where the women 'seemed to have known each other for years and years'.[111] She remains positive towards her fellow patients and resolves to 'thank people, even for their smiles and kindly nods'. Indeed, the friendships Adah makes on the ward give her the courage to leave her abusive husband. The novel highlighted the real-world impact that hospitalisation could have on an individual, with its reference to a 'new code of conduct' that Adah learned from 'staying together with other women for thirteen days', which 'was to be with her for a long time'. In the real NHS, patients similarly spent an average of ten days in hospital, providing a significant amount of time to forge relationships that might also last beyond the confines of the ward. Emecheta's novel offered a portrait of how NHS hospitals could simultaneously form a site of contestation and a space for deepening social relations between individuals of distinct backgrounds.

Class divides softened on NHS wards by the 1960s and 1970s. No patients in Cartwright or Raphael's studies mentioned these tensions when they recounted their experiences. If their questionnaires did not ask explicit questions regarding class, they nonetheless provided patients with extensive opportunities to comment on it. When patients mentioned class at all, they stated that hospital life transcended income divides. 'There is a friendliness in hospital you don't get elsewhere – no class distinction', believed one patient in a typical response of this type. 'You get to know other people's lives – see the other side of life', this same person added. Of course, class tensions did not disappear. But the seeming abatement of such divisions when compared with the service's inception tracked with broader shifts in the postwar period. By the 1970s, middle-class people generally placed less emphasis on maintaining sharp distinctions of status with their working-class neighbours and colleagues.[112] The snobbishness that some middle-class patients had expressed when accessing NHS services in *National Baby* no longer presented a serious obstacle to the service's success.

While the NHS's communal layouts and designs facilitated the bonds that many Britons forged on its wards, arguments for individual rooms struggled to be heard. E.J.R. Burrough, an administrator at the Radcliffe Infirmary, Oxford, posited that single rooms would provide greater privacy and improve standards of hygiene.[113] Burrough regretted that 'open dormitories' had become 'not only built into our system' but also 'built into our thinking and wholly taken for granted'. He used economic arguments to try and puncture this apparent bloc mentality in NHS hospitals. Burrough maintained that it would be inexpensive to convert existing Nightingale wards to twenty or more individual rooms and that savings could be made by preventing the under-occupancy of existing stock. Beds, he suggested, were more likely to be filled if there were fewer overall. Burrough also rebutted assertions that individual rooms proved difficult for nurses to supervise. If patients were isolated, he argued, then staff would prioritise pressing concerns above dispensing the inefficiencies of 'tender loving care' around a shared ward.

However, individual rooms were more expensive to construct, and this fact further encouraged the government to favour sub-divided wards. The Ministry of Health demonstrated this prioritisation in its 'Building Notes', released by a new internal Hospital Building Division, headed by the prominent architect William Tatton-Brown, who had proved an early proponent of modernist aesthetics in Britain.[114] The Ministry's 1961 missive on ward units stressed the need for patient privacy and stipulated that beds required curtains.[115] It also listed different options for ward layout: from the 'duplex' design with different sexes at either end of the same unit to a 'racetrack' model that used a central core of ancillary rooms to serve wards around the perimeter. Nonetheless, all these designs were oriented towards the sub-divided communal space over single rooms. The advice on maternity wards articulated a more individualised variant of this group-oriented trend, with recommendations for smaller four-bedded wards with cubicles, and a single room adjoined to each ward to meet the needs of mothers with ill babies.[116] As modernisation progressed, giving birth in the NHS retained its communal focus, albeit with an increased provision of single rooms for those who wanted or needed them.

The hospital wards established in Britain after the 1962 plan diverged in some respects from their North American or European counterparts. In the US, an earlier tendency towards 'hotel style' rooms and small wards in private hospitals continued.[117] Western Europe offered a less stark contrast with Britain, although there were still important distinctions. Whereas most continental nations constructed eight-, six-, four- or two-bed rooms, British hospitals increasingly opted for a larger, subdivided ward with multi-bed areas.[118] The average NHS hospital patient therefore had fewer walls between themselves and others. British planners recognised that the alternatives in Europe provided a higher degree of isolation to patients, yet staffing concerns took priority. The government's Hospital Buildings Division remarked on how the typical 'Continental pattern . . . has never extensively been used here because although it provides greater privacy for the patient, it renders supervision more difficult'.[119] Given persistent difficulties in recruiting nurses in the NHS during a postwar labour shortage, administrators were reluctant to stretch resources further by having staff work across multiple closed rooms. Open environments were more economical.

These architectural choices also created more opportunities for communal dynamics. Most patients seemed to favour what Burrough dismissed in his article as 'the jolly atmosphere of community living', and planners may have had these preferences in mind.[120] This sentiment could even be found in the letters pages of the conservative *Daily Telegraph*, with readers criticising the idea that separate rooms were the only way to ensure privacy for patients.[121] 'Surely', one reader posed, 'the communal life is to be preferred to that of the hermit?' Another reader reflected critically on their experience of 'the so-called luxury of a private ward'. 'It is infinitely nicer to share the life of a public ward', they concluded in a sharp rebuttal to the view that single rooms offered superior care. Cartwright found that only 8 per cent of patients wanted a room of their own, even when offered one for no cost.[122] An appreciation for communalism trumped interest in individualised alternatives. Respondents to Cartwright's study who stayed in a single room were more likely to feel lonely; two-thirds of the people who had not spoken to other patients had stayed in this type of accommodation. Whether middle or working class, respondents welcomed companionship. 'I was offered a room on my own, but I didn't want it', said one patient. 'I like company,' this person continued, 'If you're on your own, you think too much', adding 'I wanted something to take my mind off it'. For these patients, a room of one's own paled in comparison to the company of others.

***

The state built only six new NHS hospitals during the ten years after 1956, but seventy-one new hospitals were completed or started between 1966 and 1975.[123] In the 1970s, the Hospital Plan was slowed by the same funding challenges that later strained other parts of the welfare state. Always subject to penny pinching by both Conservative and Labour governments, the NHS's initial stock of hospitals would not be replaced until nearly the millennium.[124] However, contemporaries during the postwar era recognised that new hospitals were not the only thing that mattered. When the orthopaedic surgeon H.C. Batra arrived from overseas to take up a job at Walsall General Hospital in 1974, he observed the fits and bursts of hospital construction first-hand.[125] Initially, he was struck by an institution that 'looked terribly ordinary and Victorian with an unimpressive layout', describing the hospital's atmosphere as 'strongly reminiscent of a Dickensian establishment'. These comments confirmed the continuities that existed on the other side of the NHS's foundation. 'A senior colleague who showed me round', recalled Batra, 'tried to cheer me up by informing me that a new hospital was just about to commence building'. 'Quite naively, I took him at his word', he admitted. It took fifteen years for the promised hospital to materialise. Yet, despite the absence of a new hospital, Batra still noted smaller-scale adjustments and construction in subsequent years that meant, in his view, 'the level of clinical facilities rose steadily and the overall repertoire of each department expanded'.

Beyond brand-new hospitals, these more mundane developments often carried the load of recalibrating Britons' opinions of a health service that, as Campion's testimony showed, many held initial reservations about. The institution adapted to changed expectations and often took greater account of patients' personal relationships. On hospital wards, the NHS committed to communal spaces and alleviated the tensions around privacy that these exposed environments created through spatial readjustments. The principles of social democracy, then, could accommodate individual needs. These trends did not always meet patients' expectations and inevitably proved uneven in practice, but the NHS avoided a popular reputation as rigid or unwilling to change. Beyond the walls of the hospitals, health centres helped modernise the scattered world of general practice.

3

AT THE HEALTH CENTRE

You need to visit the doctor in 1949.[1] You walk to your local GP's house a few streets away. The earlier you set off, the more likely you are to avoid the queues that sometimes stretch into the front garden. Timing your arrival well, you sit in the converted, sparsely decorated front room that serves as your doctor's waiting area. Before the NHS, the private patients sat in a different room. Now everyone waits together in the same cramped space. The room itself has been largely left alone since the 1920s. You exchange a few words with neighbours before the doctor's assistant (also his wife) tells you to enter the consulting room. The doctor – a middle-class, middle-aged man – sits behind an imposing wooden desk. You last saw him when he visited your house two months ago to attend a family member suffering from the flu. The doctor extracts your record card from a cabinet containing hundreds of others. You tell him about the back pain you have been enduring for the last few months. He listens carefully, though occasionally glancing over your shoulder towards the other dozen patients he still needs to see before he can retreat to his kitchen for a quick lunch. The doctor tells you that the pain is merely a consequence of ageing, and he quickly scribbles a prescription for a medicine with an unfamiliar name. You do not question his prognosis. You never have. He stands up (your signal to leave), bids you goodbye, and you hurry to the chemist's in the hope of alleviating your pain.

You need to visit the doctor for the same complaint in 1974.[2] Doing so means walking half an hour to the local health centre, located in the middle of the housing estate with the newsagent and the hairdresser. You booked an appointment in advance using the telephone. The local council recently built the health centre. It is a single-storey building, constructed from a steel frame and panes of glass, topped by a flat roof. At the entrance, you join a short queue to speak with one of the receptionists behind a counter. Behind her are thousands of patient files on shelves, the occasional piece of paper peeping out of the bulging folders. You notice your neighbour ahead of you and overhear that she is here about her kidney troubles. After you tell the receptionist which doctor you have arranged to see (four GPs work at this centre: three men and one woman), and why, she asks you to sit in the waiting room by gesturing at the large, open space in front of her. Seats for fifty patients fill the room. A few minutes past your scheduled appointment time, a voice over a loudspeaker calls your name. You make your way down a corridor, passing other doctors' consulting rooms, until you reach the one belonging to your GP. He is sitting at a desk facing the wall and gestures for you to sit near him. You explain your recurring backaches. He tells you that it might just be a consequence of ageing. After you question this suggestion and explain more of your symptoms, he nods and hands you a brochure detailing a group exercise class held at the centre once a week, organised by a physiotherapist. The class may strengthen your back muscles and reduce pain, he suggests. Though sceptical, you register for the free class on your way out and begin the walk home.

As these vignettes suggest, the process of modernisation that reshaped the NHS's hospitals also took place in general practice. The everyday world of family doctoring transitioned from a domestic, hierarchical enterprise in the 1940s to a more communal, egalitarian experience by the 1970s, and overall standards of care improved.[3] These changes can be traced through health centres. Beginning in Britain during the interwar years with pioneering sites in Finsbury and Peckham, these facilities brought together GPs, nurses, dentists, social workers and public health officials under one roof. Their development after 1948 made a key part of the earlier vision of a state medical service a reality. Other than an expanded capacity to cure, these facilities' advocates also believed that they would support preventative medicine, providing higher numbers of diagnostic aids and situating public health initiatives within the everyday operation of general practice. Through their emphasis on integrating disparate services in one communal facility, supporting workers in industrial areas and helping mothers and children, health centres reflected the place of the early NHS in social democratic politics.

The NHS Acts stipulated that a network of such centres should be constructed across the UK as national policy. Given the limited funds allocated to the service in the immediate postwar years, and some doctors' opposition to being grouped together in such a way, this grand ambition was quickly shelved. However, the few experimental health centres that did get off the ground in the late 1940s and through the 1950s kept their principles alive.[4] The fact that these experimental facilities were usually made possible by local councils or charitable initiatives further underlined the contributions of figures and organisations outside of the NHS's official structure to the service's overall development. When the state more comprehensively embraced health centres under Labour governments during the 1960s, it marked a significant, if far from inevitable, moment of success for the NHS's overall programme of modernisation.

The eventual support given to health centres served as the British state's distinct contribution towards rethinking what was known as 'primary care' in international medical circles by the 1970s.[5] Under this banner, medical experts believed that health systems might be rebalanced away from hospitals and towards local communities through an emphasis on prevention rather than cure. Health centres provide a window into the successes and failures of public health in the NHS at this moment, as well as the attempts to reform the service to deal with the higher instances of chronic conditions such as cancer and heart disease. In regions ranging from Devon to South Wales to Northern Ireland, these facilities achieved high density and provided the dominant type of general practice.[6] The three-quarters of GPs who did not work in health centres usually formed comparable 'group practices', owning or renting premises from a private supplier paid for with a loan from the government.[7] In both health centres and group practices, the state demonstrated its capacities to transform medical care in communities across the UK.

But what did patients make of these changes? As in hospitals, the modernisation of general practice was not just about bricks and mortar; it also represented a social process that spoke to the communalism within social democratic politics. The expanded 'medical teams', large waiting rooms and mass appointment systems made some members of the public feel as though individual concerns were being crowded out by a tide of efficiency. These patients liked the shape of family doctoring before the NHS, where a single doctor who lived nearby treated people in a homelier environment. Some members of the public expressed anxieties about the potential loss of privacy in communal medical environments, as they also voiced about the care they received in hospitals. These criticisms were amplified from the 1960s, when the patients' movement and consumerism conjoined to empower ordinary people to critique the paternalism of modern medicine.[8] The NHS needed to manage these social concerns to succeed in modernising general practice. As in hospitals, the balance between the community and the individual lay close to the heart of the difficulties facing the health service's development. Addressing these challenges was made doubly important by the fact that general practice formed one of the most regular sites of a person's interaction with the NHS, and even with the welfare state as a whole. A trip to the health centre, then, reveals how social democratic values became embedded in specific spaces and medical practices, further illuminating how the NHS matured in its early years.

MODERNISING GENERAL PRACTICE

At the start of the NHS, general practice varied in form and quality. GPs were 'independent contractors' to the service under the terms of the NHS Acts, a concession given by Bevan due to these doctors' alarm about becoming indistinguishable from civil servants. However, this status did not hide the fact that 163 Executive Councils across Britain now oversaw their services or that the government paid them a 'capitation fee' for each NHS patient. As in the interwar years, doctors worked alone or in small partnerships out of their homes or modified commercial buildings. Though now free at the point of access, visiting the doctor therefore remained similar in feel to its operation in the years before 1948. This lack of systematic change led medical experts to debate the standards of general practice in the early NHS.[9] In one important study, a leading expert even described a surgery where the doctor saw patients 'in a hut at the end of a cottage garden, the only waiting-space being a wooden shelter with no door; here the patients stood among wheelbarrows, old wire netting, and the other accoutrements of the potting-shed'.[10]

If general practice varied in its operation, let alone in quality, it was consistently domestic.[11] In addition to practising in their own domiciles and undertaking house calls, doctors often relied on their wives for administrative and secretarial support. Traditionally gendered divisions of household labour therefore permeated family doctoring. Wives spoke to patients, took messages on the doctor's behalf, cleaned the surgery and performed bookkeeping, all typically without direct payment. When doctors highlighted this burden, they usually blamed the workload created by the NHS or the greediness of their patients rather than demand that the state recompense their wives.[12] The NHS gained from the invisible subsidy provided by women's labour.

The paternalism of postwar general practice also shaped GPs' attitudes towards their patients. As pillars of their local communities, practitioners often indulged in the maxim that 'doctor knows best', even in non-medical matters.[13] Many doctors maintained that they had a responsibility to 'train' their patients to behave responsibly. *Honour a Physician* (1959), a novel by the GP-turned-author Philip Auld, revealed this perspective.[14] The book follows ten years in the life of an embattled GP, Dr Charles Gatwood, as he and his wife are worn down by the fatuous demands of patients. Working-class patients in the novel – depicted as 'spongers', 'malingerers' and 'parasites' – demand endless sick certificates and frivolities such as medical-grade cotton wool to stuff household cushions. *Honour a Physician* stereotyped the poor by highlighting garbled speech and abusive parenting. In one scene, Gatwood pays a house visit to find that a man caused his son's death by forcing him to drink too much at a wedding. When Gatwood's efforts to 'train' these wayward patients fail, he becomes more cynical about a medical system that delivered care without direct payment. The novel closed by stressing Gatwood's heroism in persevering with the NHS rather than escaping by taking a position in private industrial medicine.

The Labour Party, alongside planners and left-wing medical reformers, thought health centres would modernise this scattered world of local doctoring. They sought to bring doctors, nurses, public health officials and other experts together in a single modern building. For Ministry of Health officials, state initiative offered an upwards path. Whereas group practices formed by small clusters of doctors had so far sprung up 'piecemeal', health centres presented, they believed, 'an opportunity to plan in advance'.[15] Their proponents cared little about challenging the paternalism of medical practitioners but wanted the state to make family doctoring more modern, coordinated and communal. Put another way, health centres represented the social democratic future.

When Section 21 of the NHS Act in England and Wales mandated that local councils submit plans for health centres, proposals soon poured in.[16] Most of these designs came from local public health officials and council architects. Manchester's Health Committee aspired to build a whopping seventy-five health centres, and it illustrated their ideal model in a detailed report: a large, three-storied modern structure with a variety of clinics on a two-and-a-half-acre site that incorporated a garden and toddlers' playground.[17] The committee lamented the 'dismal condition' of doctoring in the city, believing that it made 'the existing medical service difficult and much less efficient and valuable than it could and should be'. 'Children, our greatest national asset', they declared, 'need colourful, comfortable, and clean surroundings'.

However, Manchester's plans foundered on the rock of government finance, a fate that befell dozens of other councils. Realising that the house building programme and other industrial commitments commanded the nation's construction materials and labour for the short term, the Ministry of Health reversed the initial requirement that all councils submit plans for health centres.[18] Without financial support and legislative compulsion, the chances of growing a national network of health centres disintegrated. In Manchester, pleas for even one health centre met with a negative government response which bluntly cited the need to 'restrict building to that which is urgently necessary'.[19]

Opposition among GPs to health centres contributed to the government's reluctance to extend precious funding and materials for their construction. Many doctors felt uncomfortable sharing premises and working in larger teams. Others expressed fears that close association with local government would undermine their independence. The antagonism between parts of the medical profession and government administration which had shaped the disagreements over the NHS Acts, then, had not disappeared. In 1950, six doctors boycotted a proposed health centre in Sheffield – which the *Daily Mail* described as a 'Bevan Clinic' – because they thought it might deprive their surgeries of patients.[20] Three years later, a poll of GPs found 48 per cent in favour of the 'health centre idea', but 47 per cent opposed.[21] At this point, single-doctor practices still accounted for 43 per cent of the total. General practice largely remained a close-knit or solitary enterprise, and many doctors wanted to keep it that way.

In response, the state restricted its scant health centre funding to a far narrower range of 'experimental' projects.[22] This decision reflected both the constraints of the cash-strapped NHS in its early years as well as how professional medical opinion could sometimes align itself against the service's modernisation. Though some health centre proponents such as the Trades Union Congress (TUC) continued to lobby the Labour government to implement the original nationwide programme, others, like the left-wing Medical and Practitioners' Union (MPU), endorsed the government's strategy of experimentation by reminding members that an 'all or nothing attitude will certainly get us nowhere'.

HEALTH CENTRE EXPERIMENTATION, 1948–1960

Although few in number, the postwar experimental health centres demonstrated improved standards of care and showed that GPs working in close proximity with local government did not lose their independence.[23] These sites also implemented solutions to offset patient concerns about changing aspects of family doctoring, such as shared waiting rooms or new appointment systems. The Conservative Party – back in power after 1951 – displayed ambivalence about health centres both because of their expense and their left-wing associations. In many instances, voluntary initiative from both inside and outside Britain had to make up for uneven government support.

Between 1948 and the end of 1960, twenty-four health centres opened in the name of experiment – all but three in England, concentrated around London and the Midlands.[24] The remainder emerged in Scotland, with none in Wales or Northern Ireland. Nearly all of these facilities began on new housing estates or in New Towns and served predominantly working-class communities employed in nearby industry. All emphasised their commitment to serving families and incorporated maternal and infant welfare clinics. Health centres therefore embodied the emphasis of the postwar welfare state on supporting the working-class families who, it was hoped, might drive up Britain's manufacturing base and expand the nation's wealth.

The health centres opened in this period differed in appearance and practice, and therefore faced different problems. Built within a new council estate in North London by the LCC, the flagship Woodberry Down Health Centre (1952) counted cost, location and scale among its troubles (Figure 6). Left-wing health reformers invested great significance in Woodberry Down as a model for development. Indeed, Bevan cut the first sod for the centre in a news feature.[25] Woodberry Down's minimalist design reflected what the historian Guy Ortolano has portrayed as a typical modern welfare state aesthetic, complete with a reinforced concrete frame with handmade bricks, a flat roof and narrow windowsill bands as the only external adornments.[26] Conceived by

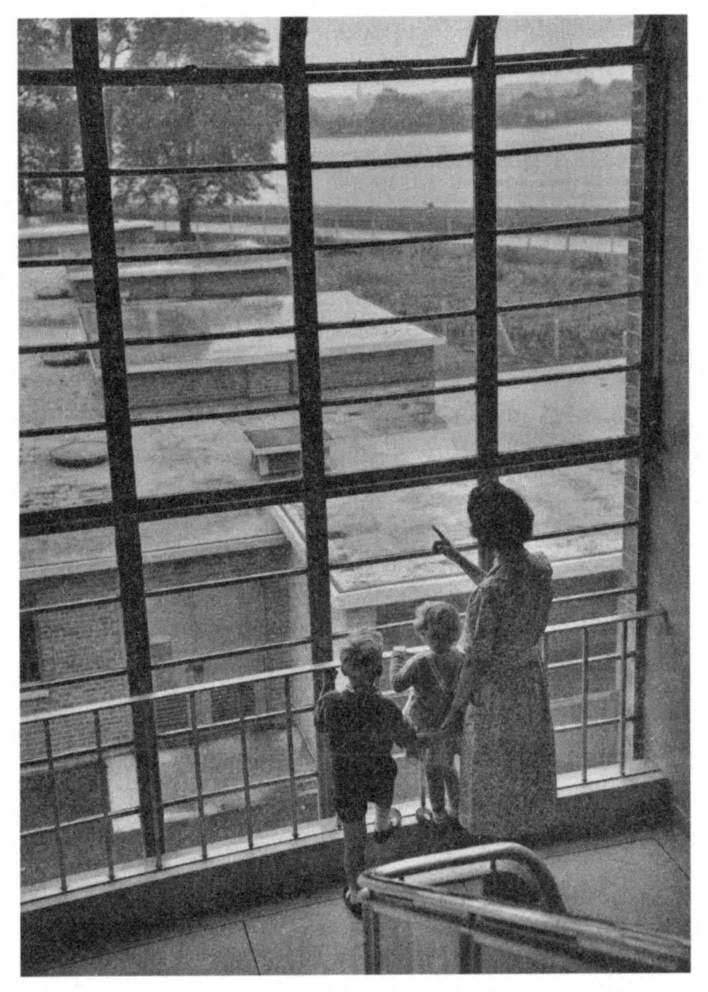

6. New health centres modernised general practice in the NHS, coordinating GP surgeries and their patients along communal lines. However, the expansive designs of early flagship 'experimental' health centres, like Woodberry Down in London, made some patients feel as if they were losing the familiarity of a visit to their local doctor.

LCC architects, such a design projected a modern form of local doctoring, worthy of the future. A playground and garden buttressed the central two-winged building that occupied the one-and-a-half-acre site. This facility came at a high price, and experts criticised its £153,000 cost.[27] Moreover, its size seemed extravagant, with one resident GP later suggesting that facilities such as an operating theatre were 'lying idle'.[28] For all the fanfare, few argued that Woodberry Down should be a model to replicate.

These complications extended to the other large purpose-built health centre at this point, Sighthill Health Centre, Edinburgh (1953). The first health centre constructed in Scotland, planners conceived of Sighthill as 'an experimental centre' and imbued it with rationalising qualities to serve 'a new housing area with a considerable population, which was not adequately served by existing facilities'.[29] Providing six GPs, a pharmacy, laboratory, X-ray department, gym and physiotherapist's room, this large facility similarly championed a centralised and technologically proficient vision of general practice's future. It exhibited a simple modern aesthetic, with concrete brick and a prefabricated flat roof made of copper on fibre. Given free rein, the architects designed a hollow-square structure, with a second-storey overhang above the main entrance. However, as with its London counterpart, the £160,000 cost raised eyebrows. One civil servant thought that while Sighthill 'contained many interesting and beautiful things', it was still 'very expensive . . . and must not be taken as a model from this point of view'.[30]

The difficulties facing Woodberry Down and Sighthill did not stop at their expense or the questionable organisation of amenities. Some patients also experienced these facilities as an unwelcome break with the past and found aspects of their location, size and design frustrating. Woodberry Down's position on the edge of the council estate may have provided pleasant views over the New River, but patients now had to travel around the park and reservoir that divided their community to reach it. Rationalising general practice through health centres could have downsides for patients, and such costs inevitably fell heaviest on those who relied on local doctoring the most: mothers with children, and the elderly. Many members of the public preferred the smaller, domestic environment of the older GP's practice to the spacious interiors of the London and Edinburgh centres. The patients attending Woodberry Down in the late 1950s first reported to a receptionist stationed within a large, bare entrance hall.[31] Attendees found such requirements made the centre 'cold' and 'impersonal', and doctors recounted that 'many patients dislike the atmosphere at the Centre, which they regard as "institutional" '. Some patients got lost in its many corridors, likely exacerbating their feelings of dislocation. As a result of these factors, local people on the estate primarily opted for other, more familiar, surgeries.

These sentiments reflected wider misgivings regarding communal general practice between the 1940s and the 1970s. Mass Observation found in a 1943 survey that 56 per cent of patients preferred to see doctors in a small practice, while 28 per cent favoured larger health centres.[32] Some of the scepticism towards health centres related to questions of privacy. Health centres could seem like impersonal and exposed environments in which to seek treatment.[33] As one working-class woman confided, 'I like my visit to be private, I don't fancy waiting in a public room, and having my illness advertised'.[34] Even by 1967, patients across Britain were almost equally divided – 50 per cent to 47 per cent – when asked whether they favoured a single-doctor practice in the practitioner's own home or a larger group practice like a health centre.[35] This uneven degree of support for the core elements of health centres presented a challenge to the NHS's plan to modernise general practice. As in hospitals, the question of privacy remained a persistent challenge.

Despite the attention that Woodberry Down and Sighthill attracted, the early postwar health centres were typically of modest size and quietly demonstrated the advantages of organising general practice on communal lines. Moreover, they developed a number of strategies designed to ease the same patient concerns directed at their larger counterparts. The William Budd Health Centre (1952) served 30,000 people on the Knowle West housing estate in Bristol, coordinating six groups of GPs, three nurses, two secretary-typists and two part-time sisters.[36] This project cost just £16,000 and was spearheaded by reforming GPs who believed that public initiative offered the best vehicle for bringing medical expertise to a working-class estate where no doctor had wanted to live. In contrast to the wasted space evident at Woodberry Down and Sighthill, all of William Budd's rooms remained in use throughout its early years. Doctors occupied the GP suites in the morning and the local authority ran public health clinics in the same rooms during the afternoons. The facility fostered professional cooperation, with doctors, nurses and other workers enjoying shared spaces such as a staff room where they could 'discuss particular patients or their families over a cup of tea or coffee'. The professional mixing that well-designed spaces engendered presented a clear advantage over most GP surgeries of the period.[37] No doctors complained that working with the local council eroded their independence, and all welcomed the incorporation of public health clinics.

Patients appreciated the William Budd Health Centre.[38] Its doctors insisted that there were 'no complaints from patients that the service becomes impersonal'.[39] Although resident GPs had an interest in making such claims, the spatial dimensions and practices of the centre give reason to believe that patients might have felt more comfortable in Bristol than in facilities like Woodberry Down or Sighthill. Based in a prefabricated, single-storied building, William Budd's smaller scale, though still distinctly modern, offered a less stark break with the past.[40] There were fewer corridors to become lost in, and the centre fostered a welcoming environment by filling its spaces with potted plants and conveniences like newspapers. The fact that patient registration expanded by 4,000 people across the mid-1950s – without a change in the estate's population – suggested the growing popularity of the centre.[41]

Philanthropy also helped demonstrate the worth of smaller centres. In Harlow New Town, Essex, health centres provided the entirety of local general practice, a unique achievement in Britain. The financial backing of the Nuffield Trust – a charitable organisation founded in 1939 to research and support medical services – combined with the ambition of the physician-turned-Labour-politician Stephen Taylor, made this depth of provision possible. Both parties established six health centres in Harlow between 1952 and 1958, as well as additional centres for industrial health and child guidance.[42] Taylor's membership of the Harlow Development Corporation ensured that he could advance health centre expansion in step with the growth of the New Town as a whole. The Development Corporation's ownership of the health centres' premises meant they could not become 'official' Section 21 centres, but they used NHS doctors and served NHS patients.

Harlow's health centres aimed to support the working-class families with children who had moved to what was known colloquially as 'Pram Town' and began with a temporary facility in Haygarth House. Announced by Taylor as 'a prototype of a true health centre, because it brings the practitioners and clinics together', this pair of semi-detached houses possessed three GP suites with separate examination rooms and consulting rooms, as well as a dental surgery, X-ray, office and a single, communal waiting room.[43] The waiting room contained a homely table and chairs, pastoralist Bruegel prints, a kitchen hatch serving tea, and French doors to give children easy access to the garden on warm summer days. These touches balanced communal doctoring with a domestic feel. They also changed minds. One patient remarked, 'I expected a health centre to be like a hospital out-patient department, but this is just like a home'.[44] The supporters of Harlow's health centres hoped they would 'provide an example to the country, and perhaps the world, of a completely integrated health service, a pattern for the future in the town of the future'. Validating these aspirations, Soviet doctors paid a visit to the Harlow centres in 1954, where Taylor used them as evidence that Britain was 'evolving from a private enterprise to a Socialist community'.

From the other side of the Cold War divide, British health centres attracted US philanthropy through the Rockefeller Foundation. Founded in 1913, the organisation had served as one of the twentieth century's most important sources of philanthropic activity in health, famous worldwide for its campaigns to eradicate diseases like yellow fever.[45] The foundation became ideologically and materially invested in the NHS and its commitment to a national network of health centres. The achievement of such a goal would, the Rockefeller Foundation hoped, provide a globally inspiring model of 'social medicine'. Advocated by leading Rockefeller figures, as well as British health reformers like Taylor, social medicine held that doctors should consider patients' wider social and economic environments when treating them.[46] These factors, its proponents held, shaped the incidence of disease and ill health. Social medicine therefore promised to integrate curative and preventative medicine. The Rockefeller Foundation believed that the NHS could practically demonstrate the value of this approach in its health centres, and it accordingly funded experimental projects in Edinburgh and Manchester.

Supported by both Rockefeller and Nuffield Trust money, Darbishire House Health Centre in Manchester proved a success.[47] The centre was based in a converted nineteenth-century hostel in the deprived Longsight area of the inner city. The Rockefeller Foundation provided a significant outlay of £31,000 during the mid-1950s to fund new examination couches, X-ray facilities and a clinical laboratory for approximately 13,000 patients – a number that the facility maintained despite initial worries that patients would not want to follow their GPs into a health centre. Although some of its clientele complained that they had to walk further than before, the practice remained busy, conducting over 3,000 surgery consultations per month and antenatal classes twice a week.[48]

The Darbishire House Health Centre also displayed an attentiveness to patients' concerns about more communal forms of general practice. For instance, each of the four GPs possessed their own waiting room, rather than sharing a single, larger room. While the Rockefeller Foundation criticised these divisions as 'inefficient', such separation met patients' expectations regarding privacy.[49] Patients could feel like they were seeing 'their' doctor even when visiting a centre staffed by a medical team. Similarly, experts in the Rockefeller Foundation, like many other medical reformers, thought appointment systems were the most efficient way to organise time in a busy health centre.[50] The use of appointments, they held, could balance the individual's health complaint with the needs of others in the community, rather than working on the basis of first-come, first-served. Patients, however, disliked appointments or found them difficult to arrange before the widespread adoption of home telephones. Some doctors, too, disapproved, and complained about patients failing to turn up as a waste of the practice's resources.[51] As a result, Darbishire House adopted a flexible approach – only 30 per cent of its attendees pre-booked consultations.[52] Most patients continued the time-honoured custom of sitting in the waiting room until the doctor became available. This situation was far from unique; one 1953 survey found that only 2 per cent of GP surgeries used appointment systems.[53] Darbishire House's acknowledgement of patient preferences regarding privacy or accessing care helped prevent local residents from being excluded, even if it would be too far to say that it embodied anything close to a 'democratic' practice. Like most other facilities of its kind, Darbishire House gleaned patient views on an impressionistic basis. Before 1960, no health centre featured a formal consultative committee to take patients' views.[54] Even in centres like Darbishire House, grounded in the community-oriented tenets of social medicine, patients had few opportunities to directly challenge the paternalism of general practice.

Nonetheless, successes in Manchester, Edinburgh, Harlow and Bristol helped stimulate revived demands for health centres at the national level. This renewed enthusiasm stemmed from a series of academic and policy studies of the earlier centres.[55] A 1960 report on health centres produced by a practitioner at the William Budd Health Centre identified Harlow, Edinburgh, Manchester and – with a touch of self-promotion – his own centre in Bristol as exemplars of the improved quality of care and efficiency fostered by cooperation among GPs. In a nationwide Ministry of Health survey of health centres and group practice, civil servants singled out these same centres for praise. With medical and government experts now more open to health centres, Labour felt the time was ripe to relaunch a national programme when they returned to government in 1964.

THE HEALTH CENTRE BOOM AND PREVENTATIVE MEDICINE IN THE NHS

Health centres swelled in number after the mid-1960s, delivering on earlier aspirations. Between 1964 and 1967, twenty-six centres opened, and then in 1968 alone, thirty-nine more centres welcomed patients.[56] By 1984, 1,378 centres had been established. The *British Medical Journal* spoke of a 'health centre explosion' as these facilities fanned out into non-urban areas, becoming more of a cross-class phenomenon.[57] Their improved services, communal norms and variable but modern design became a recognisable image of the changed NHS. They demonstrated an adaptability to local conditions, undermining any suggestion that this part of the welfare state was monolithic. The earlier social democratic vision of general practice came closer to reality and engaged with evolving understandings of public health, reconceptualised under the banner of 'primary care'.

The Labour Party drove much of this health centre expansion. When elected in 1964 under the leadership of Harold Wilson, the party ended the ambivalence of their Conservative predecessors. The Minister of Health, Kenneth Robinson (1911–1996), provided direct stimulus through the 1966 Family Doctor Charter (Figure 7). Though often overlooked, this agreement negotiated between the government and the BMA provided financial aid that encouraged doctors to work in groups and buy new premises.[58] Doctors could also claim reimbursement for up to 70 per cent of the salaries of nurses, health visitors and secretaries, which allowed staff to be more cheaply hired within a health centre. In the 1970s, Labour politicians continued to take an active approach to health centre expansion, sometimes personally intervening to construct such facilities in communities with deteriorating general practice services.[59]

The government assumed greater responsibility for the shape and practice of health centres by issuing a design guide to local authorities.[60] Committed to 'progressive family doctoring', this document provided advice on administration, finance and layout. The guide recommended an appointment system, a shared waiting area and a sizeable medical team. Receptionists should be given a commanding view of the waiting room, it suggested, and these workers needed to manage the patient records of all doctors together in a single office. The document also provided local planners with architectural designs of different health centres, though it noted that these examples 'should not necessarily be

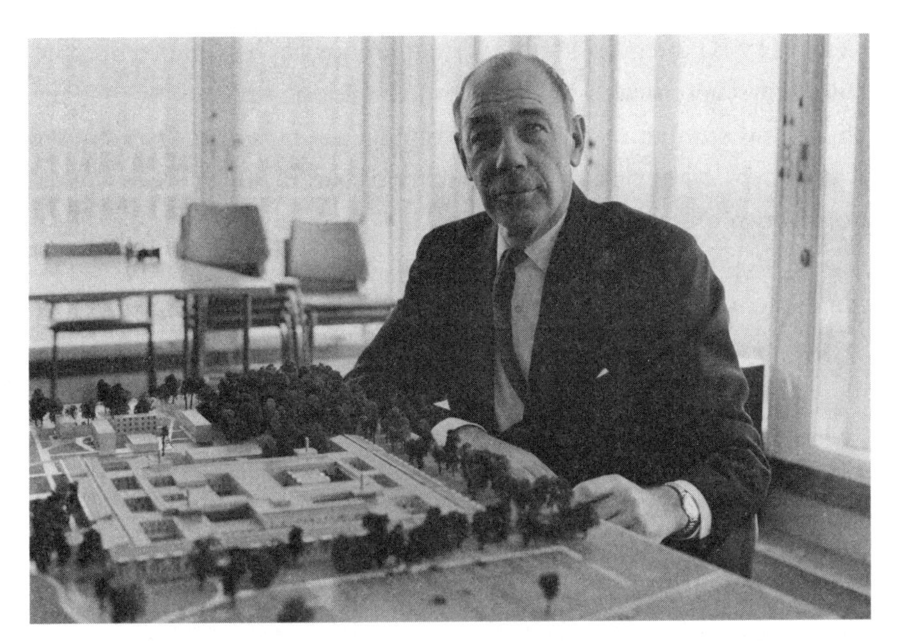

7. Labour Minister of Health Kenneth Robinson made important contributions to the NHS's postwar modernisation. At the height of a faith in state planning during the 1960s, this doctor-turned-politician continued the Conservative Party's 1962 Hospital Plan and negotiated the 1966 Family Doctor Charter with rebellious GPs.

used as model plans because health centre design is still evolving'. The central government's renewed enthusiasm for these facilities, then, did not mean a one-size-fits-all approach.

On the back of previous experiments and improved government support, health centres stretched into new locations during the 1960s and 1970s, including Wales. In the village of Dowlais, South Wales, two existing GP surgeries and a clinic had been demolished to build a new shopping centre. Dowlais Health Centre opened in 1969 and helped fill the medical gap that this urban redevelopment had left by serving a population of 17,000 people.[61] With a large common waiting room, a play area for children and a speech therapy room, the centre showcased the range of services possible within new purpose-built structures. Nearby, in the town of Merthyr Tydfil, the Hollies Health

Centre (1971) integrated four different groups of GPs, offered preventative and school health medical services and incorporated a reference library and seminar room for staff training. These two facilities ensured that 70 per cent of all GPs registered in this part of South Wales worked from health centres.

Despite the density evident in such areas by the 1970s, health centres sometimes struggled to penetrate the world of rural doctoring captured by the art critic John Berger and the Swiss photographer Jean Mohr in their book, *A Fortunate Man* (1967).[62] Part social observation, part philosophy, the publication followed the daily routine of Dr John Sassall, a rural GP in the Gloucestershire village of St Briavels, at the English–Welsh border. Berger's text was interposed with Mohr's striking photographs of Sassall's practice and his patients. Through images and descriptions of Sassall's tireless service to his community, *A Fortunate Man* provided a sympathetic portrait of the countryside doctor and confirmed their continued importance. A later cult classic among medical students, the book is structured through small moments of dedication to patients. In one scene, Sassall treats a young woman with asthma and insomnia, and intuits when having a cup of tea with her neighbours that an affair with the manager of a nearby dairy was perhaps the cause of his patient's distress. In others, he supports a new arrival to the village in securing a council house and meets with unmarried pregnant women. As these episodes suggest, Berger and Mohr wanted to show how Sassall was 'accepted by the villagers and foresters as a man who, in the full sense of the term, lives with them'.

While Berger and Mohr thought the doctor's embeddedness in his patients' community reinforced personal care, this intimacy could also cause problems. A doctor's knowledge about a patient's romantic life or housing conditions carried the risk of moralising or basing medical diagnosis on factors that the patient wished to keep private. *A Fortunate Man* overlooked these pitfalls of the older model of general practice. The authors insisted that locals trusted Sassall simply because 'he lives with them'. But not everyone would have wanted to bump into their doctor while enjoying a pint in the pub or purchasing a loaf of bread at the shops. All the same, Sassall committed to work on his own until his death, even though he expressed awareness of the transformations taking place in general practice by admitting that 'he could be consequently criticised for not joining a group practice or a health centre'.

As *A Fortunate Man* attested, remnants of older traditions in general practice persisted even as the modernising NHS changed the texture of local doctoring. Moreover, the public continued to express interest in pre-1948 customs. The popular light-hearted medical television drama *Dr Finlay's Casebook* (1962–1971) followed the trials and travails of two doctors in rural Scotland during the 1920s. As the historian Chelsea Saxby argues, the popularity of a programme focused on the facets of local doctoring that seemed to be disappearing – including regular home visits and the status of the 'doctor-as-friend' – suggested a sense of loss among the public for the medical past.[63] Similarly, the documentary *Towards a Better Life – Community Health* (1986) displayed the contrasting approaches still in existence as late as the 1980s.[64] Dr Keith Lister – a rural GP working alone in the village of Porlock, Somerset, and employed in the NHS since it began – and Dr Iona Heath – a younger GP working in a larger health centre in Kentish Town, London – offered different perspectives on doctoring and the ideal relationship with patients. Like Sassall in *A Fortunate Man*, Lister described the GP as 'a friend of the people, and he looks after them, and he looks after their health', and expressed hopes that 'patients in the village look upon me as a friend too'. Heath also provided personalised care and shared jokes with her patients in London, but imagined the GP's role in a somewhat more rationalised manner as 'offering the first point of call to make use of the services of the National Health Service'. Lister's surgery in a converted living room of a house and his self-presentation as a pillar of the community recalled doctoring from the 1940s. Heath, on the other hand, worked in a health centre with a staff of 100 people, administering to a more socio-economically and racially diverse patient population. Heath herself evidenced a greater amount of gender diversity among GPs. In 1952, only 6 per cent of family doctors were women.[65] General practice started to change from the 1960s, with about 25 per cent of all GPs being women by the late 1980s.

For all the unevenness between the past and the future of general practice across different regions, health centres still achieved high density in some rural areas. Developments in Devon, over the county border from Lister's Somerset practice, testified to a flourishing local network of health centres, spearheaded by the county council between the mid-1960s and the 1980s. Devonian planners drew explicitly on the example of the experimental health centres initiated during the 1950s, and cited the Family Doctor Charter of 1966 negotiated by the Wilson Labour government as the catalyst for change.[66] Between 1963 and 1981, forty-five health centres opened in cities like Exeter and Plymouth, small towns such as Bovey Tracey and remote villages including Ipplepen.[67] By the mid-1970s, over half of all Devon's GPs worked in health centres. Most of these facilities housed three or four doctors and a small number of auxiliary staff. Nearly all possessed communal waiting rooms, and most had a modern design with flat roofs and unadorned exteriors.[68] The majority used steel frames and large windows to provide light. Pram shelters and car parking spaces demonstrated an awareness of variable patient needs. Before this expansion, Devonian patients had primarily accessed community health services in church halls. Now, the state integrated expertise in purpose-built facilities. From coastlines to farming villages, Devonians could now see the NHS – and therefore the welfare state – transforming their communities.

Health centres like Devon's catered to a wider cross-class constituency of patients. Though pockets of rural poverty persisted, the area attracted affluent, middle-class retirees, and therefore did not experience the same degree of health inequality as inner-city or industrial areas. Devon's health centres also served a sizeable elderly population. Ilfracombe Health Centre accommodated older and disabled patients by including a ramped approach for wheelchairs.[69] Unlike during the earlier phase of experimentation, government officials no longer believed that health centres should be solely directed at the urban working class.

In both the UK and abroad, the expansion of health centres in these decades formed part of a shift towards what was now expansively described as 'primary care'.[70] By the 1970s, medical professionals and commentators began to question an older model of medicine that seemed more oriented towards curing disease than preventing it. The modern hospital's dominance within health systems – both in terms of funding and prestige – seemed to crowd out public health measures that could tackle ill health at its point of origin. This state of affairs was doubly problematic given the emergence of what the medical expert Abdel Omran famously described in 1971 as an 'epidemiologic transition', where chronic conditions – like cancer and cardiovascular disease – replaced infectious diseases – such as diphtheria or tuberculosis – as the primary causes of mortality. The best way of addressing this shift, reformers held, was integrating primary care with public health expertise through teams of professionals that could identify the initial signs of ill health on the ground, before hospitals needed to be involved at all. This global conversation reached its apex at the 1978 International Conference on Primary Care in Alma Ata, which in grandiose terms called for 'Health for All by the Year 2000'.

In Britain, medical experts arrived at similar conclusions, and the administrative structure of the NHS came under fire for being ill-prepared to address such important epidemiological shifts.[71] Medical researchers furnished evidence for how 'ways of living' shaped health outcomes. In his early research, the epidemiologist Jerry Morris, for example, found that sedentary drivers of double-decker buses in London suffered from a higher incidence of cardiovascular problems than their colleagues who regularly climbed the stairs of those same vehicles.[72] Similarly, a famous 1950 *British Medical Journal* paper by Richard Doll and Austin Bradford Hill showed an association between smoking and lung cancer. By the 1970s, reformers like Morris openly called for the NHS to give more attention to preventative medicine and epidemiological information when organising its services, as well as empowering GPs as 'Tomorrow's Community Physician'. These professionals, they maintained, could encourage their patients to exercise or quit smoking as well as oversee screening programmes aimed at helping bring a healthier future within reach.

After much debate on these questions, the Conservative government led by Edward Heath reorganised the NHS's administrative structure in 1973. This reform attempted to stimulate community medicine by replacing the original tripartite split within the service – which had separated GPs, hospital care and public health initiatives – with a framework that coordinated general practice and public health under Area Health Authorities (AHAs).[73] Family Practitioner Committees replaced the earlier Executive Councils that had overseen the work of GPs. The 1973 reforms altered the legislative status of health centres, as AHAs now took over responsibility for their planning from local councils. Modifying the leadership structure slowed the overall rate of expansion. AHAs often had to start from scratch in planning health centres, without the existing knowledge usually possessed by a local council and its medical officials. In Devon, the county council complained that the reforms had undercut the momentum behind the region's health centre programme.[74] Nonetheless, the density achieved by the 1980s in Devon suggested that the reorganisation of the NHS did not fundamentally hinder growth. In this decade, AHAs and GPs could still build health centres by applying for funding from the government's General Practice Finance Corporation. This method helped new projects – such as the Watling Vale Medical Centre, Milton Keynes (1987) – open during a later period of fiscal tightening.[75] After a faltering start, general practice displayed clear evidence of modernisation. Television programmes such as *The Practice* (1985–1986) – a medical drama set in a fictional Manchester health centre – confirmed the place of these facilities as a familiar dimension of British life.[76] But how did patients react to the boom in health centres and group practice?

PATIENTS, RIGHTS AND CONSUMERISM IN HEALTH CENTRES

In the 1970s, patients continued to express mixed sentiments about the communal dynamics that group general practice fostered. Armed with a language of 'rights' informed by the 'patients' movement', consumerism and novel mechanisms to voice discontent provided by the 1973

NHS reorganisation, the public challenged older health care norms. These currents of reform insisted that patients' personal preferences should carry greater weight in the delivery and experience of medical care. However, while mainstream consumerism gradually became dominated by free-market priorities, its trajectory in medical services was not incompatible with the state.[77] In fact, the NHS responded to consumerist impulses and developed ways of learning about patient problems. Though imperfect, the solutions enacted in the service carried important consequences. Patients did not merely come to tolerate more communal forms of medical care but could favour them. They often welcomed new, larger facilities and pooled services, appreciated novel features of group practice like receptionists, and even sometimes found an increased sense of privacy within a more anonymised form of family doctoring. In short, health centres facilitated the flowering of communal, social democratic relationships during a decade when the welfare state came under financial and ideological pressure elsewhere.

The health centre boom coincided with a groundswell of activism around the industrialised world that challenged paternalist attitudes within medical care.[78] From consumer champions to feminists, these campaigners were united by a desire to rebalance health care in favour of the layperson. In Britain, the Patients Association proved particularly important in advancing these ideals. A schoolteacher named Helen Hodgson formed the organisation in 1963, seeking to empower patients in the wake of the thalidomide scandal that left hundreds of babies disabled because of a defective anti-morning sickness drug. In the Patients Association's work to transform the NHS, the organisation drafted leaflets on 'patients' rights' and vigorously pursued media publicity.[79] It worked closely with consumer rights advocates, regularly referring to patients as 'consumers' in their activism.[80] Magazines with a consumerist bent, such as *Which?*, frequently featured articles on medicine, and the Patients Association maximised this burgeoning popular interest in understanding health services by translating it into a language of 'rights', including the right to accurate medical information or the right to complain.[81]

Paperback handbooks like *The National Health Service and You* (1965) – which billed itself as 'the first complete cradle-to-grave guide to your rights in today's Welfare Britain' – detailed these entitlements to the public in consumerist terms.[82] With regard to general practice, the volume described how to choose a surgery, change doctors and negotiate consultations to ensure an accurate diagnosis. The book demonstrated how choice and negotiation had become ever more important expectations among patients as the postwar decades advanced. Although the reach of this type of consumer activism across social classes likely remained uneven, it popularised the view that patients empowered with knowledge of the NHS's structure and services would receive better care as individuals and drive up overall standards. As the social policy expert Richard Titmuss enthused, 'educated public opinion is . . . the most powerful ally of the medical profession'.[83]

All the same, consumerist publications like these did not represent an antagonist view towards the state. *The National Health Service and You* instead lauded the NHS for ensuring that patients were, in its view, 'entitled to the world's most comprehensive medical service, divorcing the care of health from questions of personal means'.[84] It placed these benefits in a transnational perspective for the reader by describing other countries' health systems, and disparaged these overseas alternatives as closer to Britain's own arrangements before the generosity of the NHS. In a testament to the nuances of health consumerism in this period, centring patients did not mean an automatic critique of nationalised provision.[85] The individualist impulses of consumerism had many possible destinations, and not all favoured private medicine outside the NHS.

From the 1970s, feminists also sought to empower women patients in the NHS. Like its counterparts elsewhere, the women's health movement in Britain critiqued the sexism within modern medical care.[86] The control of predominantly male doctors over medical technologies like birth control or the frequent condescension that women faced from practitioners numbered among the issues that motivated feminists to call for change. At first, some feminists attempted to establish health services outside of the NHS, such as family planning clinics or therapy groups. When these grassroots initiatives largely failed, the women's health movement shifted to improving the public system by arming women with information and an awareness of their rights. Writing in 1975, Lin Layram embodied such an approach when she shared her experience of breast cancer in the feminist magazine *Spare Rib*.[87] When Layram discovered a lump in her breast, one NHS doctor at a family planning clinic dismissed the seriousness of her condition. The doctor neglected to insist that Layram contact her GP and ask for tests. It later emerged that the lump was indeed cancerous. Following her experience, Layram encouraged other patients with similar concerns to have the confidence to ask for expertise beyond the 'average clinic doctor or GP'. 'It can only be confirmed by a biopsy report and women should insist on this as soon as possible', she wrote, 'or other women should insist on their sisters behalf'. Empowering patients with information and the knowledge of their rights offered a means to change the NHS.

At the same time that consumer campaigners and feminists subjected the medical profession to increased scrutiny, some doctors had already begun to consider how to treat their patients with more empathy. The Hungarian psychoanalyst Michael Balint proved influential in stimulating this reflection on patients' needs.[88] Balint's seminal work *The Doctor, His Patient, and the Illness* (1957) posited that GPs had the opportunity to consider the 'whole' patient – unlike doctors in busy hospitals – and to understand how family practitioners were a 'medical tool' in their own right.[89] While these theories displayed hints of paternalism by prioritising the doctor, they spoke to an increased awareness of the patient's position within everyday medical encounters.[90] Beyond Balint, theorists of general practice in the 1960s paid increasing attention to emotions such as 'sympathy' to ensure a more equitable doctor–patient relationship.[91] By the point that health centres expanded across the country, then, experts, practitioners and planners were exhibiting a desire to listen to patients, who seemed, for their part, increasingly willing to speak.

Community Health Councils (CHCs) featured among the mechanisms devised by the government to deliver on these attitudinal changes.[92] As part of the wider 1973 NHS reorganisation, 207 CHCs were tasked with a range of responsibilities that included sourcing views on services, representing the interests of groups and individuals to planners, highlighting gaps in provision and promoting public health. The film *You and Your Health* (1979) billed the work of the CHCs as 'to represent you, the patient and the consumer, and the local community'.[93] This public broadcast informed patients in Wales about how to exercise their rights under the NHS. Real-life doctors and patients described how to claim compensation for side effects caused by drugs, and actors demonstrated how to press for quicker hospital appointments when referred by their GP. It also revealed how CHCs collected public opinion by depicting a survey taking place on the doorstep. 'Remember we are at your service,' the film concluded, 'our concern is your health'. For all the good intentions of the CHCs, the lack of definition about what patient representation meant and a tendency among other parts of the NHS to ignore their recommendations, undermined their effectiveness, as the historian Alex Mold makes clear.[94] The earlier aspirations for community medicine, and indeed public health as a whole, remained unfulfilled in the NHS, which was still dominated by the hospitals.

Nonetheless, CHC engagement with health centres demonstrated the valuable work that they could sometimes provide. The patient opinions collected by CHCs during the 1970s testified to familiar problems with the communal dynamics of health centres. Many of these studies showed that patients were generally happy with the new facilities in their communities, but features such as pooled, open-plan waiting rooms persisted as sources of contention. Patients regularly had to divulge sensitive information – such as their reason for visiting the doctor – to receptionists stationed near a communal waiting room (Figure 8). Though this positioning may have helped receptionists oversee the waiting area and direct the flow of foot traffic, it also lay within hearing distance of others. 'Everyone in the Waiting Room can

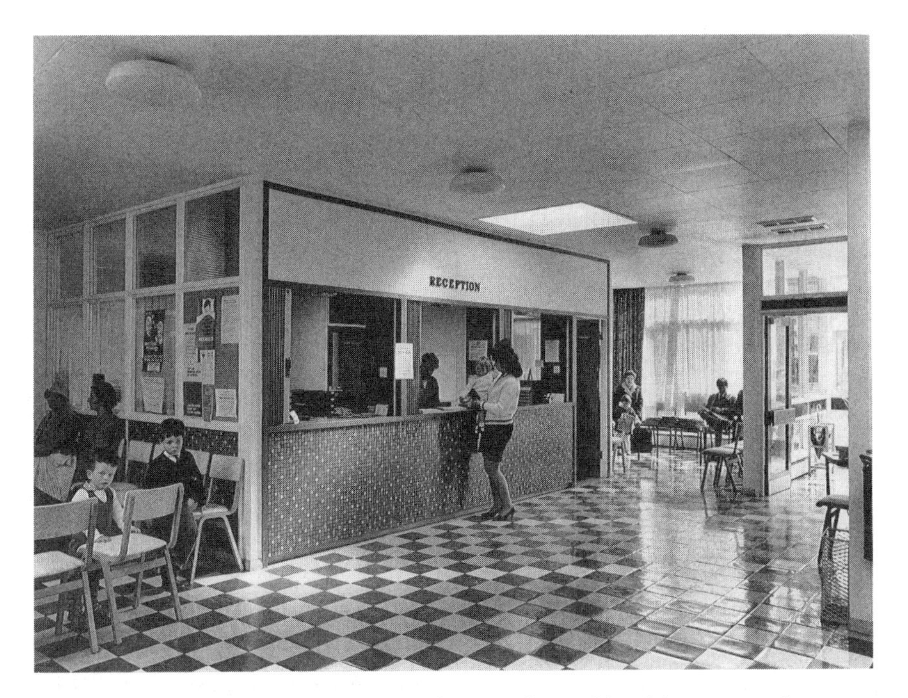

8. During the 1960s and 1970s, the number of health centres dramatically expanded across the UK, including this facility in Ilfracombe, Devon. Seemingly mundane adjustments to their designs – such as smaller waiting rooms and sound-insulating barriers – helped address earlier patient concerns about privacy.

hear what you say to the doctor', complained one patient to a CHC in central London.[95] Patients expressed similar feelings in Northern Ireland – a region that delivered 60 per cent of its local doctoring through sixty health centres by the late 1970s.[96] One patient survey showed that the vast majority of local people were satisfied with these new facilities, with 80 per cent finding them as good as or better than earlier forms of general practice. Nonetheless, 27 per cent of patients still thought that 'there was not enough privacy in the reception room', recalling the complaints made during the earlier experimental period.

Other apprehensions about privacy centred on appointment systems and the associated uptake in GPs employing receptionists. By the 1970s, seeing the doctor usually meant booking in advance. In 1964,

15 per cent of patients said their doctors used an appointment system, but by 1977 this figure stood at 75 per cent.[97] The growth of health centres and group practice facilitated medical reformers' achievement of this long-held goal, as more professionals working under one roof necessitated greater coordination of the practice's time. Health centres typically included an office staffed by receptionists and other clerical workers to manage appointment systems. However, the increased presence of receptionists attracted a significant amount of criticism from patients previously accustomed to fewer people standing between themselves and their doctor.[98] Alongside her important work researching patients in hospitals, the medical statistician Ann Cartwright found in a nationwide study of general practice during the late 1970s that 30 per cent of people said they did not like having to tell the receptionist why they wanted to see the doctor.[99] To many patients, a receptionist's inquiries about why they wanted treatment over the phone or in person seemed an unwarranted extension into the doctor–patient relationship. For their part, receptionists sometimes expressed a sense of divided loyalty between patient and doctor, with many seeing themselves as an 'umpire' adjudicating the 'rules of the game'.[100]

Though some patients criticised receptionists, many others welcomed their role. The inverse of Cartwright's findings, after all, showed that 70 per cent of people did not mind telling the receptionist about their illness. Similarly, another study of London health centres across the first half of the 1970s found that between 60 and 77 per cent of patients thought receptionists made it easier to see their doctor.[101] These patients did not just tolerate the additional layers of administration but embraced them. While the aggregated 'yes' or 'no' answers to surveys make it difficult to evidence why visitors to a health centre or group practice felt positively towards receptionists, the overall trend suggested growing appreciation of more communal dynamics.

Other patients valued greater anonymity and choice. The decline of GPs like Sassall in *A Fortunate Man* – who lived a few streets away and went to the same shops or pub – helped keep medical information from neighbours. Despite the nostalgia for intimate doctor–patient relationships evidenced by the popularity of television programmes like *Dr Finlay's Casebook*, in reality much of the public recognised the benefits of modernised general practice. The falling rates of home visits by GPs would have decreased any trepidation that accompanied a middle-class professional entering the home. Similarly, registering at a health centre with four or five doctors could expand patient choice. More doctors increased the chances of accessing women GPs who, like Iona Heath in the film *Towards a Better Life – Community Health*, formed a growing part of local doctoring by the 1970s. By the end of the decade, one study found that 33 per cent of Asian doctors in the NHS worked in health centres, compared to 19 per cent of British-born doctors.[102] This higher density of GPs who qualified overseas also provided more options for immigrants, or their descendants, who wanted a doctor from their own ethnic background or who spoke their primary language. Both privacy and choice, then, could be improved by the expansion of communalism in health centres.

By this point, the modernisation of general practice had started to exhibit at least some attentiveness to the needs of patients from ethnic minorities. To be sure, campaigning organisations such as the Community Health Group for Ethnic Minorities (CHGEM) came into existence in the late 1970s partly out of frustration with the health service.[103] 'Insensitivity to other cultural habits and Ethnic Minority Group needs generally ignored by the NHS', summed up the group in an early statement. Yet the organisation did not abandon the public service. Rather, they decided to adopt the strategy of a pressure group, 'attacking the system' from the outside and working with like-minded organisations to 'change attitude of NHS staff at all levels'. Their contributions included establishing a national 'Resource Centre' that held, among other materials, visual guides to ease medical communication with patients from ethnic minority backgrounds who spoke English as a second language. One such guide for pregnant Asian women aimed to facilitate their discussions with doctors and nurses about appetite and morning sickness (Figure 9). Though organisations like CHGEM continued to highlight the discrimination that people of colour faced as

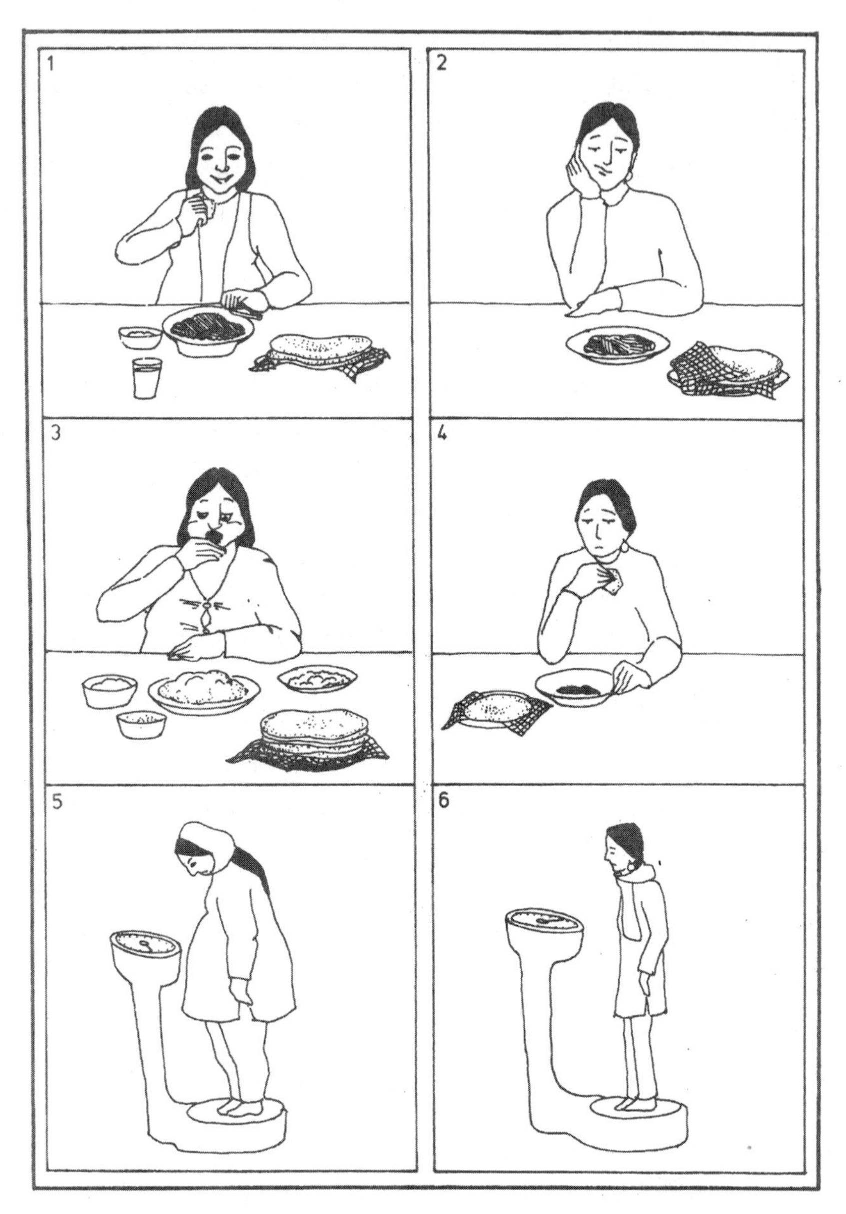

9. Organisations outside the NHS sought to make the service more responsive to a changing Britain, including greater ethnic and racial diversity. During the late 1970s, the Harehills English Language Project in Leeds devised this visual aid for issues in maternity care, such as fluctuations in appetite, to ease communication between medical practitioners and their patients who might have found it difficult to speak English.

patients in the NHS, including the persistent issue of doctors not taking their pain seriously, the efforts of such organisations helped recalibrate the health service to a more ethnically and racially diverse Britain.

The growth of patient representation committees that sourced criticisms and suggestions further helped address patient concerns in general practice. In Aberdare, South Wales, a health centre included a patients' committee from its inception in 1973.[104] This committee, formed of thirteen members ranging from a retired teacher to an industrial worker, met every few weeks. They discussed issues in the centre spanning the appointment system, car parking and waiting room decor to medical matters such as helping devise a screening process to send letters to patients on their sixtieth birthday. Patients were sometimes now given something akin to the voice that health consumer activists had campaigned for and even included within the community focus of primary care. Didcot Health Centre, Oxfordshire, took a different approach, inviting a patient representative to the general management committee for the practice.[105] The centre's GPs believed that while some patients might feel confident to speak out, 'on the whole they are frightened to say exactly what they think for fear of upsetting their relationship with their medical team, and possibly jeopardising their future care'. An elected patient representative offered, to them, the best solution. Mrs Brenda Soper – a local Citizens' Advice Bureau member – was duly elected and quickly approached by patients with concerns about 'the confidentiality of personal problems at the health-centre reception-desk'. 'This is a perennial and notoriously difficult problem', the health centre admitted, 'but renewed discussion has produced several ideas for improving the situation'. Problems such as privacy in the waiting room could be better acknowledged, and therefore addressed, by the 1970s because of this increased openness to patient criticisms.

There were no quick fixes to the concerns provoked by the communal dynamics of health centres. Patients still sometimes found receptionists intrusive, appointments systems frustrating or large waiting rooms exposed. However, experts at least began to examine these problems and pose solutions. Dr Ruth Cammock, a medical doctor and architectural researcher, highlighted the issues that patients faced in health centres and group practice in her publications.[106] *Health Centres Handbook* (1973) stressed the need for staff awareness of patient privacy.[107] It established an important architectural principle in health centre design by dividing their spaces into 'public zones', 'staff zones' and 'interaction zones'. Cammock made recommendations on how to balance privacy in each. She identified the reception area, for example, as 'the place where the patient makes his first contact with the health centre organisation – the shop-window which must reassure all comers that they can safely entrust their most private problems to its care'. Cammock suggested practical solutions to reduce anxieties around privacy. 'Each reception station should be distinct and separate', she insisted, 'so that callers are not conscious of queues on either side watching and listening to their requests'. Partitions along a reception desk for each office staff member served as a low-budget solution. Though only a small change, the adoption of such material divisions by many centres helped alleviate patient apprehensions. In 1974, one of Cammock's reports on privacy attracted the government's attention.[108] Their interest was piqued after she claimed that architects were unconcerned with 'privacy as an emotional need, nor with providing a feeling or illusion of privacy'. In agreement with many of Cammock's criticisms, civil servants included her advice about screens and zones within future government advice to local planners.[109] Such reflexivity could never entirely solve the tensions brought about by communal dynamics in health centres, but it did help promote physical alterations that smoothed the path of modernisation in general practice.

***

Though health centres suffered a faltering start due to a lack of government prioritisation and opposition from doctors, they eventually became local staples throughout the UK. These facilities stood as visible demonstrations of the NHS's ability to modernise local doctoring and reflected much of the international emphasis on primary care that had emerged by the 1970s. While hospitals still absorbed the lion's share of budgets and prestige, and preventative goals remained elusive, health centres brought this novel iteration of modern medicine into communities. On a local level, many patients appreciated new buildings, better equipment, and access to an expanded range of medical personnel and services. Over time, the advocates of health centres devised at least partial solutions to patients' attachments to older traditions in family doctoring and personal expectations about privacy.

Three decades after the service's inception, then, the process of NHS modernisation had borne fruit in its hospitals and doctors' surgeries. The supporters of the service helped embed a distinctive health system more in tune with social democratic principles. It extended government-provided medical care free at the point of use, supported families and workers, and brought different constituencies of patients together in shared spaces. Even if some of the earlier unevenness in the quantity and quality of treatment bequeathed by the institution's interwar and Victorian inheritance remained, the NHS displayed a degree of adaptability. The rising tide of individualism in the postwar decades could not only be accommodated within this predominantly state institution but harnessed to strengthen it. At the same time that these developments unfolded, the NHS's international reputation also underwent an important transition that further entrenched its place in British life.

PART II

THE NHS AND THE WORLD

4
THE ENVY OF THE WORLD

In the summer of 1959, the American medical activist and policy expert Michael M. Davis (1879–1971) boarded the *Empress of India* and began a voyage to Britain.[1] Almost as soon as Davis left port in Canada, he and his wife, Alice, began asking anyone they could find with a British accent a series of pointed questions. Their inquiries continued once they docked. The couple made time to see the new West End hit *My Fair Lady* (1956) and took in the rugged beauty of North Wales, but remained focused on quizzing the people that they encountered. Teahouses in British parks emerged as the perfect place to pose their queries, as the pair could approach unsuspecting punters sat on benches with a smile before getting out their notebooks. 'Our seatmates at the tables or on the grass knew by our accent that we were Americans', Davis later shared, 'and when we got acquainted, we usually found they were surprised by us, because they thought Americans ate lunch at expensive restaurants'. The topic of all this interrogation was the NHS. Like many overseas medical reformers and experts, Davis took extensive interest in Britain's health service. As a man on the political left, he believed that the institution might offer some lessons to those in the US fighting for greater federal government involvement in the provision of care, even if he recognised that the exact structures of the NHS could not be copied. Davis was delighted to find that the 100 British people he spoke with – from hotel maids to housewives to taxi drivers – were 'practically unanimous' in saying that they still 'wanted the Health

Service' a decade after its introduction. The public's principle reason for liking the NHS, he reported to labour organisations on his return to the US, lay in providing 'an important emotional relief from financial anxiety'. 'Our judgements of another country will be helped by humility and frankness about our own', Davis added in his call to end the comparative insecurity felt by many US citizens.

The British health service competed for the attention of foreign observers like Davis during a feverish mid-century period of reform in global medical politics.[2] An explosion of charters, plans and institutions sought to distribute health care on universalist principles in nations all over the world, old and new.[3] The International Labour Organization's Philadelphia Declaration in 1944 called for 'comprehensive medical care' as part of a wider demand for economic planning.[4] Novel ideas of 'human rights', advanced by postwar institutions like the United Nations (UN), often stressed the need to access health services.[5] In the same year that British nationalised medicine came into existence, Article 25 of the UN's Universal Declaration of Human Rights stipulated a right to medical treatment, and the World Health Organization (WHO) began its mission to raise global standards of health from its headquarters in Geneva.

Amidst this heady atmosphere of medical transformation, the NHS's supporters sought to build international influence. They did so at a time when Britain's place in the world seemed uncertain due to the abrupt end of wartime 'lend-lease' agreements with the US and the onset of decolonisation in the empire. The Cold War confirmed the US and the Soviet Union as the dominant postwar powers, and the loss of Britain's overseas territories undermined the nation's historic authority on the world stage. During the twelve months before the NHS's inception in July 1948, British soldiers left India and Palestine, and the first wave of workers drawn from the new Commonwealth arrived in London aboard the SS *Empire Windrush*.[6] From the mid-1950s, more and more nations gained their independence. Faced with such events, the proposals offered to maintain the UK's international standing ranged from stopping the tide of decolonisation with armed aggression

– which did indeed occur in places such as Kenya or Malaysia – to more peaceful strategies such as deploying British expertise in town planning or pursuing soft power through cultural mediums like ballet.[7] For the NHS's proponents, it seemed possible that the service would have impact in these latter spheres. Bevan boasted that the NHS provided Britain with 'the moral leadership of the world', and predicted that 'before many years are over we shall have people coming here as to a modern Mecca, learning from us in the twentieth century as they learned from us in the seventeenth century'.[8]

These statements masked anxiety about Britain's standing vis-à-vis the English-speaking nation that now eclipsed it in the international pecking order. Though the NHS's founders and early enthusiasts regularly spoke in terms of what the institution meant for 'the world', they in fact cared most about American opinion and closely monitored reactions from across the Atlantic. In their speeches and writings, the supporters of the NHS focused on the US above all. For their part, the views of US experts about Britain's health service fractured along political lines. On one side, the advocates of a federal guarantee to health care, like Davis, thought that the NHS provided both inspiration as well as specific elements that might be transplanted.[9] On the other side, their conservative opponents – who have received more attention from historians – perceived the service as a warning about the risks of 'socialized medicine'.[10] Many British supporters of the NHS seized on the opportunity to work with the first group by helping them try and enact a system of national health insurance. As the historian Dan Rodgers has shown, a long tradition of transatlantic exchange on questions of state welfare dated back to the nineteenth century, but this cooperation did not, as he also suggests, completely collapse after 1945 when the Cold War cast many social programmes as 'communist'.[11] The case of medicine shows continued engagement. However, even with this cooperation, US reformers proved unable to establish a right to health.[12] In the face of diverging priorities and persistent criticism from US conservatives, the aspirations among British medical activists, trade unions and politicians to hold up the NHS as an inspirational model dimmed.

Instead, these groups retreated to drawing lines of national distinction. This about-turn contributed to the emergence of welfare nationalism around the NHS back home, as the supporters of the service publicly stressed the differences between the UK and US health systems, rather than offering points of commonality. In the 1970s, many Britons were starting to agree with Bevan's view that the NHS stood as the 'envy of the world', regardless – or sometimes because of – foreign scepticism about such claims.[13]

By looking at the service from across the Atlantic, different facets of the NHS's domestic development and cultural image come into view. The service became increasingly 'British' after the 1970s, and therefore more resilient against neoliberal critique, as it enjoyed public attachment afforded to institutions understood as indicative of values essential to the nation. In contrast, free-market proposals struggled to shake off an association with the apparent flaws of private medicine in the US. But these later connections were the outcome of a historical process. It was not inevitable that Britons would automatically think about the US when they reflected on foreign health systems or the place of private medicine at home. To appreciate where these links came from, one needs to consider how welfare nationalism emerged from the ruins of an earlier medical internationalism.

THE NHS AND NATIONAL HEALTH INSURANCE IN THE US DURING THE 1940S AND 1950S

The Second World War created new opportunities for US health reformers, and many looked to Britain for encouragement. US citizens also began to speak of 'rights' in exchange for the sacrifices they had made during conflict.[14] These demands, reformers believed, could be translated into a national system of health insurance, in which workers and employers would pool their resources into a medical fund managed by the federal government. This proposed system might not replicate the European models that were being formulated at the same time, but it would guarantee universal health coverage. Like many others around the world, Americans took an interest in the publication of the British

Beveridge Report in 1942 and its promise of universal health care. Beveridge cashed in on this popularity by touring the US in 1943, where he even met President Roosevelt. As the war reached its conclusion, fears of falling behind Britain on the topic of welfare spread across the US political spectrum. The Republican Mayor of New York City, Fiorello LaGuardia, admired Beveridge so much that he hosted a luncheon in his honour.[15] In a radio address one year later introducing his own Health Insurance Plan for city employees, LaGuardia reflected that 'Great Britain seems to be far ahead of us'.[16] 'It will not be long', he informed his listeners, 'before Great Britain will have a complete coverage – a National Health Insurance System in operation'.

The comparative deficiencies of the US system only became clearer to its critics when the establishment of the NHS confirmed LaGuardia's predictions. As in most industrialised countries during the mid-twentieth century, the US relied on a mix of municipal, private and voluntary initiatives to provide medical services delivered by a profession with high disciplinary specialisation.[17] At base, access to health care depended on income. For those who could afford it, organisations such as Blue Cross and Blue Shield provided security through health insurance that Americans took out on a voluntary basis. The size of the US made accessing medical facilities difficult for many citizens. Moreover, racial health divides also blighted the US, as the legacies of slavery, experimentation on African Americans and continued discrimination within medical institutions shaped the system's overall outcomes.[18]

The health reformers on the US left during the 1940s, like Michael Davis, believed that national health insurance could cohere this uneven assemblage of medical services and raise standards of care for the poorest. Like many other reformers of his generation, including Beveridge, Davis's first exposure to health inequities came via the settlement movement, where volunteers provided youth work, adult-learning classes and legal advice to the local people they lived among (Figure 10).[19] Hailing from New York, he joined the People's Institute in 1905, organising civic clubs for the impoverished inhabitants of Manhattan's Lower East Side. During the next two decades, Davis held the position of Director of the Boston Dispensary, where he pioneered financial support for the less well-off through a 'pay clinic' where patients gave small sums to see a doctor.[20] In 1936, he established the Committee for Research in Medical Economics, an organisation that published *Medical Care* – the first journal in the world devoted to the economic and social aspects of health services. He was a busy man. In total, Davis penned

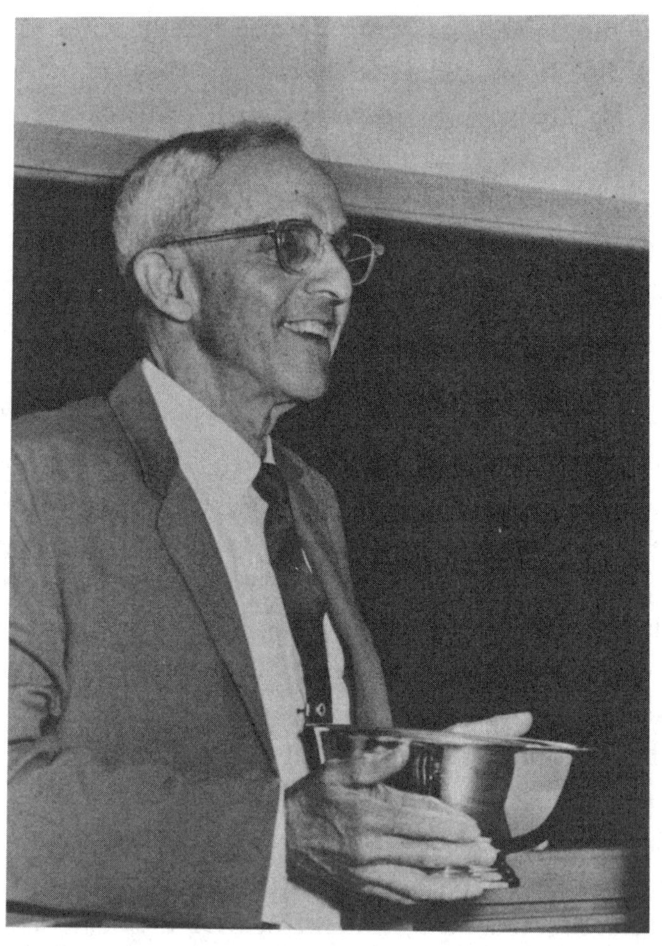

10. At the same time as the NHS modernised, many commentators and experts around the world expressed interest in Britain's experiment with nationalised medicine. The US health reformer Michael M. Davis took inspiration from the NHS when fighting to extend federal support for health care in his own country.

12 books and over 250 articles.[21] By the 1940s, he was a firm advocate of national health insurance. With one eye fixed across the Atlantic, Davis publicised the 'monumental' Beveridge Report's proposals for US audiences.[22] In a speech delivered shortly after the inception of the NHS, he observed with envy how 'All of the democratic countries of Western Europe have enacted compulsory health insurance'.[23]

The best hope of achieving this goal lay in the successful passage of the Wagner–Murray–Dingell bills, introduced annually to the US Congress for ten years after 1939. Davis possessed links with the senators involved in this legislative campaign, which aimed to establish a national health insurance fund paid for by workers and employers through a payroll tax. In 1945, President Truman announced his support for national health insurance in a speech drafted by Davis. In sweeping terms, the President told Congress that 'the health of this Nation is a national concern; that financial barriers in the way of attaining health shall be removed; that the health of all its citizens deserves the help of all the Nation'.[24] What became described as the 'Truman Health Plan' merged with the Wagner–Murray–Dingell bills and soon attracted extensive debate.

National health insurance in the US enjoyed a degree of popular support. Though the public disagreed on whether government, voluntary or private solutions offered the best future, they favoured ameliorating medical costs.[25] Many Americans expressed frustration with the medical profession and its apparent profit-making. One 1944 poll found 82 per cent of respondents agreeing that 'something must be done to make it easier for people to get medical care'. Popular books such as Carl Malmberg's *140 Million Patients* (1947) channelled this anger, questioning doctors' boasts that 'Americans are the healthiest people in the world' by pointing to class and racial inequalities.[26] Malmberg predicted that a national plan like Truman's would save 3 million lives and prevent a loss of more than $10 billion a year in productivity. 'Great Britain has already taken a long step in that direction with enactment of its National Health Service Act', he concluded in a further invocation of developments across the Atlantic.

But not all Americans were so supportive. In a political culture increasingly gripped by Cold War suspicion, any extension of federal welfare could expect to receive intense scrutiny. The proposals for systematic health care reform in the US attracted a better-funded campaign of opposition from the medical profession than in Britain. Although Bevan's battles with the BMA had proved fierce, they paled in comparison to the charge of the American Medical Association (AMA) against the Truman Plan. Founded in 1847, the AMA became not just the dominant representative body for US physicians but a political powerhouse in its own right. Foremost among their public campaigns lay opposition to external involvement in the financing and organisation of medical care – especially from federal sources. Any association between government and health care, to them, was tantamount to 'socialized medicine', a term that carried communist connotations and suffused US debate. Indeed, President Roosevelt had refrained from including health insurance in the 1935 Social Security Act primarily because of concerns about how the medical lobby might react, showing the influence of the AMA even at the height of the New Deal.[27]

Davis, like those who established the NHS, recognised that the successful foundation of universal health care depended on the ability to wield public opinion against its detractors. 'Progressive professional men cannot by themselves realize their ideals against antagonistic policies of organized medicine', Davis claimed.[28] He insisted that the 'active participation of the public' represented the 'only way' forward. In his mind, reformers had to promote 'medical-economic measures – of which national health insurance is the chief' to 'obtain lay understanding and enlist aggressive popular support'. Through such a strategy, he maintained, the AMA might be overcome.

To channel popular feeling, Davis founded an organisation called the Committee for the Nation's Health (CNH) in 1946 and served as its executive director. Over the next ten years, the CNH lobbied Congress for national health insurance, provided technical literature to interested parties and coordinated activist efforts.[29] They successfully enlisted notable figures to their cause, such as Eleanor Roosevelt, who undertook an appeal for the CNH in late 1946.[30] The former First Lady took particular interest in health reform, praising the NHS in a 1949 British public information film on polio services – the disease which had ailed her late husband – for establishing a 'right' to medical care. Despite the CNH's small membership of about 200 persons and its limited budget – $70,000 in 1949, compared to the AMA which had received double that amount from just pharmaceutical companies in the previous year – the organisation worked hard to advance national health insurance.[31]

Unexpectedly, a considerable part of Davis and the CNH's efforts involved rebutting conservative attacks on the NHS. The AMA held up British nationalised medicine as a nightmarish glimpse into the future if the Truman Plan were to reach fruition. To resist the apparent threat of 'socialized medicine', they hired the leading public relations firm Whitaker and Baxter to manage what was then the most expensive marketing campaign in world history.[32] The campaign's anti-communism, libertarianism and championing of the 'American enterprise system' made the new British health service a special target. In a speech before a meeting of the Public Relations Society of America in late 1949, Clem Whitaker claimed that 'Socialization is epidemic in Europe'. 'It has all but paralyzed Great Britain', he added.[33] Whitaker revealed that he and his partner Leone Baxter had collected information on this dangerous experiment across the ocean, including the recruitment of a special 'news observer in London to follow developments in the British socialized medical system'.

With this expertise behind them, the AMA tarnished the NHS as dictatorial. In a June 1948 issue of *Editor and Publisher* magazine, they placed an article about the onset of the British service that included a cartoon where a doctor administered a dying – or possibly dead – 'England' with medicine from a bottle labelled: 'Socialization of Everything – Doctor Quack's Cure All'.[34] The depiction of President Truman telling Uncle Sam to 'Come Uncle, take your socialized medicine' suggested the threat of the US following Britain's lead. In a pamphlet released the following year titled 'America's Vital Issue', the

AMA sketched their own history of the state's involvement in health care.[35] They began with the nineteenth-century German Chancellor Otto von Bismarck, who they claimed 'established the system to place the masses under obligation to him and make them servants of his Government'. Reworking this troubling genealogy in the immediate aftermath of war with Nazi Germany, the pamphlet traced a line to Soviet communism and concluded: 'Today, England is the tragic victim of just such a method'.

The AMA regularly invoked aid from the Marshall Plan that the UK received from the US during the immediate postwar years.[36] These funds were given to bombed-out and hungry European nations to facilitate reconstruction and prevent the spread of communism. Britain received the largest amount of Marshall Plan aid in Western Europe: 26 per cent of the total, compared to France's 18 per cent and West Germany's 11 per cent. US policymakers seemed happy for such funds to be spent on social services like the NHS, albeit only until 1950, when they exerted pressure on the British government to make welfare cuts to fund rearmament for the Korean War.[37] However, the AMA consistently adopted a different view by arguing that the UK misused such funds on the NHS. The organisation claimed that 'American taxpayers are now paying the costs' to whip up anger against what they presented as a dangerous British experiment with nationalised medicine.[38]

The NHS did not receive a friendlier welcome in the wider US media landscape. The *New York Times* ran multiple articles on the service, viewing the institution with both curiosity and condemnation, as indicated by one headline which described 'British Socialism Leveling Classes'.[39] US medical journals broadly expressed a dislike of the British scheme. *Medical Economics* often reprinted the views of British doctors critical of the NHS. 'Where British Planners Went Wrong', a 1951 article by a British surgeon, identified the service as the cause of wider moral deterioration.[40] The pursuit of 'medical Utopia' by politicians, to this home-grown critic, meant that his fellow countrymen had lost their 'freedom of action' and become a 'veritable slave of the bureaucracy'. *American Druggist*, a pharmaceutical trade magazine, expanded this theme in a special issue on the NHS and 'What it Means to America and Its Pharmacists'. Its cover featured an adapted image of the Royal Coat of Arms of the UK, replacing the motto '*Dieu et mon droit*' – 'God and My Right' – with 'CHEMIST TO THE STATE'.[41]

Far from seeing it as harmless commentary, Davis and his allies felt that such criticism of the NHS posed a threat to winning support among the US population for national health insurance. In a CNH newsletter to journalists in the labour movement, the organisation lamented how 'News of Britain's recent Health Service Act has frequently been distorted in this country', and they claimed that this 'misrepresentation' formed part of a 'systematic campaign to smear legislative proposals . . . for national health insurance'.[42] 'Correct information in the American labor press about the British Labor Government's program will help build a more enlightened attitude here toward our own National Health Insurance legislation soon to be introduced into Congress', continued the CNH, in a clear signal of the stakes involved. The US supporters of the Truman Plan accordingly tried to correct inaccuracies about the NHS. Facts, they reasoned, would turn the tide. Davis rebutted AMA claims by publishing his own descriptions of the British service which detailed its administrative dimensions and costs.[43] In CNH communications, they presented the NHS as a consensus issue in British politics by drawing lines of historical continuity between the Liberal Party's 1911 National Insurance Act and Labour's NHS Acts. The NHS represented a humane enterprise to the CNH, as well as a democratic one through its overall management by a minister accountable to Parliament. The CNH's supporters wrote to national newspapers and opinion leaders, supplying details on British health legislation, as well as statistics.[44] These efforts reflected the surprising energy that US health reformers thought necessary to expend in defending what was, after all, a foreign medical system.

MEDICAL INTERNATIONALISM

These attempts to rehabilitate the American reputation of the NHS were undergirded by help from British sources. Trade unions, medical activists and even the British state cooperated with US allies out of a shared ambition to position the NHS at the forefront of social advance. Working across borders, they hoped to improve the standing of this important model of universal health care, and thereby ease the passage of national health insurance in the US. This medical internationalism did not translate into success for the Truman Plan, but its trajectory shaped new forms of attachment to the institution at home.

In 1950, the CNH asked the British TUC for material about the NHS, writing that 'we do want to get the facts straight in order to present the truth about the program in contrast to many distortions and unjust criticism which appear here in this country'.[45] This type of correspondence was not unusual. Davis sent a similar request to David Stark Murray, one of the early advocates of the NHS and president of the SMA. He referenced attempts to pass national health legislation in the US and added that 'we would be helped if we had some first-hand comments from Britain as to how the new National Health Service is actually getting under way'.[46] The two British organisations gladly fulfilled these appeals.

The CNH and its allies also received help from the British state. British Information Services (BIS) played an important role in this regard. During the war, BIS was a propaganda organisation tasked with projecting an image of a brave nation standing alone against Nazi Germany in order to persuade the US to join the fight.[47] In its postwar role as a New York-based information wing of the British consulate, it engaged in a rather different battle. From Rockefeller Plaza in central Manhattan, BIS provided material on the NHS to the CNH, spoke to their members and checked drafts of their press releases.[48] Back in Britain, the Ministry of Health hoped to counter critical stories about the NHS written by the many visiting American journalists by arranging interviews with Bevan himself. In the first year of the NHS alone, the Ministry and the government's central Public Relations Division arranged meetings with correspondents from thirty-four different American media outlets, including *Life*, *Collier's Weekly*, the *New Yorker* and a spread of national and regional newspapers.[49] Bevan became somewhat of a celebrity in the US through these interviews, even appearing on *Time* magazine's front cover during the spring of 1949.[50]

An interview between Bevan and the editor of *American Druggist*, John W. McPherrin, illustrated both Bevan's media appeal and the motives behind the British government's desire to participate in the US battle over the NHS's reputation.[51] Though no friend of nationalised medicine, McPherrin could not help but admire the 'steel grey hair', 'sharp blue eyes' and jovial personality of his Welsh interviewee. He asked Bevan about the Truman Plan, and observed that, 'If we are going to have such a program, it seems to me that British hindsight on this subject could be much better than American foresight'. Amused, Bevan offered a lengthy critique of the 'cash motive' in private medicine that created, to him, inequity. Eventually, one of Bevan's civil servants arrived to hurry the minister to another meeting. McPherrin quickly asked him, 'Do you think this Health Scheme of Great Britain will work in America?' Halfway out the door, Bevan paused briefly. 'The method we are using to provide health for the people will spread all over the world', came the reply, 'In modern society, it is inevitable'. 'America must come to it', Bevan proclaimed, and concluded with a friendly flourish: 'Ta, Ta, Mr. McPherrin, come and see me again sometime'.

As a member of Labour's radical wing, Bevan's faith that the right to health would unfold across the globe reflected his wider political beliefs. The NHS offered a means of distinguishing Britain from the US, despite the two nations' military alliance against the USSR. Bevan regularly criticised this anti-communist foreign policy stance, as well as the reach of US capitalism abroad.[52] Indeed, he put these beliefs into action in 1951 when he resigned from the Attlee government to oppose health budget cuts – including the imposition of charges for dentistry and ophthalmic services – that helped fund rearmament for the Korean War. Bevan retained an interest in the wider world and the frontiers of social democracy, including its significance to medical politics. He followed health reform in other countries with interest, perceiving them, through British eyes, as attempts to 'launch a National Health Service'.[53]

While Bevan believed that state health services would spread across the world, he maintained that Britain played a special role. Through the NHS, the nation enjoyed 'the moral leadership of the world'.[54] In a speech given to civil servants in the Ministry of Health, Bevan argued that 'Great Britain has shown that it is still the pioneer in many things, and can show the rest of the world where to go'.[55] Bevan was not known for bipartisanship. On the eve of the NHS's introduction, he had lacerated the Conservative Party as 'lower than vermin' for its apparent failures to alleviate poverty during the interwar period.[56] Even Bevan, though, was keen to stress that the achievement of the NHS did not belong to 'any special political party' but rather 'a special quality of British genius'. Although 'the old oak has been shaken by many blasts', he reflected, the NHS showed that 'the sap is still running'. Bevan, then, articulated an anxiety-tinged sense of decline regarding Britain's international standing, but also presented the possibility for a new beginning through the nation's welfare policies.

Despite such statements about the service's 'Britishness', medical internationalism proved the dominant register at this time among the foremost defenders of the NHS. The significance of the service lay in how it might encourage other nations to enact its core universalist tenets. David Stark Murray of the SMA boasted that the NHS 'will be the envy of and model for all other nations'.[57] The SMA's journal, *Medicine Today and Tomorrow*, spoke in grandiose terms about 'turning points' in human history, describing the beginning of the service as 'the most solid and far-reaching attempt yet to free a section of the human race from fear of insecurity and fear of ill-health'.[58] The British left brought these views to the US, where the CNH amplified them. In a 1950 CNH newsletter, the organisation reiterated one visiting British doctor's belief that the NHS represented 'the most comprehensive piece of legislation for the provision of security and safe-guarding of health . . . that has ever been passed in any country at any time', which would soon become 'the basis of health schemes in all other countries in the world'.[59] The claims for universal health care, then, were building, and the NHS lay at the centre of what seemed possible on the international stage.

The links between the US and British medical left became clear during a controversy over a *Reader's Digest* article in 1950. This dispute created new defenders of the NHS at home, showing how international disagreements over the service impacted developments in Britain itself. In a piece titled 'Granny is Gone!', the President of the University of Pennsylvania, former Republican Governor and presidential aspirant Harold E. Stassen charged 'socialized medicine' with increasing Britain's death rate.[60] Topped by an image of a grave stone, the article narrated the story of a sixty-two-year-old grandmother who, suffering from lobar pneumonia, could not secure a bed in a local hospital. Despite the best efforts of her doctor, she died after being unable to access fourteen hospitals. Stassen used her tragic case to allege that once medicine became free at the point of delivery, people offloaded family members to hospitals at the government's expense, preventing treatment for the truly needy. Most troubling for NHS-supporters and their American allies was the fact that *Reader's Digest* possessed one of the largest circulation rates in the US.

Stassen's article provoked outrage on both sides of the Atlantic, and not just from the left. In the pages of the *British Medical Journal,* where two years earlier fierce editorials against the NHS could regularly be found, Sir Heneage Ogilvie – a respected London surgeon – rebuked Stassen for paying 'little more than lip service to veracity'.[61] To Ogilvie, the question was not 'whether the State takes part in the future development of a medical service, but, if and when it does so, what part it will take'. Indulging in some comparison of his own, he claimed that 'The poor American is worse off than Granny, for he gets very little unless he pays for it'. Ogilvie took his riposte to the conservative-leaning *Spectator* magazine, where he accused Stassen of responding to a 'wave of socialised-medical-hysteria' that seemingly plagued the US. The British surgeon questioned Stassen's use of statistics, claiming that he had taken a narrow one-year snapshot, which was unrepresentative of the general trend of a falling mortality rate in Britain. For good measure, he presented his own statistics regarding the infant death rate, revealing British improvements compared to the US. As editor of the medical journal *The Practitioner*, Ogilvie had his own interests in defending the reputation of British GPs and hospital doctors. However, this dispute was more than a squabble over statistics. In making his rebuttal, Ogilvie aligned himself with the NHS, illustrating how Britain's medical profession was becoming synonymous with the institution itself. The criticisms of the NHS from abroad were increasingly seen as slights against the assembled ranks of Britain's medical workers.

US health reformers amplified this controversy. The CNH reprinted Ogilvie's response to Stassen.[62] Democratic Senator Claude Pepper of Florida – an advocate of national health insurance – sent a cablegram to Bevan expressing his dismay at another of Stassen's *Reader's Digest* articles, and asked for his advice on how to challenge it.[63] For their part, the British state took considerable interest in Stassen's critiques. The Foreign Office and the Ministry of Health sourced the articles and speeches Stassen delivered to medical and political organisations.[64] When *Reader's Digest* declined a right of reply, one civil servant lambasted the magazine as 'deeply reactionary, anti-British, anti-Welfare State, with no pretension of being fair'. These comments revealed the growing fusion of national values with welfare in some quarters of Whitehall. Undeterred, the British government prepared special notes on the Stassen article and reprinted copies of Ogilvie's *Spectator* piece for distribution by BIS. The Stassen–Ogilvie disagreement drew in a range of participants. MPs placed pressure on the Ministry of Health to defend the NHS and the reputation of Britain's doctors. Labour MP Gilbert McAllister wrote to Bevan about the 'poisonous nonsense' spread by Stassen and demanded that the Minister better publicise Ogilvie's riposte.

The *Reader's Digest* dispute also attracted the interest of British citizens, who wrote to the Ministry of Health to complain about Stassen. These offers of support could come from unexpected places. One businessman with over 150 employees began by admitting that the 'taxes on my business and personal income are such that I have every personal reason to make me dead against the expenditure necessary to run the new Social Services'.[65] However, he recognised the benefits provided by the NHS to his staff, and sought to defend the institution from Stassen. Aware of 'how widely (probably throughout the world) this article will be read', he felt angered by 'such a distorted picture of our Health Service' and offered to write a letter to the *Reader's Digest* himself, if the government thought it might be helpful. The foreign attacks on the institution had structured this man's path to embracing what he now described as 'our' NHS.

Though such controversies facilitated a growing identification with the health service by the British medical profession and some members of the public, they failed to rehabilitate the institution's American reputation. The US left's efforts to salvage the standing of the British service by presenting facts met with little success in furthering the cause of national health insurance. Indeed, as the 1950s progressed, the AMA's frightening vision of the NHS further squeezed out such aspirations. Much to Davis's disappointment, the defeat of the Truman Plan in Congress and the election of Dwight Eisenhower as president in 1952 made legislative change improbable. When conflicts over tactics divided the CNH, it lost its limited financial backing and eventually disbanded four years later.[66] The labour movement in the US turned away from a federal solution and embraced private health insurance, trying to secure the best deals for their members rather than supporting a national platform that might guarantee universalism.[67] The immediate postwar campaign to achieve universal health coverage ended in failure. Despite significant cooperation, health internationalism possessed clear limits. Nevertheless, transatlantic exchanges on how to organise medical services continued, further hardening attachment to the NHS in Britain.

MEDICARE, MEDICAID AND THE NHS IN THE 1960S

After the disappointments of the Truman Plan, health reform returned to the political agenda in the US during the late 1950s. Concern over the capacity of older people to afford the increasing costs of medical care fuelled a revival of interest in the issue that again involved the NHS.[68] The presidencies of John F. Kennedy (1961–1963) and Lyndon

B. Johnson (1963–1969) witnessed a greater push for legislation to help older people as well as the poor pay for medical care. In 1965, Medicare and Medicaid amendments to Social Security achieved these two objectives, even if they entrenched the private health care model rather than transform it.[69] The British NHS played an important, albeit diminished, role in the debates surrounding this US legislation. While US reformers met with some degree of success compared to the 1940s, their British allies felt increasingly marginalised by American critiques and began to pivot towards welfare nationalism.

It was at this point that Michael and Alice Davis undertook their voyage to Britain, but other Americans also expressed a continued interest in the NHS. Paul F. Gemmill and Almont Lindsey, a professor of economics and a labour relations expert, respectively, published books on the service that – like Davis's research – drew on information gathered through field trips and interviews with the British public.[70] Several US authors corresponded with Richard Titmuss and Brian Abel-Smith, two experts in social policy at the LSE.[71] Davis worked with both men, telling Titmuss in the spring of 1960 of his determination to ensure the passage of the Kerr–Mills Act and the Medical Assistance for the Aged programme (which preceded Medicaid and Medicare). Though he predicted the AMA would oppose the bill, Davis affirmed with confidence that 'Labor will fight it with tooth and nail!'

The US population received further exposure to the NHS through popular culture. At the height of the 'British invasion' in pop music during the 1960s, teenagers with an attentive ear might have learned that the titular character from the Beatles' song 'Doctor Robert' worked for 'the National Health'.[72] Comedy sketches from *Monty Python's Flying Circus*, first broadcast in the US in 1972, sometimes played on tropes about the apparently regimented nature of British medicine. In one skit, John Cleese reprised the role of an angry sergeant major, ordering heavily bandaged NHS patients to perform military manoeuvres. If health systems like Canada's came to form an increasing share of the foreign examples invoked in formal US debate, then the British NHS persisted as a recognisable point of comparison.

The US labour movement extended a more traditional left-wing interest in the British NHS. Trade union members continued to study the service in person, conducting interviews with the British public.[73] These US visitors frequently embellished their reports with accounts of receiving treatment through the NHS, offering a personal perspective on the care available across the Atlantic. In 1958, the largest federation of trade unions in the US, the American Federation of Labor and Congress of Industrial Organizations (AFL-CIO), recounted in their newspaper how one of their members gave birth in the NHS.[74] The author on workers' education Joyce L. Kornbluh recounted her attendance of mothercraft classes, the birth of her daughter and the receipt of coupons for milk and orange juice. 'Even though we were American visitors to the country', Kornbluh approvingly informed her US readership, 'medical care including maternity services would be completely free for our whole family'.

Though Bevan died in 1960 from stomach cancer, he would have taken pleasure in how the NHS continued to inspire others abroad. The African American historian, sociologist and civil rights activist W.E.B. Du Bois recounted his own embrace of socialism in part through his experience with the NHS. In a 1960 speech to the Wisconsin Socialist Club, Du Bois compared the anti-communist McCarthyism that gripped the US with European social democracy that, to him, represented 'the most successful form of government'.[75] He suggested that his socialist politics derived, in part, from his European travels. 'One of my first experiences was in England', Du Bois recalled, when afflicted in London with 'a severe attack of intestinal disorder'. After a young GP treated him, Du Bois asked for the bill only to be told that 'there was no charge, that his services were paid for by the British government'. 'I reminded him that I was an American and that in America we were repeatedly informed that socialized medicine in Great Britain was a failure', he recounted. Du Bois remembered that the attending doctor merely smiled in response and only charged for the drugs that he had prescribed.

Many on the US left also took inspiration from the NHS through British activists and experts continuing to travel and talk about the service. David Stark Murray undertook a US lecture tour in 1962, speaking to fifty audiences, appearing twenty-five times on the radio and fifteen times on television.[76] Murray found listeners supportive of his arguments and representative of what he described as 'a tremendous public desire for a change in the health services of the United States'. Initially, the AMA refused to debate this early proponent of the NHS, and their members heckled him from the audience. Eventually, though, the organisation gave way and representatives joined him on stage in heated discussion. In keeping with an earlier belief in medical internationalism, Murray predicted that 'the people of America are going to take a big step towards a national health service, within the next few years'. A young student and activist at the University of Chicago named Bernie Sanders was so enthused by Murray's talk that he started a lifelong campaign in pursuit of such a goal.[77]

As the AMA's involvement in Murray's lecture tour suggested, US conservatives continued to perceive the NHS as both a threat and an opportunity. Concerned over the momentum gathering behind medical reform and frustrated by the growing influence of corporate insurance interests from the late 1950s, they hoped to repeat the successful tactics of the previous decade. The journal *Medical Economics* sent a group of four doctors to the UK in 1961 to examine the NHS. Upon their return, they recounted stories of overworked doctors and corruption.[78] Their report, accompanied by glossy photographs of an overcrowded waiting room, told of 'crowds of patients in drab surroundings'. Prominent medical consultant and former British subject Horace Cotton echoed this focus on the deteriorating state of British hospitals and GP surgeries in a special series of articles on the NHS.[79] Next to a cartoon of an anthropomorphised hospital begging for government funds, Cotton informed his US readership that 500 hospitals in Britain were more than a century old, yet the government had built only eight in the past twenty-five years. Such contrasts proved easy to make because of the stark differences in capital investment between the two countries. Whereas the 1946 Hill–Burton Act stimulated the construction of hospitals and other health facilities in the US immediately after the war,

Britain's 1962 Hospital Plan followed much later. The US critics of the NHS therefore exploited the gradual – and often less visible – progress of NHS modernisation for their own ends.

These attacks provoked impassioned responses. As the 1950s shaded into the 1960s, not only did the identification with the NHS intensify in political circles, but many figures on the British left also started to display a loss of faith that the service would indeed become the pre-eminent health care model for other nations. Strains of exceptionalism began to emerge. Discussion in the House of Commons to mark the tenth anniversary of the NHS in 1958 witnessed MPs from both major parties voice strident statements of support for the health service, often with US opinion in mind.[80] Future Labour Health Minister Kenneth Robinson hailed the NHS as a 'social revolution' that gave Britain 'without doubt, the finest Health Service in the world'. 'If we go abroad and, perhaps fall ill or have a minor accident', he observed, 'we are rather surprised and a little hurt when we find that there is not the same pattern in other countries, also'. Robinson claimed that a recent trip 'across the Atlantic' confirmed the 'real fear' such an absence precipitated. The Welsh Labour MP Rev. Llywelyn Williams similarly declared that during his own visit to the US he had encountered 'appalling ignorance' about the NHS. 'I am not referring to yokels in hill-billy villages in Tennessee', he clarified, 'but to people who hold eminent positions in the medical world'. During another Commons debate five years later, Williams insisted that while he was 'not a flag-waving Jingo', he believed 'that our National Health Service is the finest health service in the whole world'. In the eyes of these supporters, it now seemed that 'our NHS' was unlikely to be replicated elsewhere, and that only amplified their pride in the institution.

This swelling sense of exceptionalism around 'our National Health Service' began to grip both main political parties. With the Marshall Plan now in the past, politicians and civil servants did not need to be as cautious about US opinion regarding the service in the 1960s. Nonetheless, as most African and Caribbean colonies achieved independence in this decade, Labour and Conservatives deployed the NHS to shore up Britain's uncertain status. Stephen Taylor illustrated this trend on the left. Fresh from his experience with health centres in Harlow, he praised the US in a 1959 *Lancet* article as 'the most dynamic society yet made by man' and accepted its lead in medical research. Yet Taylor also claimed, on the basis of the NHS, that 'it is right for us to insist that in some respects we are still ahead of the Americans'.[81] 'We may think', he suggested, 'that the ordinary people of Britain get a better deal from our National Health Service than the ordinary people get in America'. Conservative Party Chairman Quintin Hogg, writing in *Foreign Affairs* five years later, lamented the eclipse of Britain by the US as the world's leading power, but similarly used welfare services as a point of superiority.[82] 'Rightly or wrongly', he explained, 'we tend to regard our social legislation, whether in the form of pensions, socialized medicine or education . . . as in advance of anything to be found on the other side of the Atlantic'. Pro-NHS sentiment, which was shaped by criticism of US medical care, had brought these Labour and Conservative politicians into agreement with one another.

The furore surrounding an AMA pamphlet, 'A Case Against Socialized Medicine' (1962), revealed a robust sense of defensiveness about the NHS.[83] Released to oppose the King–Anderson Bill which aimed to help the aged with medical costs, the document featured quotations from British newspapers about queues and overcrowding, alongside criticisms from free-market economists like John Jewkes, who was the president of the Mont Pelerin Society – a neoliberal intellectual group based in Switzerland.[84] Like other critics, the AMA also drew attention to Britain's deteriorating stock of Victorian hospitals. Their critiques extended to a set of cartoons. One depicted a man labelled 'Britain' having fallen through ice and holding a sign saying 'BEWARE' (Figure 11). Other illustrations were gendered for similar impact, with one showing a smartly dressed man – 'BRITAIN' – facing his unflatteringly depicted wife – 'FAILURES OF BRITISH NATL-HEALTH SERVICE' – with the caption, 'He Thought He Married An Angel'.

The outrage at this pamphlet eclipsed the earlier *Reader's Digest* controversy. The *British Medical Journal* responded first, following up on

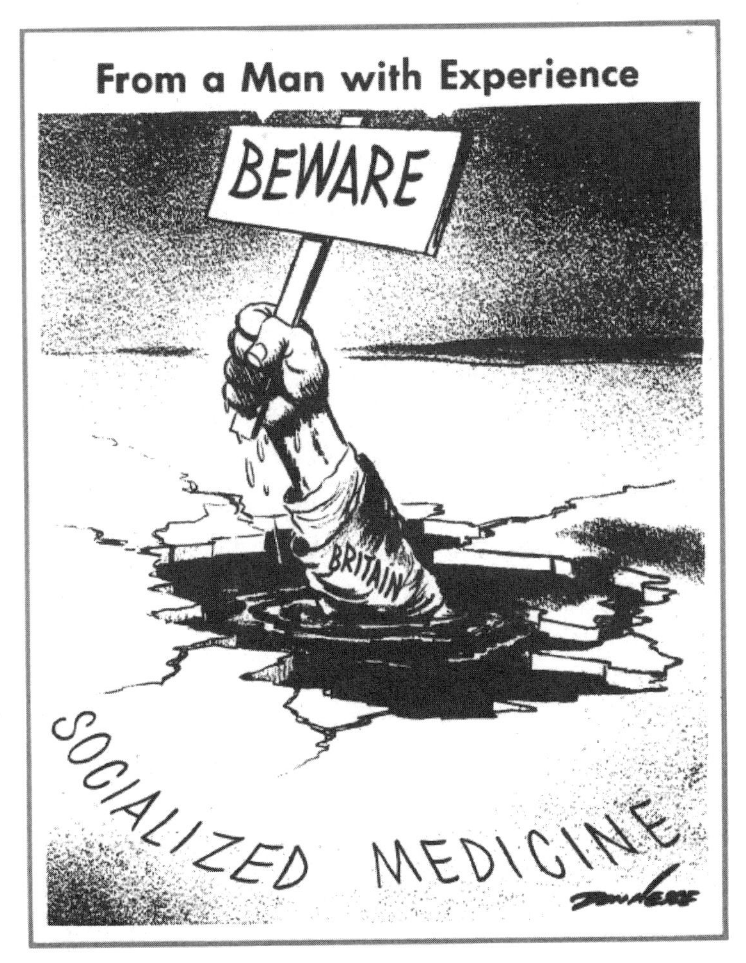

11. In order to prevent the achievement of universal health care in the US, the American Medical Association (AMA) held up the NHS as an embodiment of the evils inherent to 'socialized medicine'. Their criticisms of the NHS angered the service's defenders in the UK, who, by the 1970s, turned towards drawing sharp lines of distinction between the US and British health systems.

their other recent rebuttals of AMA critiques.[85] In an editorial titled 'A.M.A. Versus N.H.S.', they slammed the pamphlet's 'vulgarity and cheapness'. The *British Medical Journal* asserted that the AMA should be 'heartily ashamed' by their cartoons. Illustrating a developing sense of protectiveness about the NHS among some quarters of the medical profession, they counterattacked by claiming that such criticisms originated from a desire to 'distract from the weaknesses of American medicine'. 'The A.M.A. should', the editorial insisted, 'understand that they have a lot to learn from Britain and Europe about methods of providing medical services – from our successes as well as our failures'.

From this point, the dividing line between British and US medicine as defined by costs intensified.[86] *The Times* castigated the statements in the AMA's pamphlets from British critics as 'nonsense' and ended by citing the case of a New York doctor charging the equivalent of £1,400 for an appendectomy.[87] Given their opposition to the NHS at its inception, the *British Medical Journal* and *The Times* rallying to the NHS's defence was a remarkable reversal. As one medical expert associated with a left-wing organisation in the US watching the controversy remarked, 'Fifteen years ago the B.M.A. and the A.M.A. saw wholly eye-to-eye on socialized medicine'.[88] The gradual merging of the international reputation of 'British medicine' with the NHS frustrated its critics at home who wanted to distinguish between the profession and the system. This conjunction undermined their efforts to encourage doctors to imagine an existence outside of the nationalised service. As one prominent British critic pressed upon Davis before his 1959 trip: 'Remember also, that there is a tendency by both the public and the profession to confuse the "National Health Service" with "British medicine" '.[89] 'As a result', this British correspondent lamented, 'criticism or praise of the one, may be taken as a commentary on the other, and the reaction may thus be misleading'.

The British state no longer directly involved itself in foreign NHS controversies in the 1960s, or at least not to the degree that it had during the institution's inception. Yet governments still continued to respond to foreign critiques and promote the service in a positive light. By this point, budget cuts had reduced BIS in size and diminished its capabilities. Allies like Davis therefore no longer enjoyed BIS's administrative support. Nonetheless, the Conservative Party – in power between 1951 and 1964 – extended Labour's initial policy of defending the NHS's reputation abroad. Conservative Party MPs continued to request advice from the Ministry of Health about how to handle hostile questions when they visited the US.[90] For their part, civil servants gradually systematised how they dealt with the many visiting Americans inquiring about the institution in order to stem the tide of 'misinformation' at its source. After an internal effort spearheaded by public relations officials, the government kept detailed lists of journalists that the Ministry briefed about the NHS, and arranged carefully planned tours to display the service's best features.[91] Given that hostile press about the NHS reflected poorly on the Conservatives, it made sense to rebut it. They also had to recruit foreign labour to staff the service. Promoting a more harmonious image of the institution through films such as *Health Services in Britain* (1962) – jointly produced by the Commonwealth Relations Office and the Foreign Office – formed an important part of this balance of international perceptions.[92] Alongside depictions of modern facilities for the aged, disabled and mentally ill, the film featured a Black hospital nurse, helping present the service as welcoming to immigrant workers and free of racial discrimination. In testament to the continued significance of the NHS for the country's global reputation, the film boasted that 'Britain's health service has not only marked an important milestone in the history of social and medical science, it has also helped keep Britain among the most progressive nations in the world'.

The British left continued to care about US perceptions of the NHS, even if they largely shifted towards distinguishing the service from foreign examples rather than seeking to promote reform overseas. After the AMA pamphlet controversy, Kenneth Robinson wrote a four-page piece for the *New York Times* making 'The Case for Britain's Health Service'.[93] The bulk of the article focused on disproving 'a hotch-potch of myths and half-truths, concocted for medico-political purposes' and challenging accusations that Britons no longer had a free choice of doctor. Although Robinson claimed that if Americans 'want Medicare enough it will come', the prior optimism in universal health care marching across the world had largely disappeared.

NARROWED ASPIRATIONS AND WELFARE NATIONALISM

In the 1970s, members of the British left further diverged from their US counterparts on the question of how to organise medical services. When discussing the two systems, the predominant concern became drawing lines of distinction between the NHS and a model of health care premised on direct payments and insurance. Statements about the US eventually coming to embrace the British position were now rarely voiced. Though this trend began on the left, it did not stop there – a variety of British commentators and experts contributed to this atmosphere of differentiation. Moreover, members of the public also began to make claims about the NHS as a uniquely British achievement, fixed in opposition to the US. The 1970s marked the point when welfare nationalism coalesced around the health service, carrying important consequences for its later development and survival.

During this decade, the British state increasingly presented the NHS as a medical system peculiar to the UK and its political culture. With its title alone, the film *British Way of Health* (1973) expressed this sentiment.[94] Its narrator proudly informed audiences in countries that included the US, Brazil and France how, 'In Britain, ambulances, hospital care, nurses, doctors, specialists, all are free'. The film's pointed declarations that the NHS 'provides a full range of medical support and is available to rich and poor alike' reflected the left-wing politics of the film's Welsh director, Richard Marquand, who belonged to a family of Labour MPs. The three doctors speaking in the production endorsed this view with their descriptions of the service as 'marvellous'. But these medical practitioners also articulated a defensiveness about the NHS through their reminders that 'No government ever interfered with our freedom to choose where we practice, or our clinical freedom to treat as we feel we should treat'. US criticisms that the NHS was bureaucratic, monolithic and impersonal haunted such films, even as this production sought to strike a celebratory tone on the service's twenty-fifth anniversary.

Figures and organisations interested in health reform from both the UK and the US did not cease cooperation in the 1970s, but relations between them cooled. As the issue of national health insurance revived in the US during this decade, the nation's trade unions seemed less willing to invoke Britain in a positive light. The AFL-CIO publication 'The Case for National Health Insurance' (1970) took pains to emphasise that their own plan was 'not a government-operated system, as in Great Britain'.[95] As US trade unions championed workplace insurance models, they made delineations between their own ambitions and the NHS. Discussion about medical reform between Democratic presidential candidates Jimmy Carter and Edward Kennedy again referenced the British NHS. The latter even visited the UK to see the NHS first-hand and reached out to the Labour Secretary of State for Health and Social Services, Barbara Castle, for her advice.[96] Though Castle sent Kennedy details on the NHS, her private criticisms of the US as 'the citadel of freedom in medicine' revealed the pessimism of the British left when evaluating the chances of systemic change across the Atlantic.[97]

These demarcations only proliferated. In 1978, the American College of Legal Medicine debated the now thirty-year-old question of whether the US could learn from the NHS. George Godber – a former Chief Medical Officer and prominent civil servant – spoke in defence of a service he had helped create.[98] After a matter-of-fact description of the NHS's features, Godber referred to the 'basic philosophical difference between our countries'. Britain, he claimed, favoured planning and social rights, whereas the US prioritised choice and a wider variety of providers. While Godber acknowledged the superior financial resources available in the US, he insisted that the NHS exhibited 'an overall humanity'. 'Knowing as I do that I could obtain medical care of unsurpassed quality at many centres in this country, I would still rather take my chance in an unforeseen medical emergency or need for long term care in Britain than anywhere else', he added. Similarly, the following year, the Labour Minister of Health, Dr David Owen, began a lecture to the Harvard Medical School by maintaining, 'I am not trying to sell you our National Health Service'.[99] Owen then proceeded to 'set the record straight' about the NHS by correcting inaccuracies in the US media. He ended by claiming, 'I personally am proud of our health service', and emphasised his dislike of 'money barriers' in medicine. Rather than suggesting that the NHS was a model for others, he cautiously noted that 'this is a matter on which each nation must, of course, take its own decisions'.

While Owen tempered the desire to proselytise about the NHS with the tact expected from a visiting member of the British government, the Labour activist Margaret Jay faced fewer constraints when she visited the US in 1978. She began a speech to the Woman's National Democratic Club by drawing lines of differentiation between the UK and the US based on medical costs.[100] 'When we talk about the civilised "quality of life" in my country,' Jay opined, 'one of the most practical things I think we can talk about is the universal care provided for all our citizens by the National Health Service, without regard to individual means'. She attacked the 'myths' about the British service and emphasised nationalisation's benefits to medical research. Jay channelled welfare nationalism in comments on thermal scanning units initiated in the NHS, noting her 'pride' in seeing 'nuclear-powered pace-makers, which were pioneered in the United Kingdom'. 'We are very proud of the fact that 30 years ago we decided to create the world's first and most successful comprehensive National Health Service', she declared, 'and we celebrate its anniversary this year as one of the greatest achievements of life in Britain today'. Distinction, rather than shared ideals, now framed the transatlantic relationship in health reform.

The sociologist Mildred Blaxter revealed how the public were beginning to express welfare nationalism in *Mothers and Daughters* (1982), a study of medical attitudes among working-class women in Aberdeen during the 1970s.[101] Blaxter's interviews covered a wide variety of topics, including birth control, vaccination and personal health complaints. They also probed feelings about the NHS, where the US sometimes came into the picture as a point of comparison. One woman who presented the NHS as 'definitely' an improvement for working-class families also gave her thoughts on US health care. 'Considerin' them in America', she reflected, 'I mean, it costs them a fortune for hospitals now there'. To illustrate these costs, this interviewee proceeded to enumerate examples of women she knew who had moved to the US but came back to the UK to have a baby, as the plane ticket was cheaper than the hospital bills that they faced overseas. Another woman told Blaxter a much bleaker story. She started by giving her opinion that universal health care had made Britain a 'nation o' hypochondriacs'. However, despite her qualified endorsement of the NHS, she railed against the US system as an alternative by giving the account of an American subjected to intense questioning about her insurance coverage before dying from a heart attack. 'That's the American system you see,' Blaxter's interviewee summed up, 'Well, I'd never like to see that here'. These opinions reflected the emerging welfare nationalism around the NHS, a development that would have important consequences in the decades to come.

***

Davis died in 1971. Truman followed the next year. The pair had pursued the goal of national health insurance in the US during the height of a global faith in the forward march of universal health care. Both met disappointment, even if they took some solace in reforms achieved by others in the mid-1960s. Many figures on the British left initially shared this optimism and presented the NHS as the blueprint for future health systems. However, the bruising story of the NHS's reputation in the US chastened their enthusiasm, and their successors shifted to a more modest and defensive stance.

While statements on both sides of the Atlantic suggested the limiting of social democratic aspirations by the late 1970s, this thirty-year debate carried consequences for the NHS in Britain. Nationalised medicine provided a useful way to retain a sense of divergence between – and above – other nations that now overshadowed Britain by different metrics in the postwar pecking order. Even some formerly critical medical professionals, aware that 'British medicine' was now synonymous abroad with the 'British National Health Service', leapt to the institution's defence. Yet this novel source of support for the service came at a cost. The vision of the NHS as a beacon of inspiration to health reformers around the world receded into the distance. Medical universalism now seemed to stop at the White Cliffs of Dover. Some members of the public also began to think of themselves as uniquely favoured by their medical system, a nascent trend that the left would later propagate to counter proposals for market-based alternatives to the NHS. As welfare nationalism picked up pace, new arrivals from the former British Empire had to navigate its boundaries.

5

IMMIGRATION AND EMIGRATION

Ossie Fernando (1934–) always wanted to be a doctor.[1] Born in 1934 just outside of Colombo, British Ceylon, Fernando discovered an early love of biology at school (Figure 12). Pursuing these interests, he studied for five years at the Faculty of Medicine in Colombo, where both white British and local doctors donned immaculate three-piece suits to instruct their students. In 1960, Fernando graduated and entered the health service of newly independent Ceylon. Posted to the countryside, he impressed his superiors with skills in anaesthesia and aspired to become a surgeon. However, Fernando had a problem. Officials from the Ceylon Ministry of Health – who controlled the career paths of doctors – denied his request, believing that his contributions as an anaesthetist were more important. Faced with their objections, Fernando took a leap of faith. He handed in his resignation and prepared to leave Ceylon for Britain, where he hoped he could acquire postgraduate training in surgery before returning home. As the UK desperately needed doctors, the British Council speedily awarded him an employment voucher, which had been introduced by the British government the year before to control Commonwealth immigration. In 1963, Fernando boarded the P&O ship SS *Arcadia* with his wife and two young sons. Like thousands of medical practitioners in the postwar period, he journeyed across formerly imperial borders to work in the NHS. But what reception did these employees receive in Britain? And what did the reactions to their presence in the service say about the welfare nationalism now surrounding the institution?

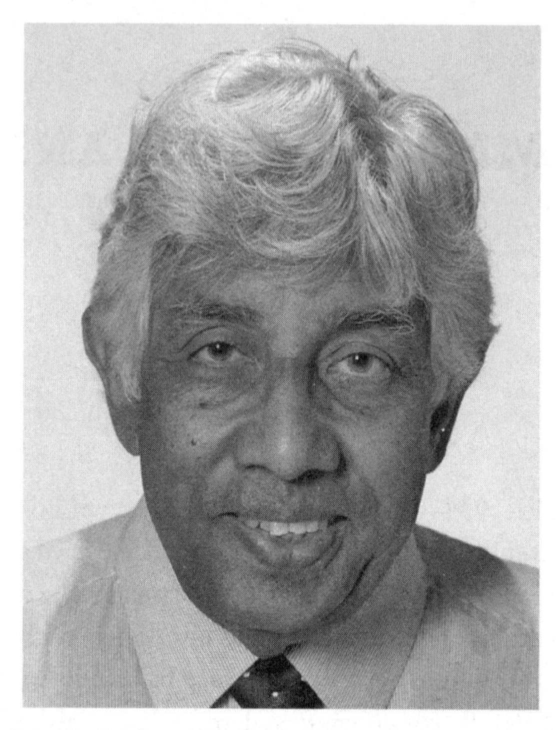

12. Born in British Ceylon, Dr Ossie Fernando immigrated to Britain in 1963 and worked in the NHS as a surgeon until his retirement. At the Royal Free Hospital, London, he helped pioneer kidney transplant surgery in the UK. Fernando numbers among the tens of thousands of immigrants to Britain who have worked in the NHS throughout its history.

The NHS would have collapsed without immigrant labour.[2] With the UK suffering from a shortage of workers, employees drawn from all over the world tended bedsides, performed surgeries and cleaned facilities. Britain did not stand alone in this respect. As other industrialised nations expanded access to medical care in the post-1945 decades, they similarly relied on the global circulation of skills and expertise to fulfil the expectations of their citizens.[3] But the flow of migrants from the Global South to the Global North carried consequences. In the case of Britain, it was also shaped by the imperial past. Newly independent countries such as India and Pakistan hoped to address health challenges among their own populations but instead lost thousands of trained practitioners to the UK, which continued to draw on the imperial legacies of shared language and medical training.[4] The attraction of health services like the NHS as a means to gain further medical qualifications or to build a better life harmed the aspirations of nations just emerging from the shadow of empire. As the NHS successfully modernised its hospitals and general practice surgeries, other medical systems in recently independent nations struggled to even get off the ground.

Although overseas doctors, nurses and other workers became a common sight in the NHS during the 1960s and 1970s, they were not always welcomed. To be sure, some migrants, such as Fernando, secured career success and plaudits for their contributions. The state and leading politicians on all sides regularly voiced support for their work. According to some of the professionals themselves, most visits to the hospital or health centre took place without overt discrimination.[5] Their ability to do their jobs seemed to matter most. Yet racism also existed within the NHS – both for overseas workers and for the immigrant patients accessing its care.[6] White patients and co-workers alike expressed prejudice against Black and Brown staff by making assumptions about their qualifications or linguistic ability, or refusing to be touched by someone of a different skin colour. Immigrants and their families were subjected to increased scrutiny by white Britons about whether or not they had the right to access taxpayer-funded health care. This discriminatory rhetoric reached fever pitch in the aftermath of inflammatory speeches by former Conservative Minister of Health Enoch Powell during the late 1960s.[7] Even as the NHS deepened many of its social democratic principles through modernisation, its universalism possessed limits.

The service's opponents blended free-market criticisms about the service's cost and state-centric structure with this popular anxiety about race. A group of doctors named the Fellowship for Freedom in Medicine (FFM) argued that 'inferior' overseas practitioners 'replaced' their white, British-born counterparts, who were leaving in alarming numbers during the 1960s for better working conditions in the US, Canada and Australia.[8] The critics of the NHS therefore redeployed the nationalism swelling around the institution for their own ends by insisting that the nation's health services should not be as reliant on foreign labour or provide care for immigrant patients. A growing sense of the service as a uniquely British achievement, then, may have helped reinforce its core social democratic values, but this belief could create barriers for those arriving from other parts of the world. To recognise these developments, the currents of opposition to the NHS should be afforded more attention than historians have tended to give them.[9] Only then can the expansiveness – and costs – of welfare nationalism be recognised. The historical origins of later neoliberal assaults on the NHS can also come into view. To see how the service became, as one politician later grumbled, 'the closest thing the English have to a religion', one must consider the apostates as well as the faithful.[10]

IMMIGRATION AND THE HEALTH SERVICE

For all the perceived or actual differences between Western countries' health systems in the postwar period, they shared one key factor: a reliance on foreign labour. Industrialised nations recruited thousands of health care professionals from overseas during the peak years of medical migration between 1966 and 1975.[11] In the case of Britain, the state drew upon older imperial networks – now rebranded in the face of decolonisation as a fellowship of equal nations called the 'Commonwealth'. Many sectors of the British economy recruited workers from these countries due to a domestic labour shortage after the war.[12] From steel plants to factories to ports, Commonwealth workers provided much-needed labour. The NHS was no exception.

Every rung of the health service's professional ladder required more workers, particularly in nursing, where estimates highlighted a shortfall of 35,000 employees as soon as the service began.[13] In response, the Ministry of Health actively recruited trained professionals from former colonies. Africa and the Caribbean became the target regions for attracting nurses, with matrons in British hospitals scrutinising references submitted by hopefuls from around the Atlantic and wider world.[14] Some future NHS employees immigrated first and then trained within the service. Dr Nola Ishmael, for instance, began her career as a nurse, leaving Barbados in 1963 to qualify at the Whittington Hospital, London.[15] 'I've always been interested in what nurses did from the books I've read', she recalled, so when 'recruitment in the West Indies was at its peak', Ishmael decided to follow many of her school friends and travel to the UK. She served on a high-dependency ward immediately after qualifying, underlining the need for such workers in the NHS. In an unfamiliar country, and often homesick, many overseas professionals and trainees relied on one another for friendship. 'We had Trinidadians, people from different countries in Africa, we had people from Mauritius, we had Bajans like myself', remembered Ishmael, adding that they all 'learnt and supported each other and I made some really good friends at the Whittington'.

Compared to nurses, doctors were less actively recruited. Like Fernando, most came to Britain on their own volition to receive postgraduate training or better working conditions in the NHS. Many migrants intended to spend a short spell in the UK but ended up staying. Fernando journeyed to a country he grew up learning a lot about, but he found it still presented its own surprises. Britain's barren winter trees, for instance, proved a shock after the lush greenery of his homeland. Luckily, he rapidly secured accommodation for his family and employment. At the Ceylon Students Centre in Clarendon Place, London, he received both an affordable place to stay and familiar meals. Fernando gained employment on his second day in the country, underscoring the demand for labour in the NHS. After working in short-term contracts as an anaesthetist, he passed his surgical exams and began duties as a surgical registrar in Croydon. In this post, he performed much of the day-to-day surgical work under the supervision of senior consultants. Having gained sufficient qualifications and training, Fernando and his family now considered returning home. However, correspondence with officials in Ceylon dissuaded him. Incessant demands for further paperwork were, he discovered, a ploy for soliciting a bribe. Jaded by these officials' behaviour, Fernando and his family stayed in the UK, joining thousands of other migrants in the postwar decades.

The presence of employees like Fernando created ethnically and racially diverse workforces in the NHS by the 1960s. Indian doctors rubbed shoulders with Trinidadian nurses and Irish GPs booked their patients in for surgeries performed by Nigerian consultants. By the end of 1965, 3,000–5,000 nurses from Jamaica alone worked in the service.[16] In 1971, 31 per cent of all doctors working in the NHS were born and trained overseas. Staff at the Mill Road Maternity Hospital, Liverpool, called themselves the 'League of Nations' in a statement of pride about the diversity within their own medical team (Figure 13). Across the NHS, these employees not only plugged necessary shortages in the everyday operation of the service but helped the institution pursue its founding social democratic promise to propel the nation into the medical future. Fernando, for instance, became employed at the Royal Free Hospital, London, in a path-breaking team that delivered some of the first kidney transplants in the UK. Though the NHS was becoming increasingly understood as a 'national' institution in the public imagination, this framing obscured the important contributions made by people who hailed from overseas.

Britain could recruit many of these professionals in the 1960s and 1970s because of older imperial legacies. In India, for instance, the Indian Medical Service had overseen the expansion of Western medical schools during the nineteenth century, and the British General Medical Council recognised the degrees that they granted between 1892 and 1975.[17] With convertible qualifications and higher wages, Britain appeared as an attractive option for South Asian medical practitioners in the postwar era, as it did for doctors in other recently independent nations. However, while the WHO supported the mutual recognition of medical degrees across borders, it expressed alarm at a transfer of expertise that 'has already handicapped so many developing countries and favoured some highly developed ones'.[18] The economist and WHO-affiliated expert Oscar Gish described medical emigration as a 'Third World Health Crisis'. In the mid-1960s, for example, India possessed 700 health centres in rural areas without trained doctors.[19] At the very moment that Britain expanded and staffed NHS health centres,

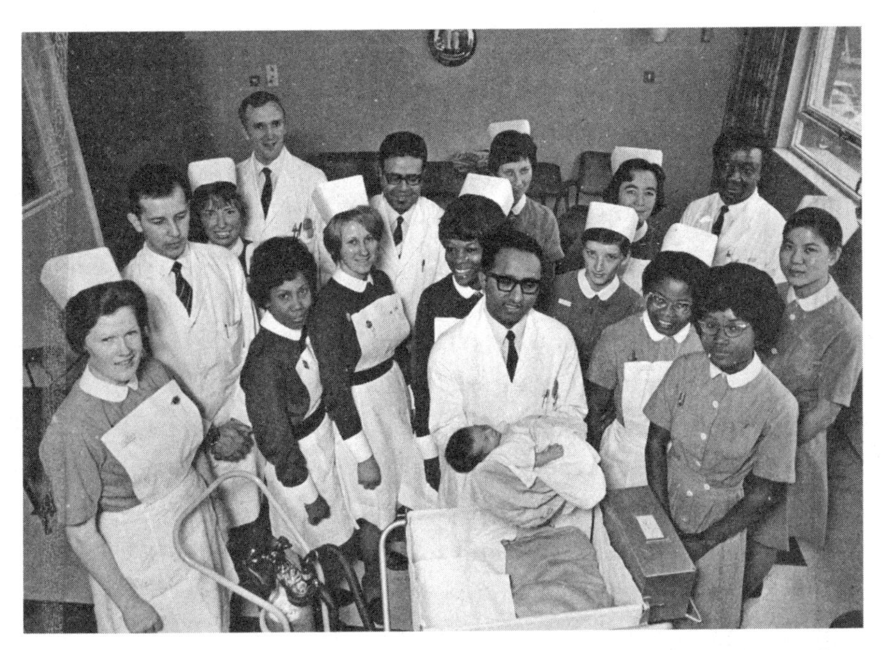

13. Staff at the Mill Road Maternity Hospital, Liverpool, in 1970. Hailing from various parts of Europe and the Commonwealth, this team referred to themselves as the 'League of Nations'.

its former colony went without. Resolving to take action, the Commonwealth Medical Association agreed in 1965 to send doctors from Britain and more economically developed countries to help train new professionals abroad.[20] These good intentions made little discernible impact. Suffering huge losses in skilled labour that might have alleviated longstanding medical challenges, countries like India introduced laws to restrict visas for foreign travel.[21] Yet these restrictions largely proved ineffective for retaining health care workers. As the Indian Ministry of Foreign Affairs summed up, 'in a free society there was no way of preventing them from leaving India or of recalling them, except with offers of higher salaries than those received abroad, and economically this was not possible'.[22]

Although British civil servants recognised the global inequality that recruiting foreign medical professionals fostered, they anxiously monitored potential disruptions to the flow of workers. Frequent rumours that the Indian government might restrict the passage of doctors provoked regular inquiries from the British state to officials in Delhi regarding their intentions.[23] A scheme in Jamaica to entice trained nurses back to the island garnered similar scrutiny. Other possible interruptions included the outbreak of armed conflict. When India and Pakistan warred over borders in 1965, British civil servants fretted that the conflict might impact recruiting doctors from the two nations that provided the most overseas practitioners to the NHS. They worried that some doctors might want to go back and help their countries, or, if they stayed, that tensions would erupt on the wards. In the end, officials were pleased to report that there was 'no evidence of difficult personal relationships between Indian and Pakistani doctors, instead there was a shared feeling of regret at what was going on; nor was there any sign of a return home – on the contrary some Indian doctors were known to have cancelled their return'.

Politicians and newspapers often singled out immigrant workers in the NHS for praise. In a 1961 House of Lords debate on labour shortages in the NHS, Stephen Taylor – now a peer on the back of his contributions to family doctoring in places like Harlow – made the blunt assessment that 'our hospital service would have collapsed had it not been for the enormous influx of junior doctors from India and Pakistan'.[24] While the Labour peer held some reservations about the capacity of these professionals to understand the culture and customs of their British patients, he concluded that 'when all is said and done we are in their debt'. As the historian Roberta Bivins has shown, the visual imagery of newspapers generally depicted overseas NHS doctors and nurses in an appreciative manner, or at least as a natural part of the service that patients would expect to see.[25]

Though many Britons embraced or at least acknowledged that the NHS relied on staff, nurses and doctors drawn from around the world, not everyone proved so accepting. An organisation of doctors that lambasted the NHS for overspending and government overreach soon began to highlight the institution's overseas workforce as a third prong to their attack. Each facet of their critique gained some traction, but they secured the most ground in fostering racially tinged fears of medical immigration.

THE FELLOWSHIP FOR FREEDOM IN MEDICINE

As the physician for every monarch from Edward VII to Elizabeth II, as well as former Prime Ministers Ramsay MacDonald and Neville Chamberlain, Lord Thomas Jeeves Horder (1871–1955) was one of Britain's best-known doctors.[26] It mattered, then, that four months after the NHS began, he founded a conservative association of doctors and interested supporters opposed to 'Mr. Bevan's travesty of a National Health Service'.[27] The Fellowship for Freedom in Medicine (FFM), as they named themselves, was not a mass membership organisation, but it still attracted over 3,000 members in the late 1950s, including professionals from all of the main teaching hospitals. Headquartered in London's salubrious West End, the Fellowship roamed across the UK. Through meetings, speeches, monthly bulletins, newspaper articles, media appearances and connections with politicians and free-market intellectuals, Horder's followers sought to restore 'freedom' to the medical sphere by ending the NHS's 'monopoly'. Their free-market economic position would eventually intersect with antagonism towards overseas workers in the service.

In its early years, the FFM advanced two principal arguments. First, they believed that the purportedly high cost of the NHS represented an inexhaustible financial commitment at the expense of British industry. Second, they argued that the service extended the reach of the state to an inappropriate degree that undermined the doctor–patient relationship and exacerbated the declining status of GPs. The NHS constituted, to them, a 'Sacred Cow', enthralling the public with false promises of 'free medicine' that obscured these deeper problems.[28] Rather than a hopeful sign of Britain's progress or confirmation of the nation's world leadership in health care, the service was presented by the Fellowship as part of the country's apparent decline in the post-1945 era. This 'declinism' about the UK's postwar standing, as the historians Jim Tomlinson and David Edgerton term it, framed discussion of subjects ranging from the economy to science, and it was usually more imagined than real.[29] Britain remained a comparatively rich and technologically proficient nation, even if it no longer held its former international pre-eminence. Yet gloomy assessments of Britain's place in the world could be politically useful, and this fact proved no less true with critical interpretations of the NHS.

In the 1940s and 1950s, the Fellowship predicted that the unexpectedly high costs of the NHS would lead to the collapse of the service, and maybe even the British economy. Initial budgeting for the service leapt from the £170 million a year estimated in the 1942 Beveridge Report to the reality of £305 million in 1949/50, and £384 million the following year.[30] Such increases undermined Bevan's belief that health spending would fall as the state dealt with a backlog of ill health. In fairness to the service's founders, the pent-up demand for health care before its establishment played some role in these ballooning costs. People who had waited years for a new set of teeth or an expensive operation came forward in large numbers after July 1948. The NHS also absorbed a marginal amount of Britain's resources, with far more of Britain's national income allocated to military spending than to the welfare state in the immediate postwar years.[31] All the same, critics of the NHS seized on the fact that its budgets – if taken in isolation – had swelled to be much larger than anticipated. In one of his many articles attacking Beveridge's inaccuracies, the radiologist and NHS-critic Ffrangcon Roberts predicted that such spending meant the service would 'involve us in national ruin'.[32] Showing the wider influence of these commentators, the prominent Austrian neoliberal economist Friedrich Hayek cited Roberts to support his own writing against nationalised health care.[33]

Horder brought these arguments across the Atlantic.[34] A bald man with round glasses, he had achieved a great deal of professional success. His public stature was confirmed by serving as the president for a somewhat idiosyncratic range of civic and political organisations, from the Peckham Health Centre to the Cremation Society of Great Britain to the British Eugenics Society. Horder sometimes displayed an ostentatiousness that aggravated his medical colleagues. As a registrar at St Bartholomew's Hospital, London, his Rolls-Royce provoked enough jealousy to force him to park it a few streets away from his workplace. Nonetheless, however much he may have annoyed his colleagues at home, the opponents of national health insurance in North America welcomed Horder with open arms. To organisations like the AMA, the Fellowship's struggles against the NHS were synonymous with their own fight against the Truman Plan. In a 1952 speech to the American and Canadian chapters of the International College of Surgeons, Horder proclaimed that the British 'experiment' in nationalising medicine had 'failed'.[35] Free-at-the-point-of-use care meant, he maintained, that 'the National Health Service is today splitting upon the rock of economics'. To ensure that his audience 'avoid the blunder we have made in England', Horder told the 5,000 doctors present not to trust politicians, to strive for unity within their own ranks and to 'explain things clearly to the public'. 'The cause is the public's cause, even more than it is yours', he insisted.

The Fellowship's 'cause' centred on returning to fee-based medical practice, which represented, they argued, the only solution to NHS funding problems. If individuals paid out of their own pockets for medical care, then demand on the public purse would lessen. Individuals, in turn, would be encouraged to take responsibility for their health, and freedom from the state would be returned to both the patient and their doctor. Vice-Chairman Reginald Hale-White presented the possibility of private medicine regaining its former status as a national good, 'flourishing alongside the National Health Service in open and fair competition, so that each can act as a stimulant to the other for the public benefit'.[36] While publicly projecting a desire to cooperate with the state service, most Fellowship members wanted private health care to occupy the larger share of the medical sphere. Pursuing this goal, they helped fundraise for the first private hospital founded outside of the NHS since 1948, the New Victoria Hospital in Kingston.[37] One of their key early proposals for expanding fee-based medicine included giving private patients access to drugs and other medical benefits without direct charge, just as NHS patients enjoyed. Granting parity with the state system on pharmaceuticals would allow these patients to withdraw from the NHS altogether and save taxpayers' money.[38]

The Conservative Party took interest in the Fellowship's concerns about NHS expenditure and proposals to support private medicine, as many sections of the party also worried about paying for the universalist welfare state. Meetings with important internal research groups, such as the Conservative Social Services Committee in the summer of 1952, to discuss 'matters of mutual interest' were regular occurrences.[39] In fact, the Fellowship proved the most frequent visitors to the Conservative Social Services Committee among all other external guests during this decade. The Fellowship also developed a close relationship with Angus Maude, the journalist, MP for Ealing South and Director of the Conservative Political Centre. They shared a belief in the threat that postwar social democratic politics seemingly posed to the middle class. One of Maude's books, *Professional People* (1952), argued that the state's insatiable need for an army of technocrats denigrated professionalism.[40] To prevent these trends in medicine, he argued, the private doctor, who embodied 'a last citadel of freedom to which all can, at need, turn for safety and self-respect', needed defending. The Fellowship invited Maude to address a meeting in 1955, where he expressed alignment with his hosts' values and claimed he 'brought a great deal of pressure on the Minister in regard to drugs for private patients'.

These connections did not force any substantial changes in policy. However, in 1953, the Conservative government established a committee of inquiry to identify ways to control NHS spending, led by the Cambridge economist Claude Guillebaud. The Fellowship expressed high hopes for the Guillebaud Committee as a chance to alter the NHS, or possibly remove it altogether, and busied themselves sourcing evidence of 'extravagance or inefficiency in the administration of the Service'.[41] The report they delivered to the committee repeated their main aims of returning prestige to general practice, ending 'free' GP services, hospital care and pharmaceutical products, and introducing alternative measures to promote private medicine.

However, the committee's report, published as *The Cost of the National Health Service in England and Wales* (1956), went in the opposite direction by giving the NHS a resounding seal of approval and praising its quality of care.[42] Claude Guillebaud's decision to contract statistical research for his report to two prominent advocates of the health service – Richard Titmuss and Brian Abel-Smith – laid the groundwork for this defence of the NHS. Contrary to the accusations levelled by the service's critics that it cost too much, these two LSE academics demonstrated that health budgets had in fact fallen in relation to GDP since its foundation.[43] The novel technique of tying health spending to national income allowed for comparisons with other countries that embarrassed the government. Britain, they demonstrated, actually received good value with the NHS. Other countries spent more on health. Titmuss and Abel-Smith's findings received praise in the mainstream press and from both main parties in the Commons, sidelining the Fellowship.[44] Horder's organisation fired back, denigrating the publication as 'mainly whitewash' and accusing civil servants of bias, but their complaints fell on deaf ears.

Outmanoeuvred by the NHS's defenders over costs, the Fellowship regrouped and turned to their second line of attack: the loss of doctor autonomy from state overreach. The many angry and disillusioned GPs in the service were fertile ground for such claims. Low levels of financial remuneration through the capitation system provoked their hostility, heightened by the demands presented by extensive patient lists in the early NHS.[45] The professional divisions between GPs in local communities and specialists in hospitals compounded these tensions. Family doctors lacked professional confidence and felt separated from hospital-based scientific medicine. Indeed, some influential hospital doctors openly denigrated their colleagues in general practice. To Winston Churchill's physician, Lord Moran, consultants and registrars simply occupied a higher rung of a professional 'ladder' than GPs. 'How can you say that the people who get to the top of the ladder are the same people who fall off it?', he remarked in a statement that infuriated many family doctors, 'It seems to me so ludicrous'.[46]

The Fellowship seized upon the grievances among GPs by attempting to revive the connotations of 'state medicine' present during the debates over the NHS's inception. Thin wage packets and hefty patient lists were symptoms, they argued, of the government's overreach in medical care, rather than something that could be solved by merely reforming the nationalised system. 'In every possible way', declared Horder, 'the status of the GP is being undermined' since family doctors had become, after 1948, 'a part of the machine'. By using this language to describe the NHS, the Fellowship mobilised a metaphor used by other conservatives during the Cold War to criticise the purportedly overbearing nature of the state in the fields of medicine and science.[47] For them, government planning relegated doctoring to just another profession. Indeed, Horder thought medicine had become 'a branch of the Civil Service', where doctors were 'no longer experts' and their new role was to 'sit and sign forms'.[48]

No Fellowship member went further with these anti-state arguments than Dr Donald McIntosh Johnson, a GP, author and MP. Johnson became the Fellowship's most vocal supporter within Parliament as Conservative member for Carlisle from 1955, and wrote multiple autobiographies chronicling his career as a doctor-turned-polemicist.[49] In the 1930s, he ran his own private practice in Thornton Heath, London, but became disillusioned with doctoring due to state interference. Clashes with the local authority over panel patients' prescriptions – provided under the 1911 National Insurance Act – convinced Johnson that government intervention fundamentally compromised GP independence. The inception of the NHS deepened his anguish. Johnson saw 5 July 1948 as a profound moment of loss, when 'my way of medical practice and that of my father before me, were eliminated overnight'. By this point he was firmly involved with Conservative politics and presented his decision to change careers as a chance 'to escape beyond the Iron Curtain of State-controlled medicine to tell my story'. Johnson described likeminded doctors as 'outcasts of the Bolshevik regime'.

The British National Health Service: Friend or Frankenstein? (1962) represented Johnson's most significant effort in linking the GP crisis to state control. The book began optimistically, presenting the Conservative government's decision to raise prescription charges and National Insurance contributions in 1961 as a sign that politicians would stop 'worshipping' the NHS as 'the Golden Calf . . . of the Welfare State'.[50] Alternative thoughts on general practice, he hoped, might now make headway. Johnson argued that the state sapped the GP of enterprise. The doctor, he diagnosed, was 'denied the undoubted stimulus of garnering money from his individual patients', and could no longer 'solace himself with escapist dreams and the consciousness of his independence'. He thought the NHS extinguished self-reliance and entrepreneurialism by compelling GPs to work in under-subscribed industrial areas, amounting to trends 'which have ground him down . . . and with it his place in the community, to . . . near medical orderly status'.

Others appreciated the connections made by Johnson between the apparent failings in the NHS, general practice and state control. Some members of the general public who harboured reservations about the NHS sent him letters. Miss Georgina Eteson from London spoke of her 'great pleasure' in reading his book that answered the questions 'we industrial workers are asking'.[51] Eteson's own doctor had left the country in 1947 in opposition to the coming NHS, and her personal frustrations with general practice centred on lack of flexibility regarding surgery opening hours and bureaucracy within the state-provided system. Other admirers included an Austrian libertarian writer called Eli Rubin, who stressed commonality between his own work on the problems of state planning and Johnson's criticisms of the NHS.[52] As these admirers demonstrated, the Fellowship was not a voice in the wilderness but sometimes channelled wider currents of opposition to government intervention in medical care.

However, matters worsened for the organisation when it eventually lost the wellspring of antagonism that they exploited among GPs. At first, things seemed to be moving in the Fellowship's direction when family doctors – fed up with low pay and lack of prestige – took radical steps against Harold Wilson's Labour government. In 1965, a number of GPs in Birmingham grew so disgruntled with the NHS that they withdrew from it altogether. The 'Birmingham Action Group' devised a subscription-based insurance scheme for patients who also left the public service.[53] Radical elements of the BMA followed suit and advanced their own plans for an alternative to the NHS, called 'Independent Medical Services' (IMS).[54] The Fellowship smelled blood. They provided funds to the Birmingham Action Group, publicised IMS and encouraged their members to donate to doctors who had displayed 'courage' in opposing the Labour government.[55] 'The way is now open', they predicted, 'for that massive alternative to the National Health Service which the country has needed for so long'.[56] However, when the BMA and the Minister of Health, Kenneth Robinson, finally came to agreement over the Family Doctor Charter of 1966, the tide turned against the Fellowship. Family doctors were now better included within the modernisation of the NHS through their access to funds for medical assistants, receptionists and premises such as health centres. The venom dissipated from the long-running crisis in general practice, and the Fellowship lost the panic and professional disillusionment that it had previously gained energy from.

Disputes over NHS costs or the place of the state in medicine brought the Fellowship few gains. Their claims were either disproven by high-profile interventions by the service's supporters or sat at odds with patients' experiences of the modernisation programme unfolding through hospitals and health centres across the country. The NHS had its problems but, to most people, it did not pave the way to financial meltdown or the creation of a totalitarian state. Nonetheless, one final opportunity for the organisation to discredit state medicine lay in a fierce debate about the emigration and immigration of medical experts during the 1960s. It was at this juncture that the Fellowship's free-market arguments conjoined with commentary on overseas practitioners.

THE MEDICAL 'BRAIN DRAIN'

As Britain recruited medical labour from abroad, the nation lost thousands of doctors going in the other direction. By the 1960s, many British-born practitioners packed their bags and left for Australia, Canada and the US for higher pay and greater prestige. Some doctors simply disliked the NHS. Joining thousands of other practitioners escaping war-ravaged European nations, they sought a new life overseas.[57] The movement of these professionals alarmed the nations that had provided their training, even though the depth of the problems it created was not as severe as in the Global South. When reflecting on the loss of the nation's expertise and labour, British commentators fretted over a medical 'brain drain' that might carry perilous consequences. The interlocked debate about immigration and emigration provided an opening for the NHS's free-market critics.

At first, no one knew just how many doctors were leaving. At the start of the 1960s, *The Times* reported that up to 700 doctors a year trained in the UK left the country.[58] Though not an exact figure, it seemed that many of these professionals were GPs driven out by the tumult within their specialism. Amidst anxiety about the implications of this exodus for the long-term health of the NHS, some parts of the media used doctors' decisions to buy a one-way plane ticket away from the service as a source of levity. Richard Gordon's *Punch* article 'The Disappearing Doctor' reworked Lord Kitchener's famous First World War recruitment poster. He replaced the Field Marshal with the sitting Conservative Minister of Health, accompanied by the caption 'ENOCH NEEDS YOU'. One *Daily Express* cartoon featured a hapless patient with a tap stuck on his toe as emblematic of the trivial demands that sent doctors – in this instance, carrying a suitcase emblazoned with 'Emigrant to USA' – scrambling for the nearest exit.

The aeronautical engineer-turned-author Nevil Shute blamed the NHS for emigration in his novel *The Far Country* (1952).[59] Shute's book followed the story of Jennifer Morton, a young woman who, on inheriting a small sum of money, visits relatives in Australia. She quickly falls in love with both the country – depicted as a prosperous, self-reliant realisation of the Anglo-Saxon spirit – and a Czech refugee called Carl, who has previously worked as a doctor but is now unlicensed. The Britain that Jennifer leaves is a drab place, scarred by both war and the rationing imposed by Attlee's Labour government. Shute himself harboured no love for postwar social democracy, and had also immigrated to Australia. When Jennifer's mother dies in the novel, she is forced to return home and help her father, who is an overworked NHS GP, enduring fourteen-hour days for his feckless patients. Jennifer is disgusted by their demands. The description of one patient, who 'came for medicine and a certificate exempting him from work because he couldn't wake up in the morning', chimed with stories in the press about the selfish behaviour that the service supposedly encouraged.[60] The novel ended with Jennifer escaping Britain – and the NHS – by returning to Australia to marry Carl, who decides to acquire his medical licence and resume doctoring. *The Far Country* offered its own explanation for the motives behind medical emigration, with put-upon European medical professionals improving their lot elsewhere.

The Fellowship was among the first to provide rigorous evidence for the ranks of Britain's doctors leaving the country. In 1961, Dr John R. Seale published an article in the *British Medical Journal* titled 'Supply of Doctors'.[61] Born in Exeter, Seale was a senior registrar at St Mary's Hospital in London and a recent visiting fellow at the Harvard School of Business. He took an interest in medical economics, especially how much different countries spent on health care.[62] Seale therefore possessed the credentials to make a splash as one of the Fellowship's most influential members. In his 1961 article, Seale warned of extensive medical emigration from Britain, with 220 doctors having settled in Canada in the prior six years alone. He also took aim at the Willink Committee on the Number of Medical Practitioners and Medical Students, which had reported in 1957 that the levels of doctoring in Britain were satisfactory enough to warrant a 10 per cent reduction in the total number of medical students.[63] By pointing to the draining away of British medical talent, he exposed the flaws in these prior recommendations. The Fellowship realised that in Seale they possessed a supporter who made a significant impact on debates over general practice, and they hailed his 'apparently tireless' output.[64]

Mirroring their wider views, the Fellowship blamed the NHS for Britain's medical emigration problems. In his pamphlet, *The Supply of Doctors and the Future of the British Medical Profession* (1962), Seale attributed the crisis to the onset of the service.[65] During the war, he demonstrated, the government expanded medical schools and encouraged training to avoid shortages in practitioners. Then, in the NHS negotiations, Seale believed that Bevan had exploited the high number of surplus disestablished doctors created by this wartime growth, forcing the profession to accept a system that they distrusted. Once doctors were inside the service, he alleged, the government deliberately denied wage increases and expanded junior positions to keep their incomes low. Seale believed that fewer students now wanted to pursue a career in this 'economically depressed profession' and that, in turn, doctor emigration increased. The NHS, to this leading Fellowship member, therefore exacerbated Britain's decline as a world leader in medical expertise.

Far from being technical discussions confined to the pages of medical journals, debates over the link between problems in NHS general practice and emigration played out in newspapers and on television screens.[66] Hoping to undermine public idolisation of the service, Seale and Donald McIntosh Johnson appeared in an early 1962 edition of the ITV programme *Questions in the House* for a feature that explored medical emigration.[67] Others joined the Fellowship in spreading their interpretation of the problem. In 1967, a British private GP named Dr Richard Rossdale returned from the US and provided a glowing account of what he had seen across the Atlantic in a television interview.[68] Rossdale praised the 'freedom' of American medicine, which, he believed, was 'getting lost in this country'. While the NHS saddled younger British GPs with form-filling, their US or Australian counterparts, recounted Rossdale, enjoyed research money and a closer relationship with their patients. Rossdale carefully navigated the growing welfare nationalism around the NHS when making these claims. He agreed with his interviewer that British doctors should show 'patriotism' and stay in the country, as medicine possessed importance 'for our so-called image', but he insisted that he would still advise any of his own relatives to leave the country rather than work in the NHS.

The Fellowship's activism around medical emigration provoked angry responses from the Ministry of Health. Prominent politicians from both main parties scrambled to defend the NHS's reputation. In 1962, Enoch Powell derided the publicity given to 'these grotesque allegations', calling them a 'slander' on the NHS.[69] The minister accused Seale of double-counting doctors who emigrated. While Seale subsequently admitted that his calculations somewhat inflated the total, few bought the government's line that a medical brain drain was entirely a malicious fabrication. In 1966, Kenneth Robinson acknowledged the problem and attacked doctors who left after training for taking the equivalent of £7,500 from 'the hard-pressed British taxpayer'. This position revised his previous stance, similar to Powell's, that emigration statistics represented 'propaganda' deployed by 'enemies of the Service'. Even Powell later admitted in his book *Medicine and Politics* (1966) that doctors were 'voting with their feet' at an alarming rate.[70] Though both men eventually accepted the problem, their initial response demonstrated an attempt to use the swelling welfare nationalism around the NHS to persuade doctors to stay.

Seale forced the Fellowship's opponents to account for evidence that discredited nationalised medicine. Brian Abel-Smith – who had joined with Richard Titmuss to spike the Fellowship's guns in their earlier statistical work for the Guillebaud Committee – published a study that broadly accepted a considerable degree of medical emigration.[71] Abel-Smith and Kathleen Gales's *British Doctors at Home and Abroad* (1964) confirmed that GPs made up the main body of emigrants, at 23.7 per cent of all professionals who had left. Of these, 59.1 per cent had previously worked in the NHS. However, their study drew different conclusions when explaining why doctors emigrated. Only 9 per cent of respondents to their questionnaire voiced objections to 'socialised medicine'. Instead, general practice's position as a 'low status occupation' explained their decision to leave. The LSE economists concluded that 'the system as it exists in Britain appears to have played some part in the decision to go to other countries where a different pattern of practice can be found'.

Seale's influence ranged beyond Britain. In 1962, he undertook a US speaking tour funded by the AMA to discredit the Kennedy administration's attempts to pass a Medicare Bill.[72] The President himself even defended his plans against Seale's interventions. As part of a lengthy speech on health reform in Madison Square Garden in New York City, Kennedy expressed his awareness that 'there is going to be a program this week against this bill in which an English physician is going to come and talk about how bad their plans are'.[73] 'It may be', he continued, 'but he ought to talk about it in England, because his plans . . . and what they do in England are entirely different'. After drawing these lines of distinction, Kennedy nonetheless reminded his audience that 'what we are now talking about doing, most of the countries of Europe did years ago'. 'The British did it 30 years ago', he added. That a sitting US President even addressed the opinions of a Fellowship member underlined how the emigration controversy marked the high tide of the organisation and reflected the force, range and impact of their critiques.

IMMIGRATION AND RACE

Back in Britain, the outflow of domestically trained doctors and the inflow of overseas-trained doctors became linked. The critics of medical immigration like the Fellowship argued that foreign-born medical experts possessed questionable qualifications, a shoddy work ethic and poor linguistic capacities compared with those who were leaving. Their claims that non-white doctors 'replaced' British-born doctors overlapped with popular criticisms about the NHS based on race. The mix of disquiet about immigration, race and medical workers created an atmosphere that led the government to implement regulatory controls over foreign workers in the NHS during the mid-1970s. If welfare nationalism strengthened the service's foundations by building support, it could also draw firm boundaries for those who worked in the institution or accessed its care.

Rather than acknowledge medical immigration's historical background, let alone its impacts elsewhere, the Fellowship framed it as a question of race. They consistently depicted British doctors as white and Commonwealth doctors as non-white, despite the blurring of these distinctions in both directions. Some non-white British doctors were born in the UK, just as immigrant doctors could be white if they came from a former imperial holding like South Africa or another European nation such as Ireland or Poland. Nonetheless, the Fellowship focused on workers of colour in the NHS, lambasting their training, interpersonal skills and ability to empathise with patients. These professionals, they charged, gained their degrees from institutions of 'indifferent quality' and spoke an unacceptable standard of English.[74]

The criticisms of linguistic ability served to emphasise not only the poor standards of care that these professionals were alleged to provide but also their foreignness. 'When doctors employed by hospitals in responsible posts are unable to communicate to their patients or relatives', Seale charged, 'this is no longer human medicine, it is veterinary medicine'.[75] To him, inferior foreign doctors in the NHS treated British patients like animals. That the vast majority of these doctors spoke fluent English mattered little to Seale, and he neglected to address their complaints in medical journals about being rendered in this way.[76] One study of hospital doctors from ethnic minority backgrounds in the North-West of England during the late 1970s found that only 15 per cent experienced language difficulties.[77] Painting all non-white practitioners as poorly trained and incapable of clear communication fit the Fellowship's broader imagining of the NHS as an impersonal bureaucratic machine. In this way, ethnicity and race conjoined with their free-market views on finance and state intervention.

The Fellowship positioned their stance on doctor immigration as a matter of free expression. 'In these days it is not done to speak of such matters for fear of being accused of colour prejudice', complained Dr Reginald Hale-White – Horder's successor after his death in 1955 – and he added that 'all sorts of things that have nothing to do with the colour question are not being said because of this fear'.[78] 'Criticism of the present conditions has nothing to do with colour prejudice', he maintained, but rather the 'lowly qualifications' of 'these immigrants' who 'can barely make themselves understood'. 'Far more important', the Fellowship's new Chairman concluded, 'is the certainty that nearly everyone would sooner be looked after by their own countrymen when

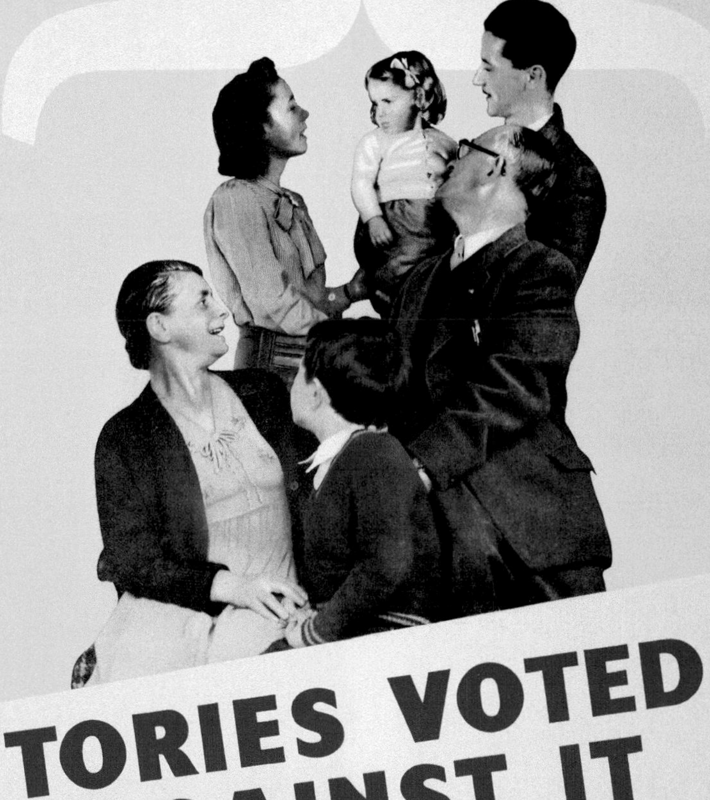

1. The early NHS foregrounded the health of children and mothers in its services and promotional material. This decision reflected the political emphasis on the family in postwar Britain and formed an integral part of the Labour Party's efforts to present the institution as a caring guardian of everyday Britons.

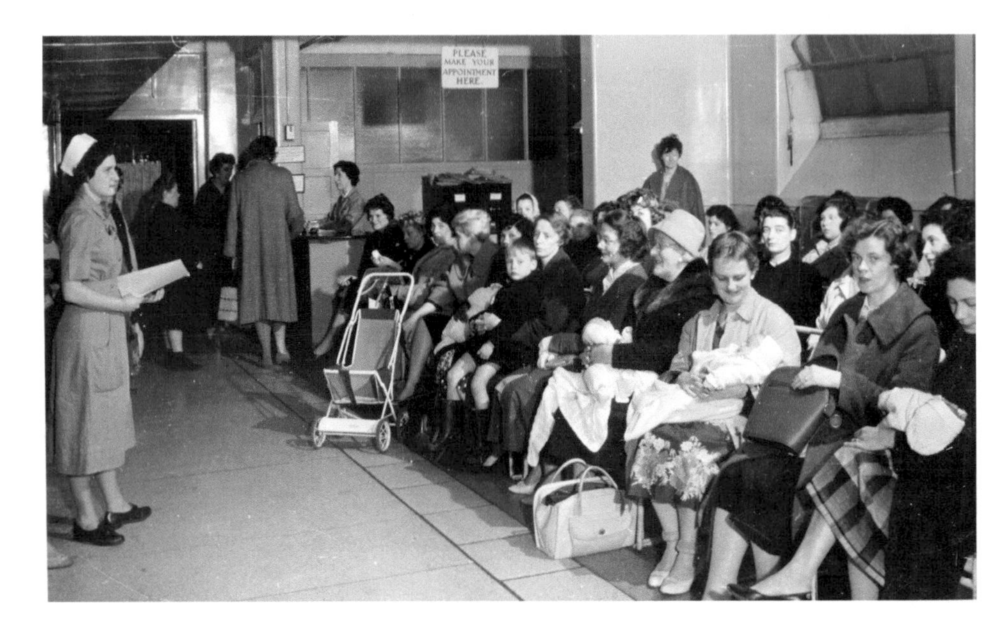

2. The facilities that patients experienced in the early NHS often dated back to the Victorian past, such as the Jessop Hospital for Women in Sheffield, which first opened in 1878. Far from a 'golden age' of spending on the welfare state, the postwar health budgets needed to upgrade older buildings or undertake new construction remained low by later standards.

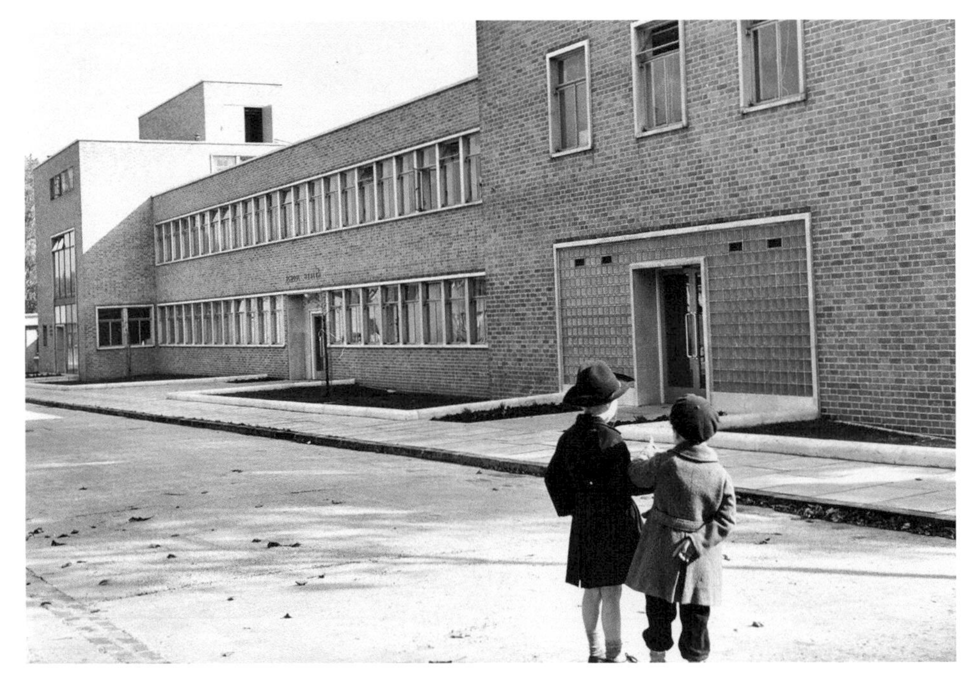

3. It took time for the service to offer new facilities like health centres, including the Woodberry Down Health Centre in London. As the service's modernisation gathered pace, it reflected a postwar faith in state expertise and planning, but it could also prove adaptable to local conditions.

The nuisance value of sound often bears little relation to its intensity.
(Report on Noise Control in Hospitals, King Edward's Hospital Fund for London)
NOISE
ALMOST ALWAYS ANNOYS

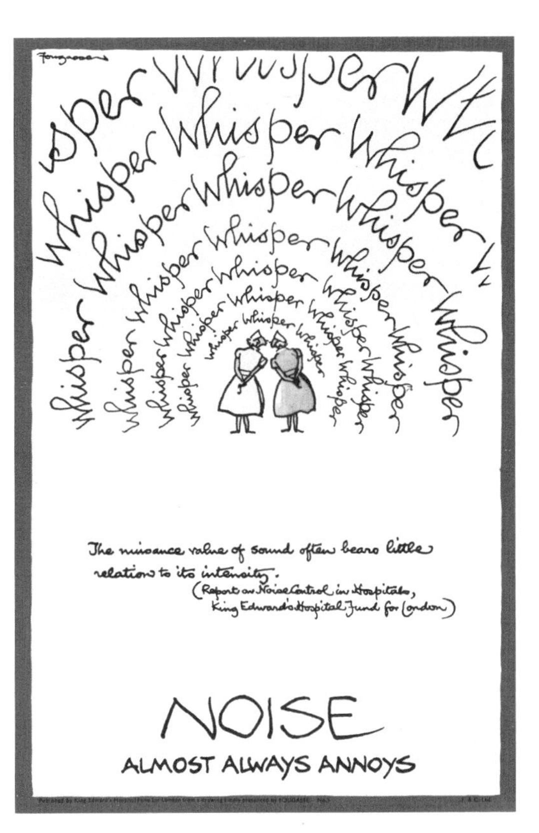

4. Organisations external to the NHS contributed to the service's development. With some success, the King's Fund – a charitable body – encouraged health service staff to pay greater attention to noise in hospitals through reports and promotional materials like this poster. Though not without limitations, the modernising NHS exhibited a degree of attentiveness to changing expectations among its patients and wider attitudinal shifts in British society.

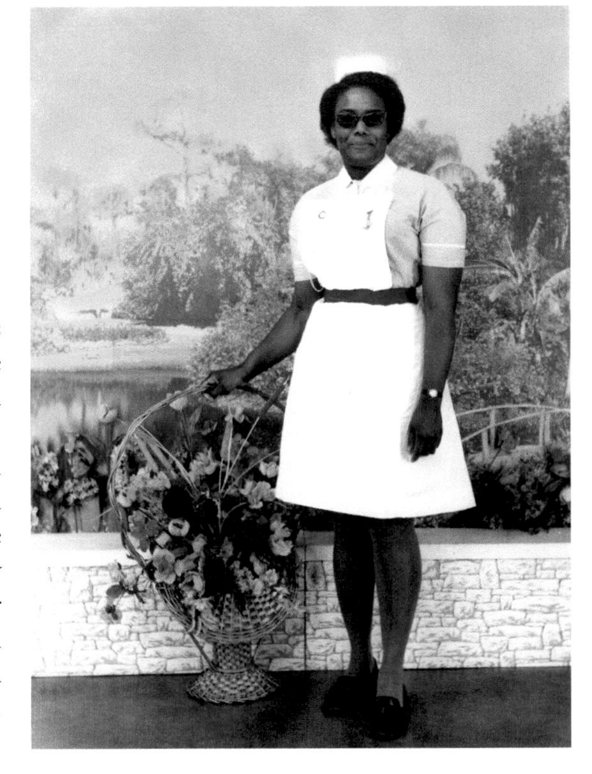

5. Immigration made the NHS's promise of universal health care possible. The service attracted employees from all over the world, and often drew on links with the former British Empire and the new Commonwealth. These doctors, nurses and ancillary workers were often praised for their contributions, though they could also be subjected to racial discrimination.

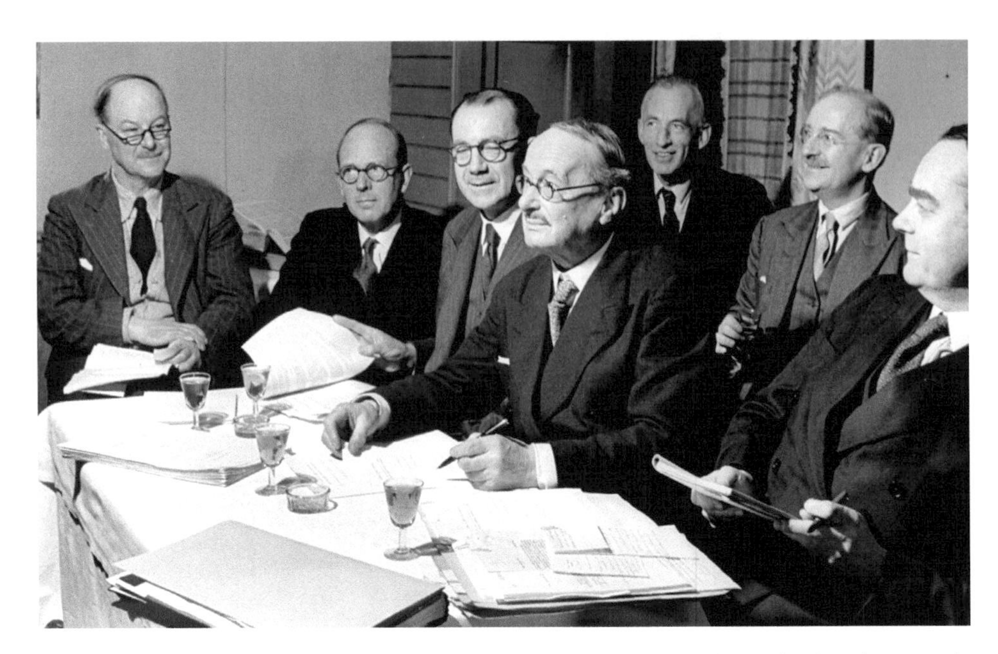

6. Not everyone welcomed the NHS. The Royal physician, Lord Horder (in the centre), formed the Fellowship for Freedom in Medicine in 1948 to oppose nationalised medicine. The group criticised the health service's costs and perceived it as a dangerous overreach of the welfare state that would lead Britain to authoritarianism. In the 1960s, the Fellowship blended their free-market opposition to the NHS with a racialised critique of the institution's reliance on overseas workers.

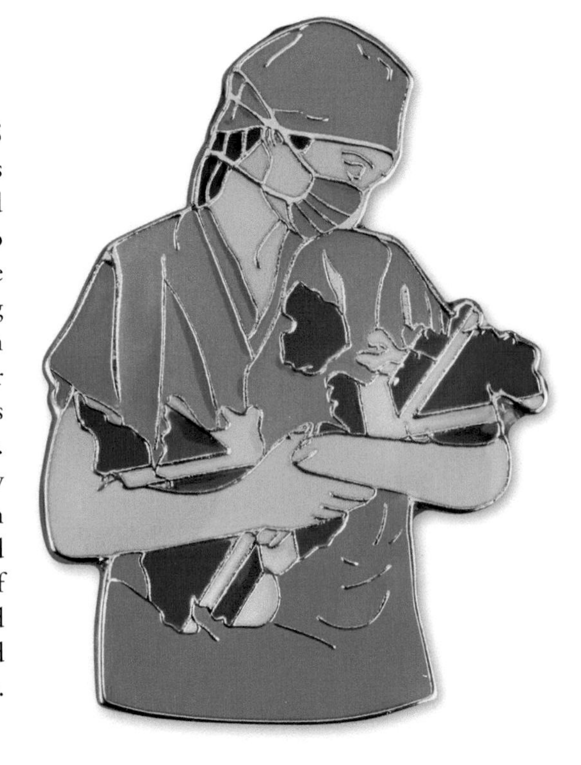

7. From the 1970s, the NHS shed much of its prior emphasis on children and family life, and became more strongly tied to national identity. Whereas in the 1940s and 1950s its left-wing supporters held up the health service as an inspiration for all other nations, now they presented it as a uniquely British achievement. This welfare nationalism grew over time – as this badge from the 2020s shows – and fostered greater public support, even if such feeling could also be deployed against the NHS's patients and workers who hailed from overseas.

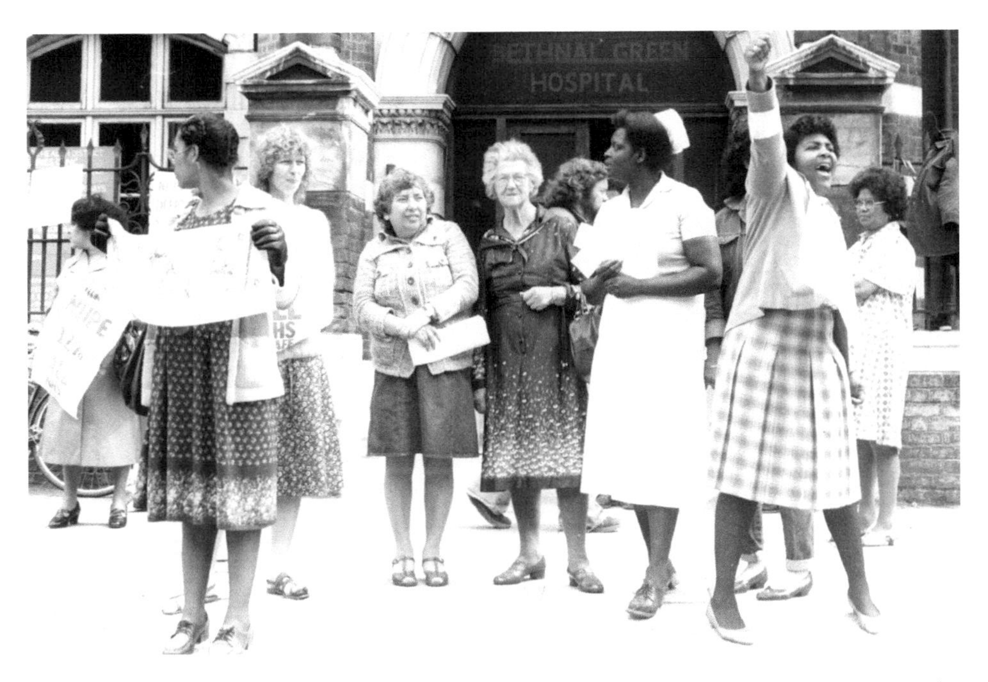

8. The economic shocks and political radicalism of the 1970s also shaped the NHS. For the first time, strikes among doctors, nurses and ancillary workers took place across the service on issues ranging from low pay to the presence of private patients within the public system.

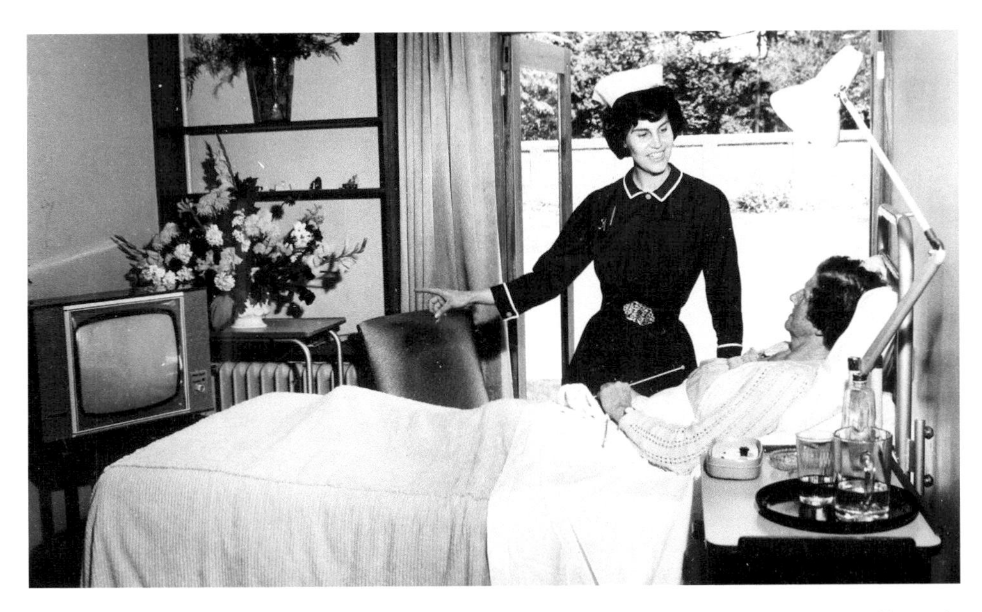

9. The turbulence of the 1970s also fuelled the arguments made by free-market intellectuals and politicians that a system of private health insurance should marginalise or replace the NHS. Organisations such as the British United Provident Association (BUPA), they reasoned, would offer more choice and privacy to patients in either 'pay-beds' within public hospitals or in purpose-built facilities outside the NHS, like the Woking Nuffield Nursing Home. These proposals were explored by Margaret Thatcher's governments in the early 1980s.

NUPE NUPE NUPE NUPE NUPE NUPE NUPE NUPE NUPE

BARKING HOSPITAL TODAY

YOU TOMORROW?

BARKING'S FIGHT MUST BE YOUR FIGHT

10. During the 1980s, trade unions fought a fierce battle against marketisation policies introduced by the Conservative Party, such as outsourcing in-house NHS cleaning work to private companies. Their struggles in the name of 'Our NHS' presented its privatisation as an imminent outcome, which proved politically effective in sharpening public focus on the service but has sometimes obscured the institution's surprising resilience.

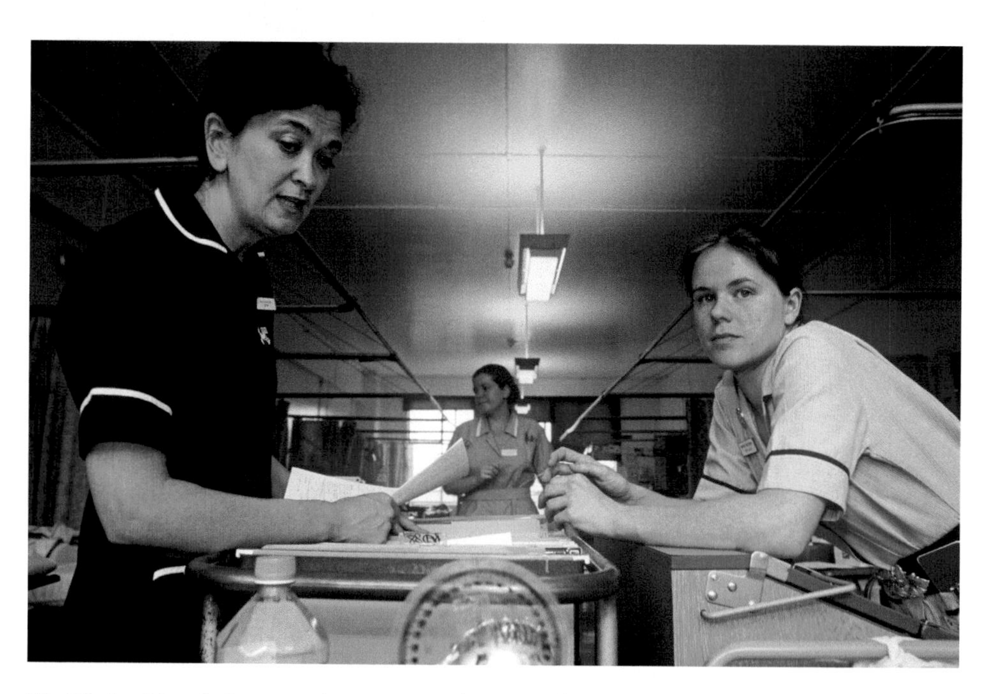

11. Under New Labour in the 1990s and 2000s, the NHS underwent a second wave of modernisation, which emphasised introducing market principles into the service. These reforms proved controversial and could sometimes result in deteriorating conditions for patients and staff. However, the party also boosted NHS spending to its highest level proportionate to GDP, revamped its facilities and reduced waiting times.

12. The popular tradition of observing NHS 'birthdays' began as an act of protest by trade unions in the 1980s. If these occasions lost some of their radical edge later under New Labour, the party still entrenched the celebration of a welfare institution and its social democratic values on a mass scale. The NHS logo on the bottom of this image – in Pantone 300 blue and Frutiger Bold Italic font – was rolled out in time for the fiftieth anniversary. It provided a sense of coherence for the service and became one of the most famous 'brands' in the world.

nhs
50
NHS
1948 - 1998

Sylfaenydd y Gwasanaeth Iechyd Gwladol
ANEURIN BEVAN
1897 - 1960
Founder of the National Health Service

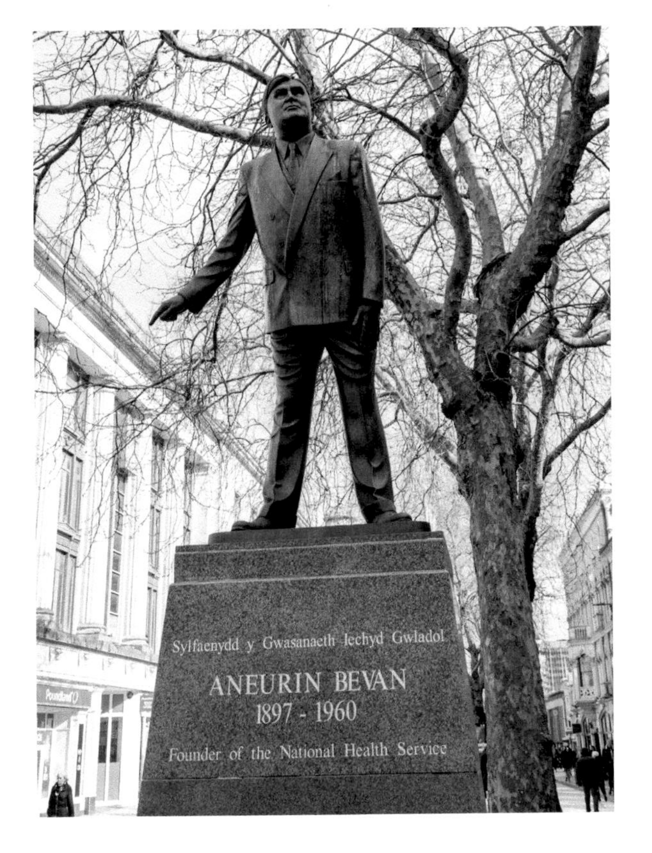

13. Aneurin Bevan (1897–1960) was a democratic socialist who rose from working in the coal mines to presiding over the legislation that established the NHS as Minister of Health and Housing in the postwar Labour governments. A charismatic – and sometimes polarising – figure, by the end of the twentieth century he was widely remembered as a 'founding father' of the NHS, with statues erected in his memory, like this one placed in Cardiff in 1987.

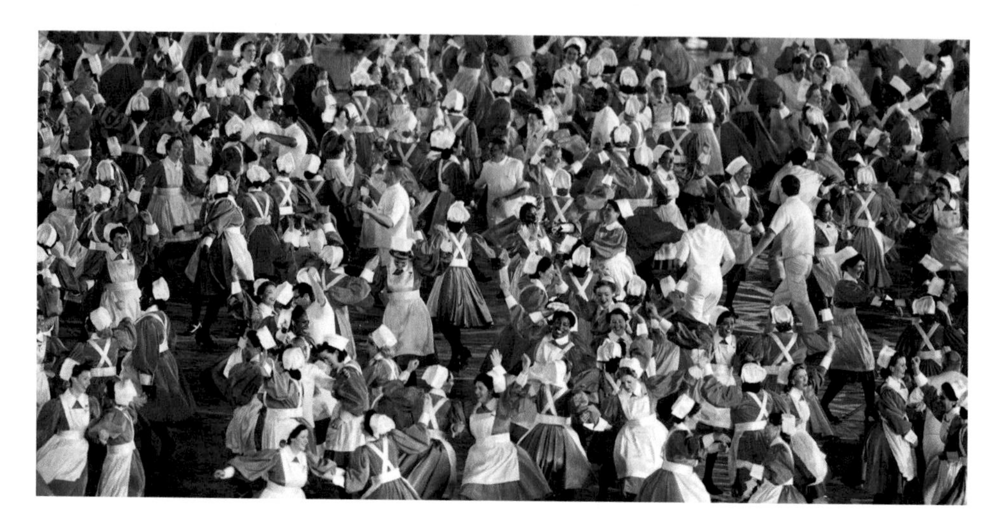

14. By the millennium, the NHS stood as a colossus in public life. Though changed from its origins during the 1940s, it had become the fifth-largest employer in the world, overtaken older rivals like education in terms of public spending, and it was celebrated like no other state institution. Moments like the Opening Ceremony of the 2012 London Olympic Games confirmed the significance of the NHS, reinforcing the findings of multiple opinion polls that it was the thing that made people 'most proud to be British'.

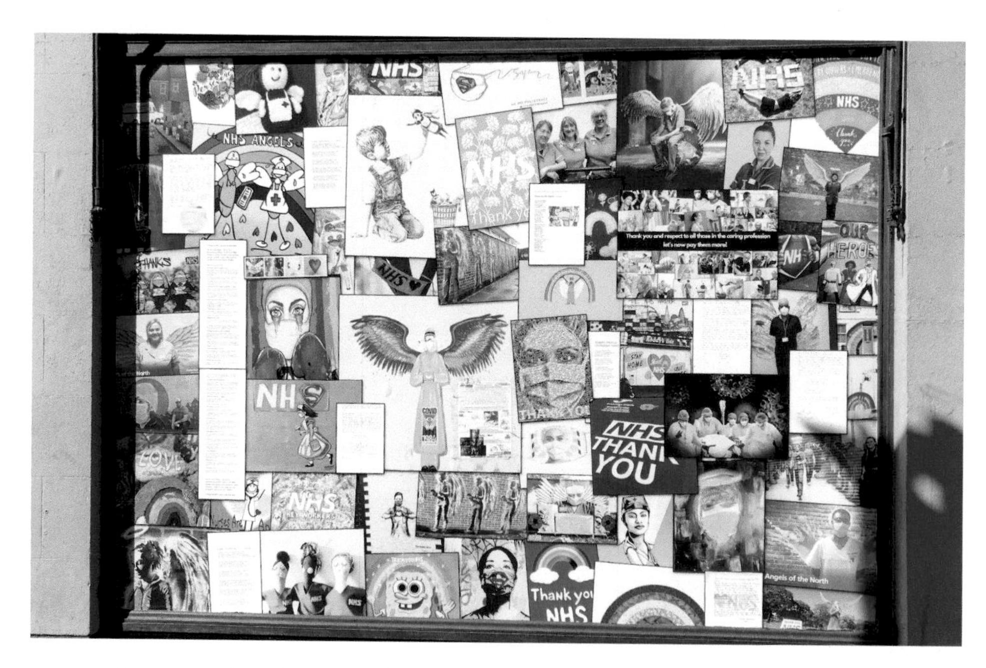

15. During the COVID-19 pandemic, celebrations of the NHS intensified, including offering the institution 'thanks' in public spaces like this street in Oxford. Poorer communities and ethnic minorities suffered a greater loss of life as a result of the pandemic, underlining longstanding health inequalities. Even though the NHS and its social democratic principles survived the twentieth century, the service could only do so much given the collapse after the 1980s of other public initiatives and institutions also aimed at reducing social inequity.

they are ill and it is a third-rate service that renders this problematical everywhere and impossible over a wide area'.

Some critics of Britain's reliance on overseas medical labour recommended that the government place greater emphasis on race in future recruitment. A Liverpool surgeon in gynaecology and obstetrics named Henry Vincent Corbett made such an argument in a letter to John Biggs-Davidson MP, a member of a group that opposed non-white immigration into Britain called the Conservative Monday Club.[79] Corbett began by making a distinction between the quality of doctors from the 'Old' Commonwealth (countries such as Australia and Canada) and those from the 'New' Commonwealth (countries such as India and Pakistan). 'Some way must be found . . . to permit settlement here if desired, of first rate white immigrants from the "old" Commonwealth', he urged. Corbett's strategy lay in offering white doctors 'suitable posts in the Junior Hospital grades on arrival, without having to apply for jobs'. Non-white doctors, by way of contrast, should be encouraged to leave after they fulfilled their training in Britain. Corbett was aware that his ideas might be dismissed as 'unfair discrimination'. 'In practice', he countered, 'discrimination must rightly be exerted on humanitarian grounds because all countries in the "new" Commonwealth are said to be hopelessly under-doctored'. In Corbett's view, the shortage of doctors in the Global South – which was, after all, caused in part by the draw of health services in former imperial powers like Britain – could be used as cover for denying their recruitment in the NHS. When civil servants considered Corbett's idea, one remarked that they could 'see some advantages from our point of view . . . in distinguishing between doctors from the old and the new Commonwealth', but concluded it was not possible.

As these remarks illustrated, the contributions of immigrant workers in the NHS could be overshadowed by their race. On the one hand, professionals such as Ossie Fernando recalled that they did not experience any racial discrimination within the service, either from colleagues or patients. What mattered, Fernando recounted, was that he could do his job. The study of hospital doctors in North-West England found that only 9 per cent of non-white practitioners experienced 'prejudice' in relationships with their patients.[80] Racism did not permeate the service to the extent that it could not function. In one overseas doctor's view, if race was the primary thing that people thought about when accessing care, 'you wouldn't have a health service at all in this region'. On the other hand, many professionals felt that such bias shaped career opportunities in the NHS. The North-West of England study found that almost a quarter of both white and non-white doctors mentioned situations where comparatively qualified people went up for the same job, but the non-white doctor did not get the position.

Professional hierarchies shaped attitudes towards workers of colour in the NHS. Some members of the public might have felt freer to racially abuse a nurse than a senior consultant. Ermine Rodgers experienced such mistreatment when working with the elderly, some years after she had left Trinidad to take employment in the NHS as a nurse during the 1960s.[81] One afternoon, Rodgers and a white colleague were asked to bathe a patient. Rodgers remembered that when her colleague left, the patient 'began abusing me about the colour of my skin, splashing the water, hitting out'. Rodgers described this experience as a rare occurrence – 'she was just an angry old woman as I know everyone is not like that'. Nonetheless, such episodes underlined the racism that could be directed at immigrant professionals in the NHS, regardless of the institution's reliance on their labour.

Further denigration of non-white medical professionals, and questions about whether immigrants had the right to access NHS care, could be found in the letters sent to Enoch Powell. In 1968, Powell delivered an inflammatory address to a Conservative Association meeting in Birmingham – later dubbed the 'Rivers of Blood' speech.[82] He argued that the degree of Commonwealth immigration into Britain was tantamount to 'a nation busily engaged in heaping up its own funeral pyre' and would inevitably lead to racial violence. Much of Powell's speech centred on the access of foreign-born persons to welfare services, which he claimed came at the expense of white Britons. The ability of Commonwealth immigrants to access 'the rights of every citizen, from the vote to free treatment under the National Health Service' squeezed out, Powell argued, worthier recipients. Despite the fact that people of colour were often discriminated against when accessing welfare services, Powell maintained that white Britons now occupied the disadvantaged position.[83] 'They found their wives unable to obtain hospital beds in childbirth, their children unable to obtain school places, their homes and neighbourhoods changed beyond recognition, their plans and prospects for the future defeated', he lamented. The NHS sat, in Powell's mind, at the forefront of a mix of welfare services that immigrants had less of a right to access than their white British counterparts, even if he omitted his own role in having boosted Commonwealth immigration when recruiting NHS staff at the Ministry of Health. Peter White, who had left Curaçao to work in the 'Mother Country' during the 1950s, put Powell's stance another way, remarking that 'he had been the minister who had gone to the Caribbean pleading on bended knees for our Prime Ministers to send workers to this country'.[84] Once the contents of Powell's speech became known outside Birmingham, Conservative Party leader Edward Heath quickly sacked him from the Shadow Cabinet for inciting racial hatred.

Cast into the political wilderness, Powell still received an outpouring of support.[85] Hundreds of East London dockers went on strike in solidarity, and thousands of Britons wrote him letters. Much of this correspondence focused on immigration, including its relationship to medical care. In 1973, Mr S.J. Turner complained to Powell about emigrating British doctors and their replacement with Commonwealth practitioners unable to 'understand our language sufficiently well to comprehend' their patients, and offered the opinion that 'there were too many immigrants in this country, and the matter was out of hand already'.[86] These types of complaint rarely, if ever, mentioned the large numbers of Irish doctors and nurses working in the NHS, underlining the significance of race, and not just foreignness, to discussions of medical immigration.[87] Descriptions of 'coloured staff' who 'sit around' accompanied one nurse's declaration, 'up Rt. Hon Enoch Powell, to hell with the blacks'.[88] 'You are of course right about the consequences of staffing the hospitals to so large an extent with staff who are not from this country', agreed Powell.

The letters to Powell also showed how, when presented with a non-white doctor or nurse on visiting their local hospital or GP surgery, some members of the public requested a white professional. NHS services could even accommodate such requests. When Mrs G.D. Shepherd from Newport, Wales, cancelled a hospital appointment to treat jaundice in early 1972 upon discovering that her examination would be conducted by an Indian doctor, a nurse helped her find a white doctor on a subsequent visit.[89] 'I feel it is quite wrong that I should be expected to go against all my principles and be examined by an Indian', Shepherd told Powell, adding – in an echo of the Fellowship's logic – that examination by a foreign doctor would be 'useless' as she would not 'have any confidence in his skill or viewpoint'. However, a different outcome occurred when James Johnson from Durham visited his local hospital to treat a rib injury. When he asked if he could be attended 'by a white person', one nurse told him he would have to take the staff who were present or leave. Shocked, Johnson left and received treatment at another hospital from a white doctor. 'I am now worried in case I might need medical attention for a more serious reason', Johnson confided to Powell, 'and I just could not allow a coloured person to touch me'. These views revealed hostility to the inversion of status hierarchies that examination by a non-white practitioner engendered. They also showed fears about the proximity between races created by medical encounters. 'What right have I under the National Health Scheme', he asked, concluding that 'It would now seem that a decent white person in this country has no rights'.

This language of 'rights' revealed the wider questioning over who could legitimately make claims on the NHS, as well as a different point of entry to welfare nationalism for those with a conservative viewpoint. The provision of social services to new arrivals in Britain ranked among the most pressing concerns in wider discussions of immigration.[90] As a result, the growing sense of popular possession of the NHS could dovetail with anti-immigration politics. After all, Powell's 'Rivers of Blood' speech testified how health care sat alongside school places and council houses as areas of controversy. His supporters were similarly incensed. One man expressed his 'fury' after reading a 1973 *Daily Mirror* article about foreign-born patients: 'Can we really afford to be so generous with our scarce medical resources that we are able to permit foreigners to take advantage of them in this way to the detriment of our own people?'[91] Another woman from North Yorkshire recounted to Powell claims from her granddaughter, who was a pharmacist, about Pakistani immigrants 'obtaining £'s worth of tablets free' and then leaving the country. When her granddaughter refused to provide more than a month's supply to one patient, their doctor – who she made sure to mention was also Pakistani – intervened to ensure that the required three months' prescription was fulfilled. These events left the correspondent's granddaughter to surmise that they had conspired to sell medicines abroad at the expense of the British taxpayer. At a point when the left fostered welfare nationalism around the NHS by rhetorically fixing it in opposition to US health care, similar feelings were engendered by conservatives through reference to immigration. As a result, the public awareness of 'our' medical resources, 'our' people and indeed 'our NHS' brought in both sides of the political spectrum.

Regulatory changes to the recruitment of foreign doctors in the 1970s and 1980s followed, in part, from this outpouring of tensions around immigrants' rights to health care and the politicisation of issues like linguistic ability.[92] In 1971, 1972 and 1975, the General Medical Council (GMC) withdrew its recognition of medical degrees from Sri Lanka, Pakistan and India, respectively. Reversing older imperial trends, doctors arriving in Britain now had to undergo an examination. The Temporary Registration Assessment Board of the GMC administered these tests, which included a language component. As with immigration policy more generally, both the Labour Party and the Conservative Party enacted legislation that restricted the flow of foreign medical workers. The Medical Act 1978, passed by a Labour government, formalised the controls on doctors predominantly drawn from the Commonwealth. By the mid-1980s, the Conservative government made foreign-born doctors prove that they were applying for a job that could not be filled by a British-born doctor. The NHS continued to depend on overseas labour – it could not function without it. Nonetheless, the legislative changes of this moment delivered on the wider cultural attitudes towards the service's overseas employees, amplified by voices like the Fellowship.

In the wake of this expanded regulation lay the practitioners. Dr A.F.A. Sayeed, from the Overseas Doctors Association (ODA), summed up the imbalance between the historic commitment of his members to the NHS and their treatment by various governments.[93] 'Our settlement in this country was not by our choice alone,' wrote Sayeed in the late 1970s, 'the successive Governments' policy or rather lack of it, for the last two decades are equally responsible'. 'Now a large number of us are settled here,' he added, 'We are part of the multi racial society'. Sayeed underlined how they had 'served and are serving the NHS with unparallel devotion, dedication and diligence, yet we were neglected too often and too long'. Sayeed's words dovetail with the historian Kennetta Hammond Perry's depiction of the position of many Commonwealth migrants in postwar Britain – people who frequently asserted a heartfelt right to belong in their new home, but who faced denials of that same sense of belonging.[94]

***

The workers who arrived in Britain during the postwar decades staffed a modernising health service crying out for doctors, nurses, porters, cleaners and ambulance drivers. As government officials understood, their labour made the NHS's promise of health for all possible. Many people recognised and appreciated these contributions. Some Britons, though, thought that their presence in the health service exemplified wider problems with the nation's new relationship to its former colonies. To them, a Black face in a white coat on a hospital ward was just as troubling as a Black face in the factory or pub. It represented the same problem. These Britons also questioned whether immigrants had the right to access the health service. The growing belief in the NHS as a uniquely British achievement, then, created barriers, which were sometimes racialised. Opponents of the NHS placed these distinctions into sharp relief by whipping up controversy over issues such as the balance between the emigration and immigration of medical professionals. The UK, they claimed, lost its home-grown talent to greener pastures abroad, as 'inferior' overseas doctors took their places. Both the Fellowship and Powellism contributed to the tighter regulation of overseas workers in the NHS, and a general atmosphere of stricter immigration controls, introduced by both Conservative and Labour governments in 1962, 1968 and 1971. In many respects, the NHS personified the history of decolonisation and immigration in Britain after 1945 – a story of both opportunity and prejudice. The economic arguments advanced by critics like the Fellowship against what they scathingly referred to as a 'Sacred Cow' had made comparatively little headway. However, new opportunities for the NHS's free-market opponents were about to open up during the political and economic tumult of the 1970s.

PART III

'CRISIS' AND SURVIVAL

6

THE LIMITS OF FREE-MARKET MEDICINE

In July 1974, three factions sat around a table at the Department of Health and Social Security (DHSS), the centre of gravity for NHS policy after the Ministry of Health's reorganisation six years earlier.[1] They met in Alexander Fleming House, South London – an impressive concrete building and the pride of its modernist architect, Ernő Goldfinger (a man famous for both his soaring tower blocks and for being the inspiration behind the Bond villain with the same name). The government made up the first faction, represented by the new Labour Secretary of State, Barbara Castle (1910–2002). Hailing from a Labour family outside of Sheffield, she was a household name for championing socialism and women's rights. Like most politicians, her ministerial career encompassed its fair share of contradictions. A radical 'Bevanite' in her youth, she had still tried to introduce legislation to curb trade unions from striking in the mid-1960s. A smoker, she now led a department fighting the scourge of lung cancer. The second faction comprised a trade union delegation from Charing Cross Hospital, led by an older woman called Esther Brookstone. Dubbed the 'battling granny' by her critics at the *Daily Mail*, this grey-haired union steward opposed the presence of private medicine in the public NHS and had shut down a pay-beds ward in protest (Figure 14). The hospital's consultants formed the third faction. They wanted Charing Cross's private patients to stay, as their income partly depended on patients paying for care. As a contest over the balance between the state and the market, the Charing Cross

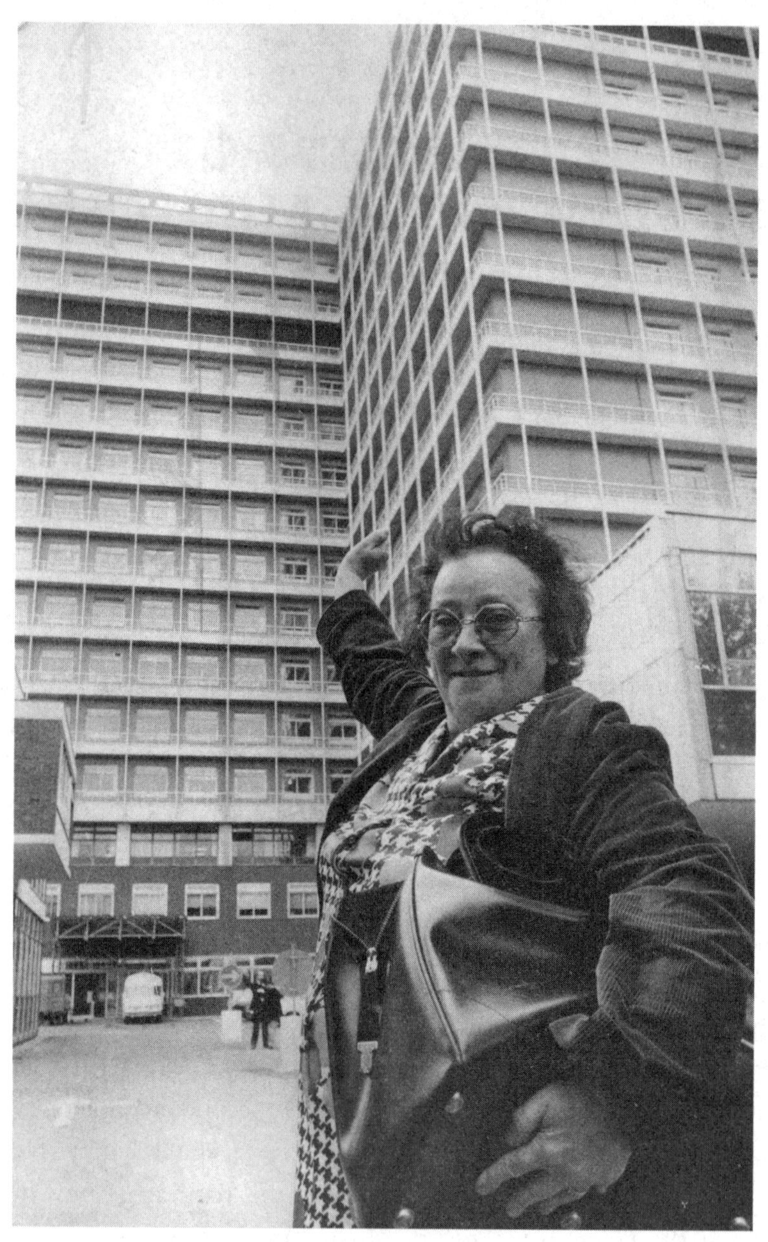

14. During the 1970s, economic shocks fuelled radical demands to alter the pre-existing balance between state and markets in the NHS. In 1974, the trade union steward Esther Brookstone closed down a ward for private patients at Charing Cross Hospital, London, to protest their presence within the public NHS.

dispute encapsulated the struggle between social democratic and neoliberal politics intensifying around the NHS during the 1970s and 1980s.

As the earlier activism of groups like the Fellowship for Freedom in Medicine confirmed, no 'consensus' had ever existed on the funding and organisation of the health service.[2] Although the state dominated the medical sphere after 1948 – and both main parties at least publicly supported this depth of government intervention – both the political left and the political right consistently pushed at the margins of the status quo. The left wanted to expand the boundaries of the NHS. Bevan, for instance, had even proposed nationalising the pharmaceutical industry and assorted private suppliers of medical equipment in order to save the service money.[3] In the early 1970s, radical left-wing supporters of the NHS like Brookstone began to openly call for the government to abolish private medicine on its wards and consulting rooms, so that resources could then be focused on public patients. On the back of trade union pressure, the Labour Party adopted this stance as official policy. However, the Charing Cross disagreement came about because the unions felt that Labour moved too slowly to purge private health care from the NHS when it returned to government.[4] The ideological disagreements that had always framed discussion about the service were moving into the open, even provoking tensions among its longstanding supporters.

The political and economic turbulence of the 1970s created the conditions for such previously marginal positions to move in from the fringe.[5] In 1973, an oil crisis shook the industrialised world. The Organization of the Petroleum Exporting Countries (OPEC) boycotted Western nations for their support of Israel during the Yom Kippur War, causing oil prices to quadruple. In Britain, the nation entered an extended period of economic turmoil as industry suffered, unemployment returned and inflation soared. Edward Heath's Conservative government implemented a three-day working week after coal miners and railway workers went on strike to secure their livelihoods. Forced into a humiliating U-turn in its battle with the labour movement, the Conservative Party lost power in 1974 to Labour, which faced many of the same problems. Labour presided over a sterling crisis in 1975, leading the government to borrow $3.9 billion from the International Monetary Fund (IMF). The decade ended with Labour crashing out of power after a wave of strikes that would long be remembered as the 'Winter of Discontent'. Battles between Esther Brookstone and the Charing Cross consultants seemed like symptoms of the malaise gripping the nation as a whole.

Margaret Thatcher exploited this sense of crisis – which was, like any crisis, used for particular ends – to secure electoral victory in 1979 and usher in a different kind of radicalism.[6] Castle initially welcomed Thatcher as a breath of fresh air. 'After all', she remarked in her diary, 'men have been running the show as long as anyone can remember and they don't seem to have made much of a job of it'.[7] Despite these words of admiration, Castle and Thatcher held little common ground in their politics. The new Conservative government initially sought to use the disruptions of the 1970s as a platform to enact a neoliberal programme in health care. They expressed no love for the NHS's social democratic principles, and were much more strident in criticising them than their Conservative predecessors. Instead, private health insurance, they maintained, would best ensure choice and self-reliance as it connected individuals to their medical expenses and encouraged purchasing services on an open marketplace. The communalism of the nationalised service, they also implied, was inferior to the sanctity of an individual hospital room or private doctors' clinic. Whereas the left wanted to stamp out private medicine, a constellation of think tanks, insurance industry leaders, medical professionals and Conservative Party politicians pursued its expansion so that the NHS might become irrelevant or even disappear altogether. Rather than 'rolling back' the state, as neoliberal politics is often depicted, these groups deployed the state to pursue this primary objective.[8] Historians have largely downplayed the long campaign to marginalise or replace the NHS out of a view that the Conservative Party embraced the service as a cheap means of keeping health spending low or that they always intended to merely adjust its administration.[9] The decades of neoliberal thinking about the superiority of private medicine over the NHS, not to mention the well-formulated proposals among Conservatives to shift the overall balance in medical care towards the market, spoke to much grander ambitions. This longer-term goal – which lay at the heart of free-market aspirations – deserves attention alongside the internal reforms to management structures or service procurement that eventually transpired.

However, the NHS would be a difficult beast to slay. The postwar modernisation of the service had, after all, met with some success by the 1970s. It was not some clapped-out or discredited state industry. Rather, this welfare institution had proved itself capable of responding to social change and enjoyed a swelling wave of welfare nationalism that entrenched popular support for its social democratic values. The defenders of the service – despite the differences within the left on issues like pay-beds – launched counterattacks to discredit insurance-based alternatives. Nonetheless, with the NHS facing its most openly hostile government to date under Thatcher, its survival hung in the balance.

THE FALL AND RISE OF PRIVATE MEDICINE

Thatcher did not pluck her vision for diminishing the role of the state in health care from thin air, nor did she act alone. She drew on a much longer tradition in free-market thinking that responded to the curious position of private medicine after 1948. Implementing the nationalised service had not led to the end of private health care. Bevan's concessions to the medical profession to secure their support for the NHS had allowed fee-based medicine to continue. Britain's GPs could still take on patients who preferred to pay for care, as family doctors insisted on being 'private contractors' rather than NHS 'employees'. Few patients, though, opted to pay. In 1952, only 2 per cent of people used a private GP in conjunction with the state service, and only 1.5 per cent relied on private practice exclusively.[10] In hospitals, private medicine clung on through pay-beds. Consultants on their rounds would talk with NHS patients on the public wards and then bustle down the corridor to speak with their private clients. This coexistence between the public and private realms rankled those on the left who had hoped that nationalisation might mark the end of what they perceived to be the grubby business of paying for medicine. But they took heart from the predictions of the service's early proponents, like William Beveridge, that in areas such as general practice the numbers of people willing to pay 'will be so restricted that it may not appear worthwhile to preserve it'.[11]

However, private medicine did not wither on the vine. Even if its leaves shrunk back after the onset of the NHS, it was able to send out new roots. Provident associations – which were non-profit mutual organisations – underwrote private medicine's revival by offering insurance that covered out-of-pocket health expenses, such as the cost of a pay-bed. The British United Provident Association (BUPA) emerged in 1948 through an amalgamation of pre-war insurance funds.[12] By the mid-1960s, it dominated a revivified private health market that, while tiny compared to total NHS provision, steadily expanded. Subscribers rose from 39,000 in 1947/48 to 252,000 in 1955/56 to 592,000 in 1965/66.[13] BUPA sat alongside Private Patients Plan (PPP) and the Western Provident Association (WPA) as Britain's largest private health insurance providers until the 1970s. In 1950, these three organisations had 56,000 subscribers, insuring 120,000 people. Numbers increased to 274,000 subscribers and 585,000 people in 1955 and, during a sizeable year of growth in 1966, climbed to 735,000 subscribers and 1,445,000 people.

Typical schemes involved a sliding scale of benefits based on a subscriber's annual contributions, determined by whether they joined as an individual or with dependents. BUPA offered a typical middle-aged person subscribing to their cheapest plan in 1962, for example, the promise of £13 13s a week to cover the expense of a private bed in a hospital or nursing home.[14] Such benefits would cost this subscriber £5 17s per annum. Restrictions applied: those aged over sixty-five were not eligible for any of BUPA's schemes and provident associations did not automatically provide coverage for the whole family. Many middle-class professionals, and some working-class people, gained access to health insurance through their jobs. One 1958 survey of 512 major companies found 98 offered such a fringe benefit.[15] By 1971, BUPA boasted that more than 9,000 companies gave access to their schemes, with many firms supplementing their employees' contributions. At the end of the decade, PPP drew approximately two-thirds of its income from group schemes and the remaining third from individual subscriptions. Regardless of where the subscribers came from, private medicine defied the predictions that it would be made irrelevant by the universalist welfare state.

The people who contributed to insurance schemes did so for a range of reasons. Some subscribers wanted to avoid bothersome delays at the GP's surgery or waiting lists for procedures at the hospital. As a health system that provided treatment free at the point of access, the NHS carried the potential for nearly infinite demand. There would always be more consultations, more medicines, more surgeries and more follow-up appointments that could be delivered.[16] The institution managed these pressures through waiting lists. Whereas health systems oriented towards the market allocated finite medical resources by how much money an individual had in their bank account, the NHS allocated finite resources by making patients wait. Bottlenecks often arose because of popular demand for access to innovations in areas like elective surgery. New procedures such as total hip replacement, pioneered in the NHS during the 1960s by John Charnley, attracted huge demand in an ageing society. By the following decade, total hip replacement carried longer waiting lists than any other operation.[17] Health insurance presented a means to shortcut the delays for a new hip, among many other procedures.

The provident associations also directed their marketing at class identities and gender roles. In the early 1960s, BUPA spent £70,000 a year on publicity, delivered by a dedicated sales team, printing plant and modern computers that were large enough to occupy an entire building.[18] The organisation's pamphlets and posters courted a middle-class, professional, male audience. One industry leader emphasised the need to direct campaigns at 'professional men', such as accountants and solicitors.[19] BUPA pamphlets focused on the 'Speed and Convenience' of private health insurance, and 'Freedom of Choice' in arranging appointments to fit around a busy work schedule.[20] The 'home comforts' advertised as part of the individual rooms that insurance usually covered included flexible visiting hours, a television and a telephone that allowed patients to 'keep in touch with your family and business'. PPP claimed to offer schemes 'for both the individual and the family man'. Though they couched their services in the language of individual convenience and personal responsibility, the private health industry banked on the appeal of the traditional masculine ideals of work and the father's role to provide for his family.

Ideas of patient privacy based on class permeated this promotional material. 'The patient wants privacy', offered the Secretary of the WPA, John Dodd.[21] In his mind, that meant as much separation from others as possible. Pointing out that most NHS wards possessed between twenty-eight and thirty-two patients, Dodd expanded: 'If you don't want to be one of the crowd, you must either pay for a private room in an N.H.S. hospital – and there aren't many private rooms – or go outside the N.H.S. altogether'. Dodd also thought that private health insurance offered 'social status' and that affluent Britons associated using the NHS with 'second-class citizenship'. 'And if there's one thing the British middle class hates', Dodd insisted, 'it's being rated as second-class'. Even if surveys showed that most Britons disagreed with such class distinctions in the NHS and favoured communal wards, a number of patients echoed Dodd's sentiments by voicing appreciation for independence and personal space. One subscriber to BUPA confided that through 'being able to be in a room of my own I have sufficient privacy in which to carry on my business'.[22] Another valued 'Quite literal privacy, restive and quiet by day and night'.

NEOLIBERALISM AND PRIVATE MEDICINE

The expansion of the private health market in the 1960s launched a charged debate among economists, social policy experts and politicians about both its future potential and its implications for the NHS. On both the political right and the political left, ideas began to emerge that pushed beyond the British norms in the funding and provision of health care that had existed since 1948. To proponents of free markets, the growth of the health insurance industry offered hope that, if nurtured, it could become big enough to replace the NHS. To left-wing supporters of the nationalised system, private health care needed to either be curbed or eradicated altogether to prevent this same outcome. The emergence of a new academic discipline in the 1960s proved crucial to this debate: 'health economics'.[23] Originating from the US and then establishing itself at the University of York and the University of Exeter, this discipline analysed where the financial resources for medical care came from and how this money might be best put to use. Health economists claimed that they could count the seemingly uncountable. From the thousands of doctors' consultations taking place across the country to the millions of pills swallowed by Britons every year, both the mundaneness and the high drama of medicine could now be tabulated and quantified like never before.

These new economic approaches showed that Britain spent less on health care than other industrialised nations. This point – laid out in pamphlets that placed the country below the likes of France or West Germany – was not new.[24] The LSE social policy expert Richard Titmuss and the economist Brian Abel-Smith had, after all, arrived at the same conclusion in the mid-1950s when completing research for the Guillebaud Report. Their work had torpedoed the FFM's argument that health spending was out of control. However, by the end of the 1960s, low expenditure on health was starting to be seen as a problem rather than an advantage. More money could shorten waiting lists for a new hip, bring in the latest diagnostic technologies or speed hospital construction. In the postwar years, medical advancement required an ever-larger number of pounds, shillings and pence. Given the low health budgets provided by both Conservative and Labour governments since the NHS's inception, the service seemed unlikely to rectify this shortfall any time soon.

Champions of the free market presented private health care as the panacea. The total money spent on medical care in Britain, they suggested, could be expanded far beyond government expenditure by encouraging individuals to dip into their own pockets and purchase health insurance. In other words, more personal spending would grow the pie that health services, as a whole, drew their funds from. The free-market think tank the Institute of Economic Affairs (IEA) served as the main mouthpiece for these arguments during the 1960s. Founded by the businessman and battery farming pioneer Antony Fisher, the IEA promoted alternatives to state planning on a range of issues, from housing to roads to broadcasting. As the historian Ben Jackson reveals, the organisation sat within an extensive network of intellectuals, politicians and business interests.[25] From its offices in a converted Georgian townhouse just around the corner from the Houses of Parliament, it printed books and pamphlets as well as organised conferences and speakers to advance its objectives. Regardless of the matter at hand, they usually believed that the market could do it better than the government. This neoliberal maxim applied to welfare services, too, and the NHS received special attention as a powerful symbol of social democratic universalism.[26] The FFM shared many values with the IEA, and indeed many members, including John Seale, who had brought the doctor emigration crisis to national attention.

Dennis Lees, an economics lecturer at Keele University, was the first IEA author to comprehensively take aim at the NHS through his pamphlet *Health through Choice* (1961).[27] Believing that the service had hitherto avoided vigorous 'economic analysis', Lees detailed the practical and moral failings of government-provided medicine. Like most other neoliberal thinkers, Lees presented health care as an exchangeable consumer product. He insisted that individual choice was paramount, rather than the pursuit of some abstract notion of 'collective provision'. As people now made choices about 'cars and washing machines', he reflected, so they should be encouraged to do the same with their health. To ensure the return of free-market medicine, Lees prescribed the transference of NHS hospitals to private providers and, crucially, the establishment of a system of private health insurance supplied by a network of provident associations. The government could facilitate this transition by giving tax relief on insurance premiums for individuals who withdrew from the NHS. Lees insisted that poorer Britons who could not afford insurance would be protected through government-issued – and means-tested – health 'vouchers' that could be exchanged for care from private providers. Rather than pushing the state back, then, he wanted the government to create and protect a new, mass health insurance market. Conscious that his proposals might be seen as a step backwards from what the NHS provided, Lees demurred that it was 'desirable to put the clock back if it is telling the wrong time'.

These radical approaches to organising and funding health services, the IEA contended, would not only bring greater choice to the consumer but also expanded budgets for the advancement of medical care. If Britons funded their own GP visits or hospital stays, then there would be extra cash to hire doctors, cut waiting lists or purchase the latest diagnostic tools. The US intellectual and later Nobel prize-winner in economics James Buchanan made similar claims in his pamphlet *The Inconsistencies of the National Health Service* (1965), which he based on research undertaken during a Fulbright Scholarship at the University of Cambridge earlier in the decade.[28] To Buchanan, the very premise of the NHS rested on a profound conflict within an individual's behaviour towards social services. On the one hand, he explained, users of the NHS demanded infinite medical resources – more consultations, more pharmaceuticals and more procedures. But on the other hand, as voters, they proved unwilling to pay for the boons of medical science through taxation. The state, therefore, simply did not possess the money to keep pace with rising consumer demand, and the nation staggered on, in his view, with a low-quality health service. In a striking reversal of the earlier conservative position during the panics over NHS spending in the 1950s, the problem now seemed to be insufficient spending on health care, especially compared to countries like the US. 'The failures of the National Health Service', Buchanan opined, 'are not exhibited by a disproportionately large fraction of British resources being drained away through investment in supplying it; the failures are exhibited by breakdowns in the quality of services themselves due to the disparity between the facilities supplied and the demands made upon them'. The American's solution to this imbalance lay in linking supply with demand through private insurance. Buchanan left the NHS behind for a celebrated career at the University of Virginia, but the IEA's assaults on the institution continued through provocative titles such as Arthur Seldon's *After the N.H.S.* (1968).[29]

The IEA felt that they enjoyed public support for their proposals. Or at least among men. In a series of opinion studies undertaken during the mid-1960s, the think tank asked approximately 2,000 married men across the UK how they felt about taxpayers financing the welfare state, how many of them used private services, and how willing they would be to use private alternatives in the future if incomes rose and taxes fell.[30] The IEA justified excluding women out of a paternalistic notion that 'knowledge about and family choice between state and private education, health services and pensions are normally made by the man of the house'. They shared the health insurance industry's faith in the masculine ideal of men providing for their families. As the sociologist Melinda Cooper has demonstrated, neoliberal figures that regularly spoke in terms of freeing the individual from the state just as often wanted government replaced by a gendered notion of familial responsibility.[31] In the IEA's studies, they found support among men for health vouchers that could be spent on the private health market. When respondents were asked if they would take a government health voucher worth £5 or £7 a year towards an estimated total cost of £10 a year spent on health care, which left a shortfall of £5 or £3 to be made up by the individual themselves, 23 per cent said they would take the £5 voucher and an additional 7 per cent the £7 voucher.

Many champions of the free market thought that rising incomes made it possible for working-class families to afford private treatment. Accordingly, confidence in the prospects of the private health insurance market drew on contemporary understandings that, as postwar austerity and rationing receded into the distance, an 'Affluent Society' had emerged.[32] As in most other industrialised nations, living standards among Britons rose across these decades. On average, weekly wages more than doubled between 1945 and the early 1960s. Though not all felt the benefits of rising incomes, consumer luxuries like domestic appliances, holidays and automobiles gradually became an integral part of everyday life for the majority of Britons. If the median male worker's earnings in the late 1960s amounted to approximately £24 per week, then seemingly most men, neoliberal thinkers reasoned, could afford to spend somewhere around £6 per annum to pay for private health insurance.[33] This view demonstrated their optimism regarding an individual's ability to always make rational decisions when spending their own money, regardless of the differing levels of information available, especially in complex areas like health care.[34]

Conservative Party politicians critical of the welfare state referenced affluence in their suggestions that most people could, and indeed should, fund their own health care.[35] The party's senior health spokesman in the late 1960s and early 1970s, Dr Wyndham Davies MP, argued that people may have to choose between 'a regular continental holiday for the family as against the regular annual, or divided, payment for a privately secured medical insurance scheme'. To him, holidays sat alongside health care as things that the population could now afford, rendering universal state medicine funded through taxation redundant. The future Conservative Junior Minister for Health and Social Security, Paul Dean MP, made similar statements when offering his opinions on the NHS in a lengthy 1968 television interview. 'You see', Dean opined in his cut-glass accent, 'I think we've got to the position in Britain now where people have got their cars, their television sets, their washing machines, their houses . . . and when they go to a public service, be it the health service or schools, they find waiting lists, bad buildings, and they're noting the contrast'. The public were waiting, Dean surmised, for a party 'to say we will build on it, consumer choice in the same sort of way that you've got consumer choice in these other consumer goods I've mentioned'. When asked by the interviewer if he had BUPA in mind when making these comparisons, Dean nodded emphatically, adding 'Yes, exactly'.

Still far from at peace with the NHS, professional medical organisations sometimes contributed to neoliberal thinking about alternatives in health care. The BMA publication *Health Services Financing* (1970) argued that Britain's poor postwar record of spending on medicine could only be improved by 'private consumption expenditure'.[36] While the association insisted that it did not want to dismantle the NHS, they argued for an expansive 'separate insurance system, paid for directly by consumers'. Underlining the BMA's connections with other critics of the NHS, the founding presidents of the IEA, Arthur Seldon and Ralph Harris, alongside future Conservative Chancellor of the Exchequer Geoffrey Howe, advised on this report's production.

In cloistered meeting rooms, the Conservative Party's Research Department more readily embraced private alternatives to health care.[37] Members included Paul Dean; the son of a British Prime Minister, Maurice Macmillan; and many of the party's most prominent free-marketeers, including Geoffrey Howe and Keith Joseph. Crucially, Margaret Thatcher was also a member. Even if the group occasionally viewed IEA-affiliated intellectuals as 'both prolix and extreme in their views', they drew up various policy statements that echoed the institute's priorities. 'We welcome the growth in private health and welfare provision', the group affirmed during one discussion, adding their rejection of 'the drab uniformity of the egalitarian doctrine'. In 1970, they declared that while Labour saw 'danger' in the growth of private medicine, they thought it was 'right and proper that people should be free to provide for themselves and their families if they wish'.[38] Thatcher's engagement with proposals to marginalise or replace the NHS with private health insurance when she later came to power was not a fleeting dalliance, but rather an extension of her longer-term membership of groups that advanced such goals.

By the 1970s, then, the increased take-up of health insurance, popular affluence and changing intellectual and political priorities had enabled alternatives to the NHS to gain currency among the advocates of neoliberal approaches in social policy. Nevertheless, their opponents on the left held their own views about what should be done with the increased take-up of health insurance. The economic tremors that were soon to rock Britain opened up this debate to a much wider range of participants and provided opportunities for both sides of the ideological dispute to make headway.

'CRISIS', PAY-BEDS AND AMERICAN DANGER IN THE 1970S

The turbulence of the 1970s carried significant consequences for the NHS. In an immediate sense, health budgets swelled as governments ramped up public spending to reverse the economic downturn caused by the oil shock, only to nosedive as the Treasury reversed position and opted for fiscal retrenchment. NHS spending as a proportion of GDP boomeranged from 3.5 per cent at the start of the 1970s, to 4.5 per cent in 1974/75, before falling back to 3.9 per cent by the end of the decade.[39] Despite this bumpiness, in general terms, the health service was enjoying more money than ever before. Nonetheless, the stop-start nature of NHS funding fuelled arguments that the service would not be able to complete important modernisation programmes such as the Hospital Plan. Space opened for the ideological debates about health insurance that had raged among experts during the 1960s to spill out into the public arena. Like in other areas of public life, the political right and the left used the widely held belief that Britain had entered a profound moment of crisis in order to experiment with what was possible in the NHS.[40] For the left, the solution lay in expanding the boundaries of the NHS alongside protecting the institution from an 'American invasion' of foreign medical corporations.[41]

For the first time, health unions started to flex their muscles and, in turn, advance radical ideological positions. Strike action of any kind rarely took place in the NHS before the 1970s. As the historian Jack Saunders notes, health workers were constrained by a deferential culture of industrial relations, with doctors at the top and everyone else below.[42] The UK's economic dislocation and internal changes within unions – such as an uptick in elected local union officials negotiating on behalf of their members – transformed this picture. The National Union of

Public Employees (NUPE), National Association for Local Government (NALGO) and the Confederation of Health Service Employees (COHSE) formed the three largest health unions and their members took direct action like never before. In 1973, ancillary workers – who included employees in hospital kitchens and laundries, as well as cleaners and porters – went on strike over low pay.[43] The following year, nurses in NUPE joined them. Though controversial given their historic image as dutiful caregivers, these nurses won public support and a pay rise averaging 30 per cent. The Royal College of Nursing (RCN) registered as a trade union in 1976, perhaps inspired by the successes of their more radical colleagues in NUPE. Even the more conservative-leaning BMA took this step in the 1970s, reversing a decades-long position that doctors should not engage in industrial action. In 1975, the BMA went on strike as part of a disagreement with the government over consultants' contracts in the NHS. No fan of unions, *The Financial Times* diagnosed the NHS with the same 'militancy bug' that, they maintained, infected Britain as a whole.[44]

Industrial action made the ideological disputes over the role of private medicine in the NHS more tangible. The left had long watched the growth of private health insurance with alarm. Sharing none of the optimism of their neoliberal opponents about its future, they foresaw declining standards for the NHS or even its demise. In the early 1960s, union branches thought providing care to patients with insurance who occupied NHS pay-beds represented a waste of resources that could better serve public patients. In 1961, the Hastings and District Trades Council voiced their unease at 'an incursion into the Hospital Service laid down by the National Health Acts'.[45] Other members of the labour movement watched on with trepidation as these 'incursions' became more common.

The stage was set for a public battle over pay-beds hitherto waged through pamphlets, economics journals and in university seminar rooms. In 1973, NUPE passed a resolution at the Labour Party conference to abolish NHS pay-beds. The party duly committed to 'phase out private practice from the hospital service' as part of its General Election manifestos in the following year.[46] This influence on Labour policy reflected unions' expanded significance during the 1970s. Trade union membership reached its peak in this decade, with more than half of all working Britons unionised.[47] New members joined from white collar professions and, particularly significant for the NHS, the public sector. White-collar membership rose by 1,379,000 across the decade. The opinions of trade unions on issues like pay-beds therefore could not be easily ignored.

The assertiveness of the trade unions over pay-beds was also driven by anxieties about US capital flooding into Britain during the 1970s. Large multinational companies, including American Medical International (AMI), Hospital Corporation of America (HCA) and Humana Inc., saw the expanded take-up of health insurance policies in the UK as a business opportunity and started establishing British outposts to take advantage. AMI ranked as the most important of these corporations, recording net profits of over $137 million in 1985.[48] In contrast to the pre-existing British provident associations, these companies pursued profit and deployed new technologies in personal finance, including the 'AMI Card', which allowed patients to pay their medical bills at a fixed monthly rate, with interest.

Whereas the neoliberal figures that advanced changes to Britain's health system revelled in their American connections, the left criticised the reach of the US medical industry. When AMI bought its first British medical facility in Marylebone in 1970, named the Harley Street Clinic, trade unions were enraged.[49] Most alarmingly for the labour movement, the Conservative Secretary of State for Health, Keith Joseph MP, met with AMI to discuss future cooperation between private enterprise and the NHS. Joseph had also hired the US management consultancy firm McKinsey to advise on the 1973 reorganisation of the NHS, underlining the growing impact of American expertise.[50] A 1973 TUC resolution against pay-beds also mentioned the Harley Street Clinic, calling on 'this present Government and future Governments to reject any proposals from the American Medical International Incorporated or the Harley Street Clinic Limited, or any other person, persons or companies, to set up private hospitals in this country'.[51] In the same year, the Bristol Trades Council voiced its concerns regarding 'newspaper reports that American companies are making enquiries with a view to taking over parts of British hospitals for the treatment of private patients'. The unions' rejection of foreign money in British health care in the 1970s therefore embodied much of the welfare nationalism around the NHS by this point. Not just a bogeyman or rhetorical foil, they felt that US capital now posed a material danger to the British health service.

The Wellington Hospital in St Johns Wood, London, exemplified the unions' fears. Established in 1974 by Dr Arthur Levin, the medical advisor for Rolls-Royce, the hospital was initially funded by capital from his business connections to the British and Commonwealth Shipping Company.[52] However, these British investors soon sold their majority share to Humana Inc., meaning that, from 1976, a US health insurance company owned the largest private hospital in the UK. Levin remained at the Wellington, while also becoming Humana's Executive Medical Director in Europe. British expertise, the company reasoned, might help crack the European market. With 265 beds, a 13-bed intensive care unit, a new CT scanner and services ranging from day surgery to open heart surgery, Humana possessed a $10 million asset that attracted a great deal of attention. During the first year of US ownership, turnover stood at £4.4 million, with a profit of £1.6 million.

Controversy regarding the Wellington stemmed, in part, from the luxuries that its predominantly foreign patients enjoyed compared to the experience of British citizens using the NHS. Prices started at £115 a day, which covered an individual room with a television and telephone, the ability to shop in a deluxe gift store, gourmet meals that included tournedos chasseur and a view of Lord's Cricket Ground. *People* magazine described the Wellington as 'the most sumptuous hospital in the world', and its clientele confirmed that reputation.[53] Both Princess Diana's father, the 8th Earl Spencer, and the star of *Lawrence of Arabia* (1962), Peter O'Toole, spent their last hours in the Wellington. In its early years, he hospital also attracted a wealthy Arab elite looking to spend oil revenues on the best of European medicine. In 1978, between 50 and 60 per cent of the Wellington's patients originated from the Middle East. The prevalence of Arab patients extended to other US-owned private hospitals in London. Of the patients at HCA's Princess Grace Hospital, 70 per cent came from overseas one year after its 1977 opening, and the hospital employed four full-time Arabic interpreters.[54] In a feature on the Princess Grace, the BBC TV programme *Tonight* noted that 'Although it's Central London, the casual visitor can be forgiven for mistaking it for the Riyadh Hilton'.[55] Given an Arab oil embargo had caused so much economic dislocation in the recent past, the management, shareholders and the customer base of the Wellington confirmed, to some observers, 'Britain's fallen place in the world, as yet another threat to its flagging economy, if not its heritage and whole way of life'.[56]

When Labour returned to power in 1974, they had to transform the unions' pay-beds concerns into policy. To be sure, key members of the government, like Barbara Castle, shared their apprehensions about the mix of international influences that seemed to encircle the NHS. However, the unions felt that the government moved too cautiously. In tense meetings with NUPE, Castle responded to demands to end private practice in the NHS 'as quickly as possible' by insisting that while 'no difference in principle' existed between the government and the unions, 'phasing out private practice from NHS hospitals had to be implemented in an orderly way after negotiation with those affected'.[57] In no mood for ponderous negotiation, many union branches undertook strike action against private wings in NHS hospitals. Brookstone's charge against the Charing Cross Hospital pay-beds became the first site of such labour unrest in 1974.

The drama at Charing Cross caught the attention of the award-winning filmmaker Lindsay Anderson. Rising to fame on the back of a satire of the British public school system in *If. . .* (1968), he continued the story of his protagonist, Mike Travis, in *O Lucky Man!* (1973). The trilogy's final instalment, *Britannia Hospital* (1982), took aim at unions in the NHS.[58] While Travis's story culminates in a bizarre Frankenstein's monster transformation, much of the film follows tensions between trade unionists, private patients and hospital administrators preparing for a visit from a member of the Royal Family described only as 'HRH'. Phyllis Grimshaw – an unsubtle caricature of Brookstone – heads a shutdown of Britannia Hospital to oppose the preferential treatment of private patients. However, Grimshaw quickly buckles once promised the opportunity to hobnob with royalty. Among her members, kitchen workers and porters still refuse to serve the pay-bed patients their meals. The private ward's irate occupants include an aristocratic gentleman, an African dictator and a cabbie having a hip replacement. The union instigators eventually follow Grimshaw's example by betraying their principles for fleeting personal gain. For their part, the hospital's administrators agree to the unions' demands to expel private patients in an attempt to restore peace for HRH's visit. Albeit through a somewhat confused political message and absurdist visuals, Anderson had brought the battle over pay-beds to the silver screen.

Back in the less glamorous corridors of the DHSS, the issues raised by the Charing Cross dispute still had to be dealt with. The delays in abolishing pay-beds stemmed from internal divisions within the Labour government. Castle's subordinate, Minister of Health Dr David Owen, feared that removing private beds from the NHS might precipitate their rapid expansion outside of it. Though distasteful, keeping the private sector within the boundaries of the NHS, he reasoned, meant that it could be controlled. Cautious civil servants felt similarly, and warned that 'sizeable competition from a private practice sector at this stage and in this atmosphere could do grave harm to the NHS itself'.[59] As a more moderate politician, Owen regularly disagreed with Castle. He shared, though, her fear of US capital. Owen remarked on the 'risk that private hospital care would be increased if private hospitals came to be run by an aggressive profit-making firm owned, for example, by American hospital or nursing home chains or by pharmaceutical firms'.[60] In correspondence with Castle, Owen advised his boss that Labour did not always need to keep the unions onside, and that 'we must now accept that there are far larger issues involved than the

Manifesto or our loyalty to our supporters'. 'I do not believe I exaggerate by saying', he continued in a reference to negotiations with consultants, 'that if we get the policy wrong there is a real risk that hospital doctors may impose a system of item by service payment and become independent contractors to the NHS on somewhat similar lines to the family doctors'.[61] In response to these concerns, Castle and her advisor Brian Abel-Smith agreed that coupling pay-bed abolition with licensing legislation to control the private sector promised the best way forward.

The pay-bed issue also formed part of the Labour government's attempts to tackle stubborn health inequalities in the UK. By the 1970s, even supporters of the NHS expressed frustration with the service's inability to eradicate the differences in health outcomes between regions and social classes. Richard Titmuss lamented how 'the higher income groups know how to make better use of the service'.[62] The sharp-elbowed middle classes, he showed through statistics, received 'more specialist attention; occupy more of the beds in better equipped and staffed hospitals; receive more elective surgery; have better maternity care, and are more likely to get psychiatric help . . . than low-income groups – particularly the unskilled'. In 1971, the GP Julian Tudor Hart published a famous *Lancet* article theorising these imbalances as an 'inverse care law', which posited that 'the availability of good medical care tends to vary inversely with the need for it in the population served'. Put another way, communities suffering from a high degree of poor health too often lacked the quality of care required to address such problems. The use of techniques in health economics by Titmuss and Tudor Hart showed how the discipline was not just deployed to try and discredit nationalised medicine but could form the basis of proposals to improve it. Indeed, the Labour government took the numbers showing health inequality seriously enough to establish a Resource Allocation Working Party (RAWP) in 1975 that introduced a new formula to distribute NHS funding based on need rather than historical precedent.[63] For the critics of pay-beds, the abolishment of private medicine in the NHS would free up precious resources that could then be redistributed to poorer communities.

However, the insurance industry and significant parts of the medical profession were not persuaded by these justifications to abolish pay-beds and instead launched a popular campaign against the government. In spring 1976, the BMA, BUPA, PPP and the Association of Independent Hospitals formed an organisation called 'Independence in Medicine'.[64] The campaign sought to combat social democracy's threat to, in the words of BUPA, 'the individual's right to enjoy freedom of choice, which was at the very root of BUPA's creed and thinking'.[65] In language that echoed that of the FFM, the campaign even claimed that Labour's measures would result in 'the justification for the watch-tower, the searchlight, and the Berlin Wall'.[66] They placed advertisements in national newspapers and emblazoned pamphlets, posters, car stickers and badges with their slogan 'Patients Before Politics'. 'General practitioners' surgeries are an ideal outlet,' they told their members, 'We urge you to display the posters in your waiting room, to give out the leaflets, and to leave the lapel badges so that young people can pick them up and wear them'. 'If the public does not see it, we have wasted our efforts', insisted the BMA. The campaign enjoyed some success. Opinion polls found that only 42 per cent of people supported abolishing pay-beds in late 1974, dropping further to 20 per cent by mid-1976.[67] Seemingly, most people did not want pay-beds removed from the NHS.

The dispute between the Labour Party and the medical profession carried a high cost to change just 1 per cent of the NHS's total beds. In 1976, after negotiations between doctors and the government, Labour eventually succeeded in enacting legislation that abolished pay-beds. The newly established Health Services Board slowly phased out these beds from the NHS in the late 1970s, reducing them from 3,444 in 1976 to 2,533 in 1979.[68] But this reduction proved a pyrrhic victory. The new Labour Prime Minister, Jim Callaghan, sacked Castle upon taking office and rendered the pay-beds policy rudderless. The government did not append licensing legislation to regulate the private medical sector, provoking exactly the expansion that Castle and Owen had predicted earlier in the decade. Pushed outside of the NHS, with their previous acceptance inside the service seemingly no longer a viable path to future growth, private medicine sought to go it alone. The sector now better aligned with the ambitions its neoliberal boosters had invested it with during the 1960s. On 3 May 1979, one of these early supporters, Margaret Thatcher, became Prime Minister.

THATCHERISM AND THE NHS

Thatcher's Conservative governments (1979–1990) began with a radical antidote for the poisons of inflation and trade union acrimony that they claimed had plagued the 1970s. The cure lay in markets. They sold nationalised enterprises like British Gas and British Telecom to private shareholders, defeated organised labour during the 1984 miners' strike and deregulated the stock market in the 1986 'Big Bang'.[69] Through these changes, Thatcher pursued a moral project that sought to foster self-reliance.[70] Accordingly, the Conservatives also aimed to 'residualise' the welfare state by making it the crutch of the very poor, rather than a set of services regularly accessed by all Britons.[71] Welfare, in their view, needed to be selective rather than universal.[72] The government privatised council housing, widened the gap between in-work and out-of-work incomes, and introduced harsher methods of managing the unemployed.[73] Thatcher shifted the nature of the welfare state and aspired to accomplish the same thing with what was now its flagship institution: the NHS.

Expanding private health insurance stood at the centre of their initial aspirations. As the most openly critical government of the NHS in the service's history, they seized on the disarray caused by Labour's botched solution to the pay-beds dispute. In anticipation of the 1979 election, the internal Conservative Health Study Group had privately argued that the NHS was 'better discarded altogether and a fresh start made in the light of knowledge accumulated and experience gained'.[74] Tempering these claims in their election manifesto, the Conservative Party still insisted that 'standards are falling' in the service and diagnosed a 'crisis of morale'.[75] The party resolved to 'end Labour's vendetta against the private health sector' and, significantly, suggested the need for 'greater reliance for NHS funding on the insurance principle'.

Through her time as a member of a Conservative health group in the 1960s, Thatcher understood the origins of her party's position. She expressed no affection towards the NHS. In her first speech as Prime Minister in the House of Commons, she took aim at its social democratic universalism by warning that there was 'no such thing as a free service in the Health Service'.[76] Thatcher regularly chastised her ministers if they used the NHS and expressed confusion if they did not opt for private treatment. Whereas former Prime Ministers like Clement Attlee made a point of using the NHS, even just for publicity, Thatcher thought receiving health care from the state set the wrong example. When suffering from a tear in the retina of her right eye in 1983, she chose the Princess Christian Private Hospital in Windsor and made sure to publicly stress the advantages that her BUPA insurance plan provided (Figure 15). In her memoirs, Thatcher later derided the NHS as 'a monolithic state system' and mused that if the service were to be started again 'one would have allowed for a bigger private sector – both at the level of general practitioners . . . and in the provision of hospitals; and one would have given much closer consideration to additional sources of finance for health, apart from general taxation'. As the NHS was a massive state employer with a monopoly on its sector of the economy, it followed that Thatcher would treat it like any other nationalised enterprise. Indeed, the Thatcher government proved reluctant to revive the funding increases that the service had started to enjoy in the early 1970s, squeezing its budget – despite the rising costs and demand for medical care – from 4.4 per cent of GDP in 1980/81 to 3.8 per cent in 1989/90.[77]

The further growth of the private health insurance industry after the pay-beds dispute buoyed Thatcher and fellow supporters of the industry. In the first three years of her premiership, the proportion of the population insured through private schemes rose from 5 per cent to 7.3 per cent.[78] Between 1979 and 1985, the number of private hospitals increased by 35 per cent, and the number of private acute beds provided outside of the NHS expanded by 54 per cent. Much of this expansion was fuelled by US capital, somewhat confirming the fears on the left in

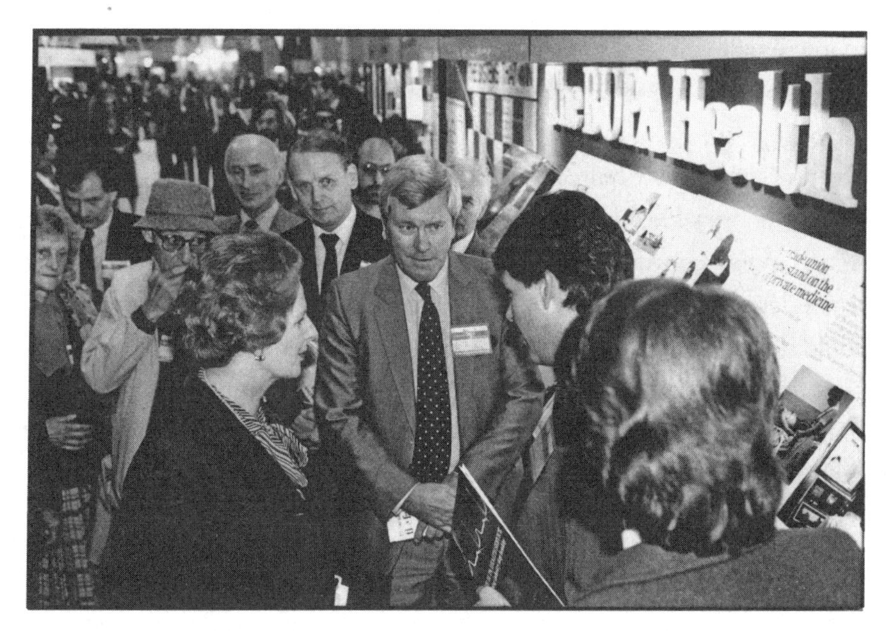

15. The febrile atmosphere of the 1970s also encouraged the proponents of private health insurance. In the previous decade, Margaret Thatcher had belonged to health policy groups within the Conservative Party who believed that organisations like BUPA should form the basis of an alternative medical system to the NHS. After becoming Prime Minister in 1979, Thatcher considered ways to make this goal a reality.

the 1970s about its involvement in British health care. In 1979, US companies owned three hospitals (including the Wellington), but by 1986 they owned thirty-one.[79] With Labour's pay-beds policy separating private medicine from the NHS, US corporations injected the necessary capital to help establish new private hospitals and rooms for patients taking out insurance plans. As the British Insurance Association observed in a meeting with the government, 'The Americans were willing to take greater short-term risks to break into a market but demanded an ultimate return on capital'.

The Conservative government used legislation and parliamentary instruments to engineer an expansion in the take-up of health insurance, following a neoliberal approach to governance, revealed by the historian Quinn Slobodian, where the state protected markets from interference, including from unions.[80] Instead of phasing out pay-beds, the 1980 Health Services Act halted their removal from NHS hospitals by abolishing Labour's Health Service's Board. In the same year, the government signed a new contract with the BMA that allowed all NHS consultants to undertake private practice, whereas beforehand only 'part-timers' could do so. The Chancellor of the Exchequer's budget the following year provided all workers earning less than £8,500 per annum a tax exemption equal to the value of the private health insurance premiums paid by their employers. The government also allowed British businesses to use these premiums to offset corporation tax and relaxed town and country planning legislation to encourage private hospital construction. Taken together, Conservative efforts sought to use the state to create a private health market large enough to rival – or even overwhelm – the NHS.

In 1981, Patrick Jenkin, now Secretary of State at the DHSS, established an inter-departmental committee to examine the 'various ways in which there could be a significant shift from public sector to private insurance financing'.[81] Through its two special advisors, Hugh Elwell, a former General Manager of BUPA, and Michael Lee, founding member of the management consultancy firm Lee Donaldson Associates, the committee tapped into private sector expertise and a broader free-market intellectual ecosystem. It assessed the existing marketplace, spoke with independent hospitals and provident associations, monitored the press and undertook statistical analysis. Civil servants submitted their final report in 1982 with a predictable degree of caution, peppering it with statements like 'market disciplines operate very imperfectly in health care'.[82] All the same, they recommended ways to encourage the population to 'opt out' of the NHS. Newspapers headlines like 'Tories to Unveil New Health Care' and 'Thatcher Backs Shake-up for NHS Finance' showed how these debates grabbed public attention.[83]

Thatcher's government took inspiration from both US and European health systems. As in the 1960s, the advocates of free-market medicine continued to look enviously at the greater dose administered in the US.

Thatcher herself liked the US health system as a model to work towards, in keeping with her admiration of the country exemplified by a close relationship with President Ronald Reagan.[84] The economist staffed on Jenkin's committee undertook a nine-month study of the US to source 'relevant American experience'.[85] Visiting US academics also brought their expertise to Whitehall, giving papers on their country's health arrangements. Nonetheless, the government also took inspiration from health systems in continental Europe. France emerged as an important focal point, with some Conservatives seeing its state insurance fund and higher direct patient contributions as an appropriate middle ground. Junior health minister in the DHSS Gerald Vaughan visited France in late 1979 to see how their health care worked for himself. On his return, he tried to calm fears that changing NHS finance meant 'an automatic return to the pre-Bevan and pre-Beveridge era when ability to pay conditioned individual access to necessary treatment' by arguing that 'We only have to look across the Channel to see health systems operating which are based on social insurance, and which not only give the care they need to all income-levels but do it without long-waiting lists'.

While the details remained to be settled, the proponents of free-market medicine felt that at long last a different future lay within their grasp. Hopes began to rise within the Centre for Policy Studies (CPS), a free-market think tank with direct links to the government established by Thatcher's mentor, Keith Joseph, to 'think the unthinkable'. One member prophesied that 'In 3–4 years time demand for private medicine will be threefold'.[86] Whereas Patrick Jenkin cautioned in the same meeting against thinking 'one leaps straight from present system to "Brave New World"', and argued that a more 'evolutionary route' with 'stepping stones' represented a better strategy, he shared much of their excitement. In the early stages of their time in office, the government welcomed data from Lee Donaldson Associates stating that between one-fifth and one-quarter of the UK's population could be privately insured by the mid-1980s.[87]

A scandal surrounding a policy document leaked to *The Economist* in 1982 hampered the pursuit of the 'Brave New World' in medicine envisioned by its neoliberal advocates.[88] Drawn up by the Central Policy Review Staff (CPRS) and discussed by Thatcher and her Cabinet, the document outlined 'radical options' for trimming back the role of the state in health care. It proposed direct charges for NHS patients, a means test for treatment, a system of compulsory private health insurance for individuals and their dependents and the mass privatisation of state-owned hospitals. 'Even though a free state service would be retained for the uninsured and possibly for the non-working population', the missive noted, 'for the majority the change would represent the abolition of the NHS'. 'This would be immensely controversial', the CPRS warned, in a statement of the obvious.

Despite the ensuing 'storm over secret think tank report', as the *Observer* described it, the document in fact offered nothing more controversial than the proposals contained in the pamphlets, policy statements and speeches produced by various neoliberal thinkers and Conservative Party politicians since the early 1960s.[89] Thatcher's later recollection that she was 'horrified' by proposals that she insisted 'had never been seriously considered by ministers or by me' belied their longer trajectory, as well as her prior contributions as a member of Conservative health policy groups, where she would have regularly been exposed to such ideas .[90] All the same, with one eye on the next General Election, Thatcher felt strong-armed into publicly distancing herself from 'the abolition of the NHS'. On stage in Brighton at the Conservative Party Conference, she claimed 'the National Health Service is safe with us' and subsequently shut down the CPRS.[91]

Yet one misstep was not enough to totally quash long-held ambitions to replace the NHS with private health insurance. Even with the CPRS consigned to the scrapheap, the CPS continued to put forward similar proposals to ministers. The *Economist* leak shook the confidence of some CPS members and raised questions about whether 'the Prime Minister's "disowning" of the report means that the door has been shut in our face as well'.[92] Yet, as the use of scare quotes in this statement suggested, the CPS recognised that Thatcher might not be so easily deterred from their mission to undermine the NHS, and she merely sought to present an image of acquiescing to popular demands. The 1983 Conservative Party General Election manifesto still included statements like 'We welcome the growth of private health insurance in recent years', alongside rejections of 'Labour's contention that the State could and should do everything'.[93] As one CPS member commented, 'The Group may well have to "go to ground" until the row dies down, but the door remains open'.[94] Michael Lee stated that he 'couldn't see what all the fuss was about'. 'The debate has just taken off – now's the time to take the initiative, and win the debate', he enthused.

Regardless of the enduring optimism among its supporters, systemic change in health care escaped the Thatcher government. Civil servants tasked with finding ways to implement the vast structural changes needed to shift Britain to a private insurance-based medical system often thought such a move impossible. The exact costing of treatments and services – necessary for any private insurance-based system with itemised billing – proved hard to gauge in a country where payment for medicine had been pushed to the margins for three and a half decades. Officials struggled to assess how much a coronary bypass or a hip replacement should cost, making meaningful comparisons between the public and private sectors difficult.[95] This reluctance illustrated some degree of path-dependence within Whitehall – shifting from a public health service to a private insurance system was an immense undertaking.[96]

The administrative difficulties in changing the funding and organisation of personal medical services contrasted with the position of public health under the Thatcher government. As the historian Peder Clark makes clear, policy approaches to preventative medicine had undergone a turn towards 'personal responsibility' by the late 1970s.[97] The emphasis that public health experts placed on 'lifestyle' in causing adverse medical outcomes could dovetail with a neoliberal idea that an individual's ill-health resulted primarily from personal choices, and not structural factors like poverty. According to this line of argument, the role of the state lay in empowering individuals to address their own health problems, rather than launching extensive interventions in the name of the 'community' at large. During the late 1980s, for instance, the Conservative government displayed such an approach in its 'Look After Your Heart' campaign, which emphasised the importance of the individual to take personal responsibility for their health and to exercise regularly.[98] The extensive newspaper and television advertising that underpinned this government initiative may have targeted working-class people mainly living in the North of England who experienced higher rates of heart disease, but it did not substantially address the income inequality that also lay behind a lack of exercise, smoking or drinking. It primarily fell upon individuals to improve their lot. The 'public' did not completely disappear from 'public health' in this decade, evidenced by official responses to the HIV/AIDS epidemic that often spoke – in fearful tones – about the threat to the community as a whole. However, campaigns such as 'Look After Your Heart' marked a change from the more community-centred framing of preventative medicine during the early decades of the NHS. In contrast, the Thatcher government enjoyed no such successes in promoting similar notions of personal responsibility in how patients accessed general practice or hospital treatment.

All the same, administrative inertia did not provide the whole answer to why neoliberal aspirations floundered regarding private health insurance. Changes within the insurance industry itself also played a part. The US money that fuelled the boom of the late 1970s and early 1980s eventually destabilised the sector. Companies such as AMI and Humana may have built new hospitals and expanded the number of private beds, but these increases exceeded demand. By the middle of the decade, in some parts of the country occupancy rates stood as low as 60 per cent.[99] Private beds lay empty, personal televisions remained unwatched and French cuisine stayed in the kitchen. British private insurance providers began to resent their US rivals. BUPA tried to continue recruiting customers in an increasingly competitive market by keeping its premiums low, despite spiralling medical inflation between the early 1980s and the early 1990s. BUPA consequently made its first loss in 1981 and posted a record shortfall of £63 million in 1990. Deregulation, foreign capital and rising medical expenses caused volatility to the private health insurance market, forestalling its capacity to assume the role that the supporters of neoliberal politics envisioned for it.

Distaste for US medical culture was not confined to British insurance industry executives. An additional blow for neoliberal ambitions lay in how their favoured alternatives grew to be associated with the inequity of US medicine.

PRIVATE HEALTH INSURANCE AND WELFARE NATIONALISM

The backlash to the *Economist* leak vividly illustrated that public opinion about private health insurance mattered. To have any chance at challenging the supremacy of the NHS, its neoliberal proponents needed to make fee-based care attractive to the average Briton. The Conservative Party enjoyed success in popularising market values in other policy areas, particularly housing, where they packaged the ability to buy one's council house as a step towards self-betterment. Similarly, when the government sold off state industries, they promoted stocks and bonds as a means of bringing the market to the masses.[100] Could medical care offer another opportunity for citizens to become model capitalists? In 1979, the Conservative Health Policy Group had thought 'the first step in reform is to persuade people that reform is necessary', though they conceded that 'entrenched attitudes and modes of thought among some may prove difficult to alter'.[101] As this note of caution suggested, the public's attachment to the NHS could not easily be undone, built as it was over the previous decades and, after the 1970s, imbued with nationalist characteristics. Indeed, supporters of the health service launched their own campaign against private medicine that drew strength from welfare nationalism. The efforts of activists and cultural figures on the left to present health insurance as fundamentally unequal and foreign to the British approach to funding and organising medical services proved an effective counter-attack in the battle for hearts and minds.

The think tanks who supported the expansion of private health insurance like the CPS recognised the urgent need to change public opinion, and they did not just preach to the converted. Even trade unions, they thought, could be enticed to openly endorse a health system based on insurance if its advantages to workers were made clear. 'This is where sympathetic "down market" press – e.g. *The Sun*, *News of the World*, etc can be invaluable in helping communications', one CPS member offered when reflecting on the media.[102] 'We need to provide plenty of material to demonstrate what we are providing is really the kindest system', insisted another. Ministers agreed with these assessments. In one CPS meeting, future Secretary of State at the DHSS Norman Fowler urged that the group must 'show ordinary people what the advantages of alternative systems really were'.

The insurance industry's focus on male breadwinners proved to be the first obstacle in convincing a changing Britain of the advantages of insurance. To be sure, many men continued to appreciate the focus on the duty of a man to provide medical care for his family at personal expense rather than relying on the state. One subscriber believed that he immediately 'saw the benefits of private medicine after we took it out'. 'When my wife was in hospital', he continued, 'the children could visit at any time, watch cartoons on the telly'.[103] For this man, self-reliance, choice and paternalism conjoined to make private insurance attractive. However, social change in the 1970s and 1980s put pressure on this paternalistic ideal. Increased rates of divorce, single-parent families, cohabitation and women's employment all undercut the health insurance industry's emphasis on married men.[104] The industry made some efforts to adapt its advertising to these social changes. One BUPA leaflet featured a concerned-looking woman in a smart suit with the caption, 'When you're building a career the last thing you want to go wrong . . . is you'.[105] Yet such advertisements drawing, in this instance, on the shifting image of the professional woman were outnumbered by those with a persistent focus on men. A more typical BUPA pamphlet from the late 1980s deployed imagery of the stock market 'Yuppie' of the period, equipped with squash racquet and coiffured blonde haircut. In light of this narrowly imagined customer base, and its supporters' inability to widen its appeal, most subscribers to private health insurance remained middle-aged professional men who voted Conservative.[106]

As the 1980s progressed, health insurance became widely discussed as both unfair and, crucially, 'American'. Television programmes about US health care by left-wing reporters, directors and producers deliberately fostered this association.[107] *I Call It Murder* (1979), a documentary fronted by the socialist filmmaker Jack Pizzey, explored the harshness of US medicine at Cook County Hospital, Chicago.[108] Pizzey captured footage during a two-week stay in the hospital, where he filmed by day and slept in the basement by night. Like most of the public hospitals in US cities, Cook County received less funding, fewer accolades and higher patient numbers than its private counterparts. It also served a predominantly low-income Black community on Chicago's South Side. Aired when Thatcher first came to power, and again in 1982 after the *Economist* leak, the film drew its title from a doctor's one-sentence response to Pizzey's question of how she would describe the plight of the US's public hospitals. The programme showed patients suffering from alcoholism and drug addiction, as well as gunshot and stab wounds. This violence sat alongside a bleak financial picture. Cook County Hospital suffered from budget cuts in the 1970s and 1980s and eventually closed in 2002. 'The principle of pay or die runs so deep in American medicine that even at Cook County patients sometimes arrive convinced that it's no-pay no-cure', the narrator told viewers, in a message that money lay at the heart of US health care. This line played over a poignant scene of a man in pain opening up his empty wallet to show he could not pay. Even forty years later, Pizzey still vividly recalled how he was 'appalled' at how 'in the NHS you would get treated and in America you wouldn't'. Though a widely held view later, it was only during the 1980s that Pizzey's interpretation of the distinct differences between the two countries broke through into the mainstream.

I Call It Murder drew attention to racism to underline the harshness of a medical system premised on payment. In one scene, Pizzey accompanied a police officer to survey what the documentary described as the 'ghetto' that surrounded the hospital, speaking to Black members of the local community who lived in 'America's private third world'. Back in the hospital, its racially mixed staff told Pizzey about the health challenges facing their patients. 'It's not a nebulous concept to say that racism has an effect on people's health', argued one doctor. She explained that conditions like hypertension were 'sixty times higher among non-whites than whites' and added that 'when you ask yourself why this happens and what racism means, well this is one area where it's clear to see what it means'. Commentary on race would have interested to British audiences who increasingly saw racism as a dividing line between themselves and Americans. After the Civil Rights Movement and its backlash in the 1960s, Europeans more commonly perceived the US as a racist society.[109] Britons, too, now frequently thought of the US as a land plagued by violence, guns and racism. This view often obscured racial inequality within the UK, clear to see in moments like the 1981 Brixton Riots or sometimes in institutions like the NHS itself. Nevertheless, the vivid illustration of these cultural themes in documentaries such as *I Call It Murder* reinforced the message that private health insurance meant discrimination along lines of both class and race.

The government fretted over the impact of *I Call It Murder*, worried that it would make the task of changing public attitudes towards private insurance even more difficult. After its first showing in 1979, Patrick Jenkin asked his civil servants to gauge the public's reaction. Once they watched the programme, Jenkin's subordinates reported that its tone was 'rather emotive' and believed it was 'clearly designed to give the impression that an insurance based health system could operate at the expense of the poorest members of the community'.[110] However, with virtually no cultural output framing private health insurance in a more favourable light, the government could do little to challenge such depictions.

Building on the momentum of *I Call It Murder*, programmes that focused on the costs of US medicine multiplied across the decade. Typical of the genre, a Yorkshire Television production titled *Sick in Sheffield, Broke in Beverly Hills* (1982) followed a group of Californian doctors examining the NHS in the less sunnier climes of the North of England, capturing their pointed reflections on how many people in the US could not afford medical care.[111] Another feature on the popular news magazine show This Week, Right Wing Medicine (1988), billed itself as 'A report from America on the free market models that are finding favour with Mrs. Thatcher'.[112] Illustrating the involvement of prominent left-wingers in these productions, the programme was fronted by Margaret Jay, the Labour activist who had delivered the boastful speech about the NHS to the Women's National Democratic Club ten years earlier.

Through such programmes, the NHS's supporters encouraged the public to equate private medicine with US consumerism. Channel 4's *Kentucky Fried Medicine* (1988) appeared as a three-part series that extended the themes set out in *I Call It Murder*.[113] The programme was co-produced by the filmmakers Yvette Vanson and Tony Wardle, who had received acclaim for their documentary work on the 1984 miners' strike. For this production on the NHS, they began with images of Las Vegas, Taco Bell and other fast food restaurants. 'America', opened the narrator to a blues soundtrack, 'home of free enterprise and the market economy – where entrepreneurs move easily between fried chicken, hamburgers and health care, using similar marketing techniques for each'. These lines took aim at the neoliberal idea of medicine as just another consumer product. The narrator told viewers in the second part of the programme how 'right-wing think tanks . . . are all advocating elements of private medicine based on the American model'. Vanson presented these comparisons as deliberate and an expression of her socialist views. 'What we wanted to do', she explained, 'was say, look at America, there's the model you're talking about, this is the free market – that's what health care like that is'. The Americans in the programme brought this point to life, recounting their stories about insurance coverage denial or bankruptcy from medical bills. Vanson and Wardle encouraged them to speak directly to British viewers. One older woman pleaded: 'Keep what you have, keep the free care. You don't know what you've got. You've got something we need here'. Another participant whose medical expenses caused a breakdown in her marriage reflected that she would 'say to any country thinking of getting a program like the United States to think again'. 'It's cruel, it's heartless', she concluded.

Britons seemed to heed the warnings issued by Vanson and Wardle's interviewees. The association between private medicine, US inequality and the Conservative government's intentions hardened within the public imagination. One 1993 study of opinion regarding private health insurance noted how 'a strongly voiced fear was a development of an America-like system'.[114] The vast majority of people invoked the US in critical terms. 'By taking out private health insurance, you are running down the NHS,' suggested one respondent, 'We'll end up like America with people ill and unable to afford insurance'. Another, reflecting on government encouragement to 'opt out' of the NHS, boldly stated, 'I wouldn't want a system like America'. 'No I don't want a system like America,' repeated a different respondent, 'I've lived there and doctors are purely financially motivated'. Such statements showed a popular embrace of the left's argument that American medicine was unfair and motivated by profit alone. Regardless of the Conservatives' interest in both European and US health systems as alternatives, the public had seized on the latter as the antithesis of the NHS, further demonstrated by the letters to local newspapers that asserted 'we DON'T want that health system here'.[115] The binaries created by welfare nationalism between the UK and the US had only become more prevalent.

Multiple opinion polls also revealed swelling support for the existing means of funding the nation's medical care. A survey for *The Economist* in 1984 found over 80 per cent of Britons supported the premise of the welfare state.[116] Across the next two years, nearly 85 per cent of people thought the government 'definitely should be' responsible for providing 'health care for the sick'.[117] A mere 1 per cent combined thought it 'probably' or 'definitely' should not possess such responsibility. As these numbers confirmed, arguments that individuals should assume primary responsibility for their health care had gained scant popular support. Rather than warming to neoliberal aspirations for funding and organising medical care through private insurance, the public grew more unconvinced. When pollsters asked which areas deserved more government spending, health trumped all others by far. In 1983, approximately 37 per cent of people opted for health, about ten points ahead of education, but in 1989 this number soared to roughly 61 per cent of people, now more than forty points ahead of education.[118] Although British voters returned the Conservatives in General Elections in 1983, 1987 and 1992, it was in spite of the party's approach to the NHS, not because of it. With little public support, ambitions to replace the health service with private insurance floundered.

***

For all the intellectual and political energy poured into it, the neoliberal dream of Britain becoming a nation of private health insurance subscribers lay in tatters. The private health insurance market proved more unstable than anticipated, and the NHS displayed structural resilience. Moreover, the widespread adoption of private medical insurance never became an appealing prospect in the public's eyes. In fact, its popular reputation went backwards in the 1980s after supporters of the nationalised system deliberately associated it with the inequities of US medical care. Welfare nationalism therefore carried consequences, shaping attitudes to what was desirable and what was not. By the point that major private health insurers returned to recording healthy profits in the late 1990s, the Conservative Party neared the end of its time in office.[119] They no longer possessed the political capital, or the will, necessary for a concerted effort to shift Britain to a private health insurance model.

These developments provoked anguish and disappointment among the proponents of private health insurance. One of Thatcher's short-lived ministers in the DHSS, Ray Whitney, concluded that his former boss relished 'her reputation as a slayer of dragons' but had shied away from 'battle with by far the most menacing of the dragons that survived'.[120] The US loomed large in Whitney's analysis of the Conservative Party's failure. 'We are happy to read stories from America of the poor being denied medical treatment, of the middle-class being bankrupted by hospital bills and of rapacious doctors piling up their millions', he noted. These horror stories about the US merely served, in Whitney's view, 'to provide solace when we contemplate our long hospital lists or any other signs of the strains afflicting the NHS'.

Conservative Chancellor of the Exchequer Nigel Lawson's famous statement that the institution comprised 'the closest thing the English have to a religion' arrived in this same moment of disappointment for neoliberal politics in health care.[121]

On the back of this defeat, the Conservative government reasoned that if the service had to exist, then at least it should be marketised in order to make it more 'efficient' and cost-effective. The 1983 Griffiths Management Inquiry signalled the ascendency of general managers in the NHS modelled on the private sector, who often assumed authority over and above clinicians and local administrators.[122] Their most important reform in this regard was the introduction of an 'internal market' in 1990, which separated the parts of the NHS that paid for care from the parts that provided it.[123] The BMA vehemently opposed the internal market, marking a pivot by this professional body towards defending the NHS after decades of oscillating between indifference and outright hostility. After the policy began in 1991, 'NHS Trusts' now bought health care from 'providers', such as hospitals. Inspired by the US economist Alain Enthoven, the internal market followed the neoliberal tenet that standards in public services could be driven up through competition. However, this reform marked a retreat from their earlier aspirations. *The NHS Reforms: Whatever Happened to Consumer Choice?* (1990), revealed the IEA's view that the internal market constituted little more than a dysfunctional consolation prize.[124] Nonetheless, these policies formed part of a different battle, one which focused on the influence of markets inside the nationalised system. If fortress NHS could not be besieged from without, perhaps it could be compromised from within.

7

PUBLIC SERVICE, PRIVATE CONTRACTS

On a summer's day in 1984, nearly 2,000 people gathered outside Hammersmith Hospital in West London.[1] Trade unionists, health activists and sympathetic members of the public had come to show their support for the hospital's cleaners on the first day of a strike. One year before, the Conservative government had pushed local health authorities to employ private contractors for services such as cleaning in order to save money and clamp down on trade unions. When managers at Hammersmith Hospital seized the opportunity, the in-house cleaners protested through strike action. As in many parts of the NHS, these employees were ethnically and racially diverse – many had immigrated to work in the service during earlier decades. Now they fought to save their jobs. As the strike progressed later that summer, hundreds of people assembled in the local common, Wormwood Scrubs, bearing placards in another display of defiance (Figure 16). After three months of contentious struggle, the cleaners' industrial action ultimately met defeat, but not before it marked a new phase in the NHS's history. Many of its participants carried banners or wore clothing emblazoned with a word that would haunt the service for the next four decades: 'privatisation'.

From the 1980s into the new millennium, both Conservative and Labour governments sought to push the NHS closer to business principles.[2] This process of 'marketisation' included efficiency drives, internal competition, enlisting private capital to deliver public medical services

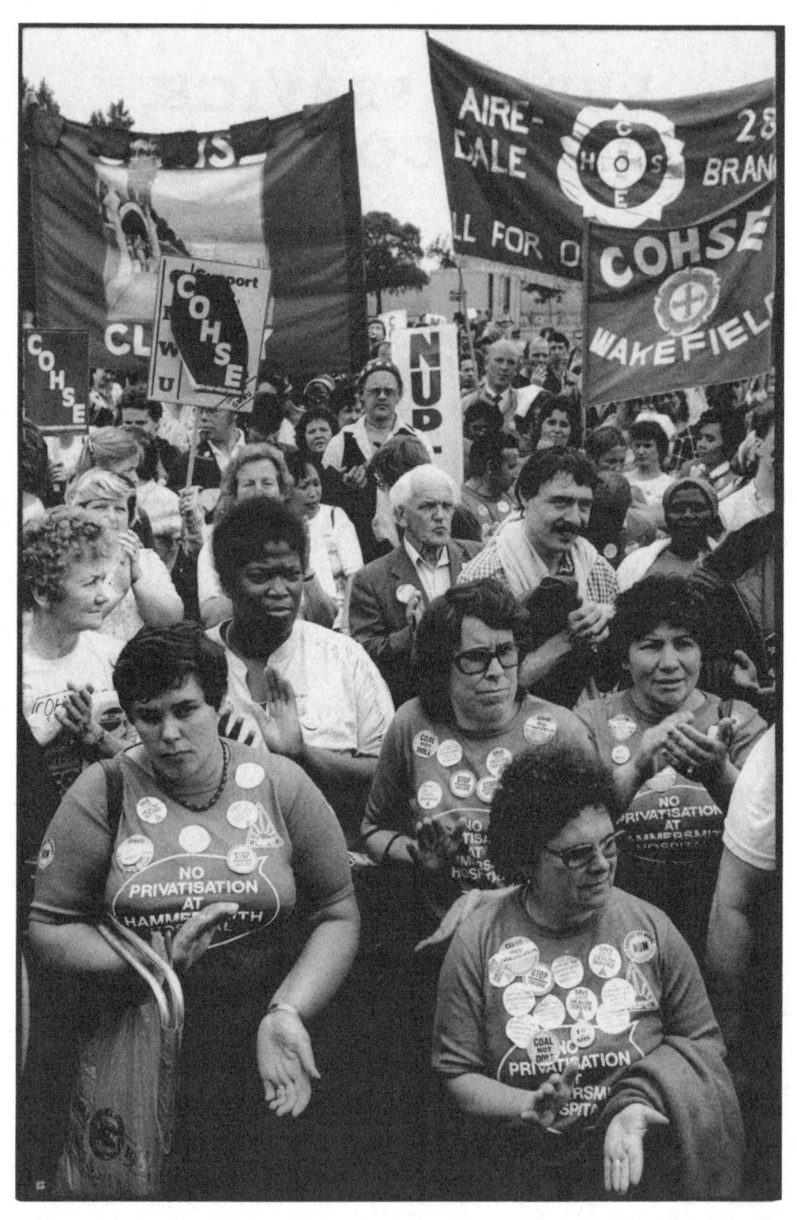

16. The supporters of the Hammersmith Hospital cleaners' strike situated their industrial action as part of the fight against 'privatisation', a word that entered common currency when discussing the NHS from the 1980s.

and facilities, as well as expanding patient 'choice' beyond the NHS. The enmeshing of a state medical system with markets was not unique to Britain. The World Bank and the IMF both insisted on such transformations to health systems as the twentieth century came to a close.[3] This package of health care 'reform', as policymakers described it in neutral terms, signalled a neoliberal adaptation to the reality of higher public expenditure on medicine. As in nearly all industrialised nations, health care spending soared in Britain, from approximately 5 per cent of GDP in 1990 to just over 9 per cent by 2010.[4] Governments raced to meet higher public expectations about medical treatment, as well as the rising costs of the expertise, pharmaceuticals and technologies it relied on. These funds were needed to pay for increasingly complex computing equipment, an expanding range of pharmaceuticals like statins, and novel medical tools such as MRI. Nevertheless, free-market intellectuals, politicians and business interests believed that the systems delivering health care should be marketised. The emphasis on competitiveness and efficiency at the heart of this process drew on a belief in the virtues of the private sector and its capacities to inspire and support better public services. In this way, neoliberal health politics shifted – from calling for the NHS's replacement with private health insurance between the 1960s and mid-1980s to advancing proposals that reshaped the service's internal workings thereafter.

In the drive towards health care marketisation, Britain displayed some notable characteristics. During the mid-1980s, it was the first country to mandate compulsory competitive 'outsourcing' for its public services (meaning, employing private providers to undertake some of the essential duties of taxpayer-funded social services).[5] The introduction of the NHS 'internal market' in 1990 formed an early attempt to restructure a public health system along the lines of a purchaser/provider split, with taxpayer-funded administrators procuring medical services from predominantly taxpayer-funded suppliers. By the millennium, the UK was also the first to craft distinct mechanisms that channelled private money to construct public medical facilities like hospitals on a large scale. These policies rarely brought the utopian outcomes that their neoliberal boosters projected, and in fact could lead to debts, scandals and deteriorating conditions for NHS patients and staff. What the political scientist Andrew Bowman and his colleagues describe as a 'franchise state' handed out public money to private contractors, financiers and their political enablers.[6] These interest groups made handsome profits from the NHS, sometimes – though not always – delivering contracts to a questionable standard that challenged the purported superiority of market principles. At the same time, many of the NHS's workers fought for, and associated themselves with, the institution's social democratic ideals like never before – a development that would prove vital to rallying others to its defence.[7]

But did marketisation equate to privatisation, as campaigners and a growing body of scholarship warned?[8] The two can be usefully distinguished as the difference between an ongoing process – with variable results – and a completed outcome.[9] 'Privatisation' emerged in the changing political landscape of the 1980s and 1990s, when governments transferred the ownership of state infrastructure – such as the National Coal Board or British Rail – and parts of the welfare state like council housing to private hands. It referred to a more-or-less wholesale shift of resources from the public to the private sector. But the popular use of 'privatisation' in relation to the NHS proved slippery and shifted in meaning over time: in the mid-1980s, the term was invoked with reference to outsourcing, but by the millennium it was also applied to the use of private money to construct health care buildings. Predictions of the imminent betrayal of the service's founding principles escalated from this point onwards, wrapped in a shroud of 'crisis'.

Though politically useful in sharpening public attention, the many forecasts of privatisation often overlooked how the NHS's social democratic values and longstanding communal practices of care had endured, or even deepened. The expanding reach of markets in the NHS carried a number of adverse consequences for its employees and patients, but it could be overstated when compared to the continued significance of the state or the persistence of communal norms within its medical spaces. Moreover, such claims also underplayed the NHS's historic cooperation with a plurality of external health providers. After all, the service was never wholly a 'state' system but had always relied on engagement with charity and, indeed, the private sector. The supporters of the NHS forced reversals in marketisation. Yet the fiery language of privatisation stoked the fears of activists and trade unions. The media amplified their concerns, splashing newspaper articles and television features on the NHS under the banner of crisis. These claims intensified during the period of austerity in public spending that followed the 2008 financial downturn, when Conservative-led governments placed unprecedented restrictions on annual NHS budget increases. Who, then, would come out on top in this recast struggle between social democracy and neoliberalism: public service or private contracts?

OUTSOURCING IN THE NHS

As free-market dreams of a nation of private health insurance subscribers faltered in the mid-1980s, outsourcing emerged as an alternative strategy to challenge the existing practices of nationalised medicine, such as hospital work. Why, neoliberal think tanks and Conservative politicians began to ask, should public services be entirely delivered by the state? The government, they begrudgingly accepted, could continue to guarantee health care, but private companies should at least bring more efficiency to its day-to-day operation. Far from being value neutral, 'efficiency' meant competition and cutting costs. In a pamphlet titled *Reservicing Health* (1982), the Adam Smith Institute – a free-market think tank which had also championed private insurance – lamented that Britain still spent far less than other nations on new hospitals or technologies such as CAT scanners.[10] Like other neoliberal think tanks in prior decades, they insisted that the government should avoid increasing the NHS budget to address these shortfalls. However, the institute did not – in this instance – fall back onto arguments about replacing the nationalised service with private insurance. Rather, they argued that savings might be made in NHS expenditure on 'ancillary services' in hospitals, such as cleaning, laundry and catering, if private contractors provided these workers instead of in-house NHS employees.

Inspired by how US hospitals spent less than their British counterparts on housekeeping and porters through such employment strategies, the institute believed savings could be passed on to patient care. The speedy enactment of these proposals harmed NHS workers at the bottom of its professional hierarchy, employees who were often women, belonged to an ethnic minority or lived in a deindustrialising area that relied on public sector employment.

Since wages had always comprised the largest part of NHS expenditure, critics of its swelling budget targeted pay packets. In 1951, the service employed 410,479 people.[11] That figure stood at more than 1 million by the mid-1980s. If paying for the NHS's army of medical professionals swallowed 58 per cent of its annual budget in 1950, in the early 1980s about 70 per cent of its budget covered these costs.[12] Even though ancillary workers benefited little from this overall expansion and remained underpaid when the high inflation of the period was taken into consideration, their industrial action – such as a nationwide strike in 1972 – rankled the NHS's critics. Outsourcing, for its supporters, offered the advantages of reducing the service's wage bill, which would help restrict overall NHS budget increases, as well as curb the power of trade unions after a decade of unrest.

The proponents of 'contracting out' looked to the hundreds of small firms that provided cleaning, catering and laundry services across the UK.[13] Many of these companies had first emerged as Britain deindustrialised, with the centres of employment in factories and heavy industry closing their doors and replaced – or sometimes not replaced – by work in places like retail outlets or offices.[14] Deindustrialisation was a gradual and uneven process. Nonetheless, whereas in 1957, 48 per cent of the UK population worked in industrial employment, by 1998 this number had fallen to 27 per cent. The world of assembly lines, coal mines and smokestacks that the NHS had been first conceived in, and indeed had matured in, was giving way. This emerging 'service economy', as it was often described, provided expanded opportunities for companies in sectors like cleaning. From factories to schools to airports, their predominantly female workforce earned low pay on part-time contracts.[15]

By the 1980s, a crop of dominant contractors absorbed about a third of the total market. Their names and market position shifted year-by-year due to mergers and takeovers, but many had grown alongside the expansion of office and retail work. Though some NHS hospitals already employed their services, these companies hoped government compulsion would provide further inroads for business.

The cleaning industry won influential allies. According to the political scientist Kate Ascher, its leading firms all donated to the Conservative Party in the early 1980s.[16] The Association of British Launderers and Caterers (ABLC) – a trade body that represented larger firms – set up a unit to lobby the government for further public service contracts. Thatcher met ABLC and other trade representatives at the 1983 Conservative Party conference.[17] In his investigative journalism, Mark Hollingsworth alleged that many such organisations and individual firms hired the public relations company Michael Forsyth Associates to help secure government work.[18] Founded by the Conservative Westminster County Councillor and future MP of the same name, the firm arranged lunches and briefings between the government and the contracting industry. Born in Scotland and having entered Tory politics immediately after university, Forsyth pioneered outsourcing local services such as refuse collection while on the Westminster Council. As the author of the Adam Smith Institute pamphlet *Reservicing Health*, he now endeavoured to advance these market-oriented principles on a national scale within the country's largest employer.

Legislation quickly followed from the energies of these free-market think tanks, private companies and politicians. In late 1983, the DHSS issued a circular that instructed Local Health Authorities to put cleaning, catering and laundry services 'out to tender' within three years.[19] This instruction meant that private companies would now compete with all in-house NHS workforces by bidding for these contracts. The winners would be selected on the basis of the lowest cost, rather than non-monetary factors such as existing knowledge of a hospital or ties to a local area. The government sought to further engineer the expansion of this market by promising to refund Value Added Tax (VAT) on any contracts secured by private suppliers. In the wake of this top-down and rapid introduction, the UK emerged as the first country to enforce competitive tendering for its public health services by law.

Outsourcing resulted in job losses and deteriorating working conditions within the NHS.[20] When a contract moved outside the service to a private provider, it usually meant the loss of wages or pension for the workers who moved with it. The government abolished the long-standing Fair Wages Resolution, which ensured companies hired on government contracts maintained pay and conditions commensurate with agreements in the public sector. Private firms were now free to drive down wages and other employment benefits (costs that comprised at least 70 per cent of most contracts). One study of seventy-nine private contractors in the mid-1980s found only one that provided a pension scheme.[21] 'Contracting out' usually shredded prior arrangements for holiday pay, sick leave, annual leave and the bonuses that made the low wages among the service's cleaners tolerable. Tens of thousands of workers simply lost employment altogether. In 1980, the NHS employed almost 260,000 ancillary workers, but by 1995 this number had been slashed to 123,000.[22] As one domestic employee lamented: 'Dedicated colleagues have left the health service after ten or fifteen years loyal service – they've been forced out really. We all feel very, very degraded'.[23]

Women felt these impacts most keenly, as they provided the majority of catering, cleaning and laundry labour within the health service. Of all cleaners in Britain, 75 per cent were women, and the onset of NHS outsourcing therefore meant more women lost their jobs than men.[24] One Northern Ireland study found that 45 per cent of women's full-time jobs were lost compared to 17 per cent of men's.[25] If women kept their positions, 87 per cent of these workers now received lower wages, compared to 67 per cent of men who retained their jobs. When a company secured a cleaning tender, it fulfilled that contract through a locally based team.[26] Recruiters sometimes interviewed women in their homes, scrutinising their living space for standards of cleanliness.[27] Low hours and wages meant that these workers usually held down one or two other jobs to support their families. In places like London, such employees were often Black or Asian, causing existing racial economic inequalities to be exacerbated when they lost their jobs.

The impacts of outsourcing also fell hard on deindustrialising areas that relied on public sector employers like never before. Given its status as the largest employer in the UK, and indeed Europe as whole after the 1980s, it mattered when the NHS shed jobs. As the historian Gabriel Winant has shown in his research on the US medical system, women were frequently propelled into health care jobs in regions where heavy industry and manufacturing declined.[28] *Halifax Laundry Blues* (1985) uncovered the anxiety that outsourcing provoked among women relying on NHS cleaning wages to make up for their husbands' lost income in the parts of Britain undergoing comparable deindustrialisation.[29] This television documentary centred on the General Hospital Laundry, which had supplied the area's local hospitals for nearly a century. The women who worked at the facility, nestled in a former hub of the Industrial Revolution in rural West Yorkshire, cleaned and folded almost 65,000 pieces of linen a week. Surrounded by the din of laundry spinners and steaming equipment, they took pride in work that involved sorting through soiled clothing and sheets by hand. 'Though it might sound silly', one woman shared, 'these poor folk can't help being ill, someone has to do the job'. Despite their commitment to patients, the government insisted that Halifax's laundry contract go to a private firm. The fact that the existing in-house NHS team offered a cheaper tender for the contract made no difference. With the General Hospital Laundry set to close in 1987, its workers voiced their anger on the documentary. 'We know we can do it a lot better, and for a lot less, we just honestly can't understand it', said one expectant mother and new homeowner. Other employees expressed worry about finding a new job in an area suffering from high unemployment. 'I do have sleepless nights about it', admitted one woman who was now the main breadwinner in her household, 'because you've always that thought about where are you gonna get your money from, to pay your mortgage, to pay your bills?' These women took great risks to at least retain their jobs until the end of the NHS contract. With no money being offered by the government for equipment repairs, they took matters into their own hands to keep the laundry operational. The documentary showed women in their fifties clambering on top of heavy machinery, shoving their hands into moving parts to administer ad hoc fixes. Like many other NHS employees in a similar position, they had been left high and dry by the government's embrace of markets.

Trade unions recognised the threat posed to the pay and conditions of the workers at the bottom of the NHS's professional hierarchy and began to campaign against 'contracting out'.[30] The policy also had ideological dimensions, launching the first battle of the TUC against what they described as 'privatisation' in the NHS. Outsourcing would not bring efficiency, they argued, but rather served as a vehicle to 'assert the primacy of market forces in the arena of social welfare at the expense of the social values of care and concern which underpin the Welfare State which provides common social entitlements for all citizens'.[31] The TUC insisted that private companies were unreliable and not necessarily cheaper, and that their business resulted in poorer standards for NHS patients. Individual trade union branches catalogued the shortcomings of private contractors and used this information against them.[32] By the end of the 1980s, they discovered that one in four private catering, cleaning and laundry contracts had recorded failures for issues like poor hygiene.[33] One contractor, the TUC claimed, employed children under sixteen, while another asked patients to wash their own underwear in sinks on the ward. The TUC provided literature and training sessions to help local trade unionists win bids for services against their rivals in the private sector.[34] These activities, they declared, would 'defend and improve our health service which, despite this government's best efforts to undermine and dismantle, is still the envy of the world'.[35]

Strikes remained the most potent weapon in the arsenal of trade unions, demonstrating the contributions of ancillary labour to the success of any NHS hospital. The implementation of outsourcing provoked a wave of opposition by the largest health unions: NUPE, NALGO and COHSE. Strikes mainly took place in London, with the most dramatic occurring at Barking Hospital in 1984.[36] Crothalls – a private cleaning company – had provided the contract for seventeen years, paying NHS rates and respecting established conditions. However, with the government's reforms, they tendered for the same contract but with a 41 per cent total cost reduction. To meet this target, the company eliminated approximately 900 weekly cleaning hours. The women who remained working for the firm at Barking alleged that they had their wages cut by a third and holiday pay reduced by a week, and that they lost all sick pay. Slippages in cleaning standards had followed, claimed the TUC. The trade unions exposed dirt and infestations of cockroaches that led an independent report to conclude that there was 'no evidence of any overall system of organised cleaning, such as is essential in a hospital'.

Eighty-four Barking cleaners went on strike. Through the cold, rain and heat, these women maintained a twenty-four-hour picket for sixteen months. On nightly broadcasts, *Thames News* told a national audience how mothers such as Christine Copeland relied on her cleaning income to support her family.[37] She travelled from home half a mile away each day to join the picket. When asked why she made such a sacrifice, Copeland told them, in her East London accent, that 'the patients in there deserve a better service than what they're getting'. Anger at the deterioration of their own working conditions blended with concern for NHS patients. The Barking cleaners marched to the headquarters of the parent company which owned Crothalls, daubing the building with graffiti that demanded they get 'OUT OF THE NHS'. Strikers clashed with the workers bussed in to replace them, police forcibly removing women who blocked the road. When one Crothalls manager – in a smart suit and tie – was photographed roughly dragging a striking cleaner out of the way at a picket, trade unionists put the image on their posters with the caption: 'MEET THE BOSS'.[38] NUPE initially promoted the strike as the front line in the fight against privatisation. The union's leadership were inspired by the Barking cleaners' victory at an employment tribunal which ruled that these workers had been unfairly dismissed – a ruling that Crothalls appealed. However, in 1985 the hospital renewed its contract with the company, regardless of the striking cleaners' efforts to be reinstated. NUPE, perceiving the fight as lost, withdrew support, and the strike collapsed.[39]

As the Barking defeat testified, NHS strike action took place in difficult years for trade unionists and the labour movement as a whole. The Thatcher government weakened trade unions by limiting closed shops, ending secret ballots and banning secondary picketing (meaning, picketing somewhere other than the employee's primary place of work). Its most spectacular, and violent, victory over organised labour came with the 1984 miners' strike, an episode that seemed to symbolise the end of union influence on national politics. Large-scale manufacturing fell away across the UK – exacerbated by the Thatcher government's economic policy, which prioritised managing inflation over ensuring high levels of employment – and contributed to a reduction in overall trade union membership, which fell from its height of over 13 million members in the 1970s to just over 8 million by 1995.[40] NUPE, NAGLO and COHSE were no exception to this decline. Separated from prior hubs of union activity, they struggled to recruit among the growing ranks of outsourced workers. With little access to spaces like hospital breakrooms, such employees often felt disconnected from their colleagues still employed by the public sector. As one woman testified: 'All the cleaning jobs I've done, and I've worked in a few . . . You are never included in anything. You're never put in the union with them'.[41]

Yet despite the gloomy assessments of some members of the labour movement, outsourcing in the NHS was still easier said than done.[42] Indeed, its free-market proponents expressed frustration with the extent and pace of change in the NHS. Outside of the South of England, the policy encountered health authorities who, out of a combination of internal opposition and trade union pressure, refused to consider external contractors. Most Welsh, Scottish and Northern Irish health authorities did not comply with the government's insistence that they consider private companies.[43] The Tory Reform Group – an association of moderate Conservative MPs – criticised the government for not mandating that health authorities choose private contractors when tendering services.[44] As a result, market forces could not save an institution the Tory Reform Group described in welfare nationalist terms as 'the best health care system of its kind in the world'. 'The trade unions', they complained, 'from the start pounced on the word privatization and equated it with the worst aspects of free market capitalism'. 'Private contractors were portrayed as robber barons', grumbled the group. Contractors, too, grew tired of these administrative difficulties and reputational slights, and some stopped bidding for public sector contracts.[45]

As these flashes of irritation suggest, NHS ancillary workers achieved some success against the government's designs. Trade unions forced several cleaning companies to withdraw from the health service by exposing declining standards of hygiene or highlighting the lack of experience among the staff that replaced in-house teams.[46] Other victories included getting contractors to pay NHS wages. If a company paid these higher wages to prevent strike action, they sometimes met the ire of their free-market proponents.[47] Workers, unions, activists and health authorities sceptical of the benefits of outsourcing combined to minimise this policy's reach. At the end of the 1980s, in-house NHS teams had won 77 per cent of all catering, cleaning and laundry contracts since the introduction of competitive tendering.[48] Moreover, the scale of outsourcing did not dramatically expand in the 1990s.[49]

Union victories could take a long time. At Hillingdon Hospital, domestics and catering workers went on strike for five years between 1995 and 2000. Trade unionists alleged that the company who secured the contract to provide these services had sacked fifty-six workers after they refused to accept a £40 per week pay cut.[50] Led by the radical shop steward Malkiat Bilku, these women began an arduous campaign to get their jobs back. Subjected to racist abuse on the picket line, Bilku drew strength from the support the strike received from the US, Germany and India, as well as from prominent figures such as Winnie Mandela. 'They know we are low-paid workers,' Bilku said of the private contractors, 'They know we are mostly Asian workers'. 'But the point isn't that we're Asian, black, white, women or whatever,' she added, 'This is a struggle of workers against greedy bosses'. Describing their fight as 'defending all working-class people and the National Health Service', these women took the firm to an employment tribunal and won, and then repeated the feat against a second company who took over the Hillingdon Hospital contract. The threat of privatisation, as they understood it, facilitated their public identification with the NHS's universalism. They secured these victories despite a lack of consistent support from UNISON (now the largest public sector union, after NUPE, NALGO and COHSE merged in 1993), which deemed the strike unwinnable.[51] In the winter of 2000, Bilku led the cleaners back to work, after winning maximum compensation for unfair dismissal.

By the new millennium, outsourcing and private competition shifted the way labour operated within the NHS in a more marketised direction. The ancillary workers who lost jobs or struggled with reduced pay packets testified to the cut-throat nature of its introduction in hospitals fifteen years earlier. Although the health service had not always treated these workers well prior to outsourcing, this policy exacerbated existing professional imbalances within the service. It also sometimes created falling standards in the facilities that patients relied on for care. However, for all the intellectual and political energy thrown behind outsourcing, its limited reach did not amount to the 'privatisation' of the NHS. Workers sometimes successfully resisted its advance, and they did so in the name of a health service that was popular, universal and still public. The balance of the market within the institution underwent further shifts, though, once the Labour Party returned to office.

NEW LABOUR AND NHS 'MODERNISATION'

As the party that founded the NHS, Labour returned to government in 1997 to high expectations. After the acrimony and squeezed budgets of the prior two decades, the party raised the stakes during the General Election campaign when they claimed that there were only '24 hours to save the NHS'.[52] Rebranded 'New Labour', the governments of Tony Blair (1997–2007) and Gordon Brown (2007–2010) believed that the salvation of public services like the NHS lay in 'a new political consensus of the left-of-centre, based around the key values of democratic socialism and European social democracy, firm in its principles but capable of responding to changing times'.[53] The 'Third Way' – as they described this ideological position – accepted many Thatcherite legacies, including the privatisation of state industries and restrictions on trade union power.[54] These compromises were necessary, its leaders insisted, to adapt public services to the realities of a deindustrialising Britain, 'globalisation' and social changes that included the expanded presence of women in the workplace.[55] Detractors on the left, including the prominent cultural theorist Stuart Hall, remained unconvinced and derided New Labour as 'Thatcherism with a human face'.[56]

However, New Labour's stewardship of the NHS did not mark a straightforward continuation with the 1980s, despite the party's qualified embrace of markets to help deliver health care as part of a revamped programme of 'modernisation'.[57] Even if New Labour expressed a more relaxed attitude to the private sector than 'Old Labour', it nevertheless extended the social democratic tradition of using the state to pursue universalist goals in communal environments, while repudiating what they saw as the 'selfishness' of the Thatcherite 1980s.[58] New Labour rejected the neoliberal view that health care was a consumer product and instead reaffirmed it as a right. They also ramped up welfare nationalism among the wider population, showcasing the service to prove that they were still, at heart, a Labour government. By the end of their time in office in 2010, NHS spending stood at its highest level, the service had expanded its employee numbers and frontiers of care, and the public signalled their satisfaction with the institution to an unparalleled degree.

For New Labour, the NHS's universalism still represented the best means of organising a health system. Its leading figures buried private health insurance and even more mixed European systems as viable alternatives. In a major 2002 speech setting out the party's intellectual position, Gordon Brown attacked the 'pure free market position' that medical care represented 'a commodity to be purchased like any other'.[59] The long-standing neoliberal aspirations for Britain to become a nation of health insurance subscribers buying treatment on an open market place would never work, Brown maintained, because consumers had 'less information and less expert knowledge' to make such choices than they possessed when buying other products. Following the tradition of welfare nationalism established on the left during the 1970s, Brown held up the US as the leading example of the perils of private health insurance. Its inefficiencies and harshness confirmed the model's unsuitability. The alternative of social insurance – in which employers and employees made compulsory contributions to a fund that paid for health care, as in France and Germany – created, he maintained, a 'two-tier' system between those who could afford to make such payments and others who relied on government support. Brown concluded by insisting that 'the NHS system of funding is demonstrably the modern rational choice'.

Testifying to this faith in the fundamental social democratic principles behind the NHS, New Labour invested unprecedented sums of money in the service. During their thirteen years in power, its total budget nearly tripled.[60] These increases fulfilled Blair's 2000 commitment to raise UK health spending up to the European average. He announced this ambition to the surprise of the Treasury during an interview on a weekend television programme, dubbed 'the most expensive breakfast in history'. By 2010, the NHS absorbed 8.8 per cent of the nation's GDP, compared to only 4.4 per cent in 1997. Health enjoyed an ever-larger slice of public spending, now roughly equal to both education and defence combined. Staff numbers ballooned by 36 per cent across this period, standing at 1,251,909 full-time equivalent workers across the UK by 2010.[61] The NHS had become a colossus of public life – the world's fifth-largest employer, behind only the US Department of Defense, the Chinese People's Liberation Army, Walmart and McDonald's. These numbers confirmed that the service was at its most expansive after the 1990s, not in the supposed high point of the welfare state before Thatcher took power.

The generosity of the government towards the NHS had limits. In 1999, it introduced the National Institute of Clinical Excellence (NICE), creating a powerful agency that offered clinical guidance in England and Wales on decisions like the provision of drugs and medical technologies.[62] Through NICE, New Labour presented standardisation as an effective means to finally address the unevenness in the quality of treatment across the UK, discrepancies that were starting to be known as a 'postcode lottery'. However, NICE also brought the NHS's rationing of care into the spotlight, with certain treatments deemed too expensive to provide universally. 'If we spend a lot of money on a few patients, we have less money to spend on everyone else', explained the agency's first chair, Michael Rawlins. These comments provided a further example of the longstanding challenges in the NHS of balancing community needs with those of the individual, now recast around issues such as access to life-extending cancer medication. In 2007, for instance, controversy arose over NICE's preliminary decision to not prescribe the drug sunitinib. During the same year, a fifty-seven-year-old man from Plymouth with metastatic renal cancer attended a NICE board meeting and recounted that, while he still endured a great deal of pain, 'the quality of life this drug gives me is priceless'. His testimony revealed the anguish sometimes caused by maintaining the NHS's commitment to universalism in a system with finite resources, even after New Labour's funding increases.

Nonetheless, in general terms, loosening the purse strings brought results. In-patient waiting times – long the bugbear of the service, and some of the inspiration for the private insurance boom during the late 1970s – fell from a mean of thirteen weeks in 1997 to just four by 2009.[63] New Labour also expanded the service's parameters. The launch of NHS Direct in 1998, for instance, gave the English public access to a twenty-four-hour nurse-led telephone information service, with similar organisations set up in the other nations of the UK. Designed to relieve pressure on GPs and hospitals, NHS Direct received the most calls from people wanting information about out-of-hours health services and from parents of young children.[64] It became the largest telehealth service in the world. The government worked to deepen the responsiveness of the NHS to public opinion through a proliferation of public surveys. In another first, town halls were held around the country where local people gave their views on its future. A thousand people attended such an event in Birmingham in 2005.[65] Although the extent to which these opinions shaped policy is difficult to establish, the NHS attempted to foster a higher degree of civic participation than seen in the past. When New Labour left power in 2010, public satisfaction in the NHS stood at its highest level since records began, a dramatic improvement on its recorded lowest point when they had entered government thirteen years earlier.[66] The persistent narratives of crisis sometimes overshadowed these longer-term developments.

However, in the eyes of New Labour, more money for the NHS needed to be coupled with 'modernisation'. In the postwar decades this term had primarily meant marshalling the powers of the state to change relationships between staff and patients, as well as upgrading facilities. In the 2000s, it referred to blending public services with market principles. Blair described his mission as the introduction of 'twenty-first-century business concepts into the heart of the service'.[67] The traditional universalist goals of the NHS would now be achieved through different means.[68] This stance reflected the ideals of the New Public Management (NPM): an approach to running public services that prioritised competitiveness and efficiency, assessed through targets, to deliver the best value for money for 'customers'.[69] Targets in the NHS – such as improving in-patient waiting times – created a great deal of trepidation among the service's workforce. The most serious metrics were colloquially known as 'hanging targets' or 'P45 targets', ominously named after the capital punishment and the paperwork British workers received after being fired, respectively.[70] Some employees found ways to 'game' targets – such as racing to meet certain metrics at a crucial point in time, and then letting performance fall away. The historian Eve Worth argues that targets and managerialism devalued the expertise of workers in welfare institutions like the NHS and led to a loss of their autonomy, particularly among women employees, who comprised 63 per cent of all public sector workers by 1997.[71] The influence of NPM brought New Labour close to the pro-business orientation of social policy undertaken by the Conservatives during the 1980s and early 1990s, often carrying adverse consequences for the increasingly feminised workforce that staffed this key part of the welfare state.[72]

The government's emphasis on modernisation heralded other changes to the relationship between the NHS and gender by the end of the twentieth century. Indeed, the reformulated language of modernisation largely replaced the older associations in social democratic thinking between the NHS, families and industrial output. Earlier in the century, the Labour Party had presented the service as offering particular support to the health of mothers and children. The transformations to family life in the decades since the 1940s – such as the rise of single-parent families, or the expanded presence of women in the workplace – required that the left rethink the NHS's role. During the 1970s, feminists had also critiqued the patriarchal logic behind the postwar welfare state and its assumption that women would become stay-at-home mothers and not take up paid employment.[73] Even if New Labour still aimed its welfare policies at 'working families', the party adjusted to the fact that these families took a different shape than in the past. As the historian Colm Murphy reveals, politicians including Harriet Harman and Patricia Hewitt successfully advanced a distinctly gendered interpretation of modernisation within New Labour, which was supportive of pluralised families and female participation in the workplace.[74] Moreover, Britain's diminished manufacturing base meant that the productionist ethos of the NHS also assumed less importance in social democratic thought. Faced with deindustrialisation, the left no longer primarily saw the service as a tool to boost the health of workers who, in turn, ensured higher levels of industrial output or a growth in manufacturing exports. With many factories permanently closed, such associations seemed out of step with a changed Britain. By the 2000s, then, the NHS did not represent a mechanism to principally help mothers, children and industry. To New Labour, the service now served as a test-case for demonstrating how to modernise public services, alongside – in the tradition of welfare nationalism – an institution that represented the seemingly unique qualities of British political culture.

Five different Secretaries of State at the Department of Health drove a dizzying array of reforms in New Labour's pursuit of NHS modernisation. Though difficult to encapsulate, these changes sought to remould the institution so that it better catered for competition and choice. If the party abolished the internal market introduced by the Conservatives, its eventual replacement by Primary Care Trusts (PCTs) continued the emphasis on administrative autonomy and competition by equipping them with similar powers to commission services from health providers.[75] An important initiative in this regard was *The NHS Plan* (2000), which started from the premise that, while the fundamental universalist principles behind the health service were sound, the institution functioned as a '1940s system operating in a 21st century world'.[76] 'We live in a consumer age', the document professed, and therefore public services needed to be 'tailor-made not mass-produced, geared to the needs of users not the convenience of producers'. The argument that the NHS was ever a 'monolithic' entity was as wrong-headed as it was self-defeating for any supporter of the institution. It ignored how the health service's evolution had indeed been driven by centralised government planning – and sometimes served professionals over patients – but still exhibited a degree of reflexivity to local circumstances and personal preferences. The postwar development of hospitals and health centres illustrated this interplay. Yet, for New Labour, claims about the NHS's rigidity served as a useful springboard for 'modernisation' – a phrase used an eye-watering 106 times by *The NHS Plan* in nearly as many pages.

The NHS Plan heralded several changes designed to integrate the institution within markets and charitable organisations in the name of 'partnership'.[77] From its inception, the NHS was never entirely a state system and always possessed relationships with voluntary bodies and private suppliers. The volunteers staffing League of Friends' shops in hospitals – let alone the private companies that constructed those same hospitals – did not spring out of the ground in 1997. They had always formed part of the mix. However, the channels for integration between these spheres formalised in the 2000s. As Blair's longest-serving Secretary of State for Health, Alan Milburn drove such initiatives forward.[78] During the 1980s, Milburn had held Marxist views and led a spirited trade union campaign to stop the Thatcher government closing the Sunderland shipyard. When it failed, he not only learned, in his own words, 'that life's a bitch' but converted to Third Way politics as a more pragmatic means of achieving left-wing goals. In 2000, this polished New Labour advocate signed a 'concordat' with the private sector.[79] The agreement asserted that there should be no 'organisational or ideological barriers to the delivery of high quality health care free at the point of delivery to those who need it, when they need it'. Barbara Castle's clashes with the private sector over pay-beds in the 1970s seemed far in the distance. Blair and Brown instead provided NHS patients with a choice of health provider – whether within the NHS, or in the private or voluntary sectors.[80] Depending on location and the condition of local waiting lists, a person wanting a hip operation, for instance, could visit their NHS GP and then be referred to a private hospital for the procedure at no direct cost.

The issue of 'choice', then, had shifted from its postwar framing: it did not just mean options for patients within the NHS, but also options outside of it. Technologies like computers and the internet further reshaped the practicalities of choice in British health care. After 2006, for example, a patient seeking a surgical procedure within a hospital could consult a government-run website called 'NHS Choices' that provided information on waiting lists and clinical quality to inform their decision-making. For their part, patients – when asked in the government's extensive consultations – did not oppose the government's 'choice agenda', even if they generally cared more about face-to-face experiences with health professionals than such technicalities of the NHS's organisation.[81] Despite this qualified public support for a diversity of health providers as a plank of the service's modernisation, the policy made an uneven impact. By 2010, for example, one English study found that only 3 per cent of local health budgets went to independent providers.[82] The persistent barriers faced by external organisations to secure such contracts included concerns over the quality of care that they provided and disadvantages in the bidding process compared to large public sector bodies. As a consequence, the NHS still delivered the overwhelming majority of health care in the UK.

Outsourcing persisted in the NHS under New Labour, but conditions somewhat improved for the workers employed by private contractors compared to their counterparts during the 1980s and early 1990s. The government enacted several measures that better protected the low-paid employees that provided many essential services in the NHS. The introduction of a minimum wage in 1998 placed firm limits on companies who cut workers' wages to win an NHS contract, which had created such disruption in places like Barking during the 1980s. During the initial battles over outsourcing in that decade, health service unions like NUPE pressured the Labour Party to support this legislation.[83] Described by one trade unionist at that point as 'a glimmer of hope on the horizon', minimum wage regulations had now become law.[84] Similarly, the implementation of several European Union (EU) directives through the Employment Relations Act (2004) supported parental leave and holiday entitlements, regulated hours of work and improved trade union recognition. These protections for workers caused some companies to complain about maintaining the 'competitive edge' (a claim somewhat undermined by the industry's continued healthy profits, helped by its links to the public sector).[85] While some companies did not always adhere to this legislation, the conditions of working in the NHS for a private contractor improved on the 1980s thanks to government intervention. New Labour's initiatives reflected much of their broader approach towards the NHS. If they believed that markets were necessary and useful in improving public services, the party still gave the state the central role in delivering resources and protecting the interests of the community as a whole.

THE PRIVATE FINANCE INITIATIVE

The use of private capital to build new medical facilities became New Labour's most controversial change to the NHS. As the principal means of financing the largest building wave in the history of the service, this approach determined much of the feel of the institution as the 2000s progressed. Pioneered in the UK and then exported to other countries (including Chile, India and several Eastern European nations), the Private Finance Initiative (PFI) had emerged under the Conservatives in 1992.[86] Announced with little fanfare by Chancellor of the Exchequer Norman Lamont, it aimed to secure private investment for public sector projects – such as roads, bridges and hospitals – which would then be paid back through long-term loan payments. The policy offered the double advantage of winning votes by expanding public services, while keeping the money to pay for them off the Treasury's balance sheet. Few investors took the opportunity at first, apprehensive about the capacity of public sector bodies to repay the loans. New Labour changed their minds. Perceiving this form of 'public–private partnership' as harmonious with their modernisation agenda, the party passed legislation that ramped up its scope and guaranteed the debt. PFI, and its sister initiatives, soon became, in the words of Milburn, 'the only game in town' for any health authority looking to construct new facilities in their communities.[87] The policy provoked further waves of activist opposition to marketisation in the NHS, which equated it with the service's 'privatisation'.

NHS hospitals had already changed during the 1990s under the internal market, introduced by the Conservatives at the start of the decade. At this point, many health authorities across the UK relied on the construction and upgrades from the postwar drive towards modernisation, their concrete or prefabricated designs serviceable if appearing less up to date than in prior decades. In fact, such authorities were fortunate. Many others continued to use the large numbers of outpatient buildings, hospital wards and surgery theatres that this earlier programme had not been able to replace. In 1997, the average age of an NHS building was still older than the service itself.[88] Regardless of a hospital's exact composition of buildings, government reforms introduced under the Conservatives reshaped elements of their organisation and feel in the years leading up to the rise of PFI. In 1994, the government had declared that public money would not be allocated for new construction until health authorities explored private capital first.[89]

While the amount of money procured in this way remained small until the later growth of PFI, this announcement signalled that funding for future building projects would be drawn from outside the service.

As part of the efforts to bring more private money into the operation of the NHS, the Conservatives had also urged hospitals to explore different streams of income generation.[90] Many hospitals subsequently leased the management of their car parks to private companies. The fact that staff and patients had to display a purchased ticket on the dashboard of their vehicle to go to work or access treatment became a long-running point of contention in the service, particularly in England where charges for parking were higher than the rest of the UK.[91] The doctor and comedian Adam Kay later quipped that the pricing system 'must have been dreamt up by someone who realized their chances of winning the lottery more than once were pretty skeletal, and thought there must be another way to raise a similar annual revenue'.[92] Retail units grew as a common component of NHS hospitals. Shops and cafés populated their thoroughfares, serving staff, patients and visitors alike. Indeed, these spaces became a prominent feature of hospital design in this decade. Hospitals, the Conservative government had even suggested, 'should consider involving a specialist managing agent or retailing group' when designing a new main entrance to maximise these opportunities.[93] The pre-packaged sandwiches, plastic-wrapped flowers or bunches of grapes that these retailers sold for profit in NHS hospitals formed a low-level, but noticeable, sign of how commercial values seeped into the everyday operation of the service.

The comedy writer and architectural commentator Ian Martin observed many of these changes with a wry sense of humour when staying as an in-patient at the Royal Preston Hospital during the mid-2000s.[94] Opened in 1981, 'long before the NHS internal market and private sector partnerships could automatically be blamed for cheap, horrible environments', it displayed the typical commercial dynamics introduced at the close of the twentieth century. One minute after the hospital café opened, Martin wheeled himself down for coffee, thanking God for 'this little bit of grubby capitalism in the hospital reception area'.

'Hospital milling-around areas are all like this now – corporate', he reflected, noting even a boutique store that sold designer clothes. The corridors were plastered with what he described as 'the usual smattering of execrable local art', framed mission statements and pie charts 'proving that 90% of patients think the food's OK'. Martin detailed 'Peeling roofs, blank surfaces, a design methodology inspired by urban fringe outlet centres', saving his scant praise for the dedication of the NHS staff who treated him. Again, the identification of markets as a creeping menace produced a public recognition of the contributions of the staff who ensured the service's universalism.

PFI accelerated hospital marketisation. Whereas in the postwar decades the funds for construction came out of the health budget negotiated by the Minister of Health each year from the Treasury, now the government approached a consortium of bankers, private equity firms, builders and service operators to raise the money on the state's behalf. In return, the consortium received a contract to design and build a facility like a hospital and operate the supporting facilities. Outsourcing often became folded into these contracts, with companies promising to provide services like hospital catering or cleaning as part of the longer-term deal. The mid-2000s represented the peak of PFI, with New Labour pushing a flurry of agreements between local NHS Trusts and private interests. After 2010, their Conservative and Liberal Democrat successors initially supported the policy, unimaginatively rebranded as 'PFI 2'. By 2015, the Treasury had signed off on 125 health projects in total, ranging from brand-new hospitals to smaller ventures like a new ward block, with a value of almost £12.4 billion.[95] In 2018, the Conservative government finally abolished PFI, citing its expense during an era of public spending austerity in the wake of the 2008 financial crisis. Although new contracts dwindled before the policy's official end, at this point it had funded roughly £13 billion in construction.

Despite PFI's eventual demise, the NHS was locked into a long-term relationship with private capital, whether hospital administrators, patients or the public liked it or not. There would be no parting with PFI until at least the middle decades of the twenty-first century. Most NHS Trusts became saddled with associated debts for an average of thirty years. The longest contract, signed in 1998 by Oxleas NHS Foundation Trust, would run until 2050. As with so much else in the service, decisions made in one historical moment would reverberate for decades. Inevitably, some NHS Trusts struggled to balance PFI loan payments within their operational budget. The Queen Elizabeth Hospital, Woolwich, opened as a flagship PFI project in 2001, but only four years later the NHS Trust responsible reported itself 'technically bankrupt' because of repayments.[96] In a familiar pattern, the deal meant that costs at the hospital were £9 million a year more than an equivalent hospital built with government money. The difference would not be spent on the Queen Elizabeth Hospital's patients, but rather on paying the shareholders of the private company with whom the Trust has signed the PFI agreement. Overall, the cost of borrowing from the private sector to fund health projects was 2.5 per cent to 5 per cent higher than public sector borrowing.[97] The public could not scrutinise PFI deals because of financial confidentiality. Imbalances often only later came to the surface when NHS managers sounded the alarm in the media. Though figures such as Gordon Brown repeatedly insisted that PFI lay in the 'public interest' by facilitating 'a proper sharing of risk and access to private service managerial expertise and innovative ideas to secure better public services', the poor value for money it provided led to its ultimate abandonment.[98]

In the wake of this murky world of contracts signed in closed rooms and politicians obfuscating their true implications lay the hospitals. These new additions possessed their own design aesthetic and changed the way that the NHS looked. Often fronted by grey or white cladding, a wall of green-tinted glass, and topped with a wavy roof, PFI hospitals sprung up all over the UK.[99] Architects complained about being shut out of important decisions in designing early PFI hospitals, with the contractors holding most of the power.[100] The cheap 'design and build' format that contractors preferred lacked any of the civic-mindedness of postwar modernist architecture, with exteriors usually resembling a conference centre or large car salesroom than a public health care environment. Sensing a rising tide of disappointment about the new

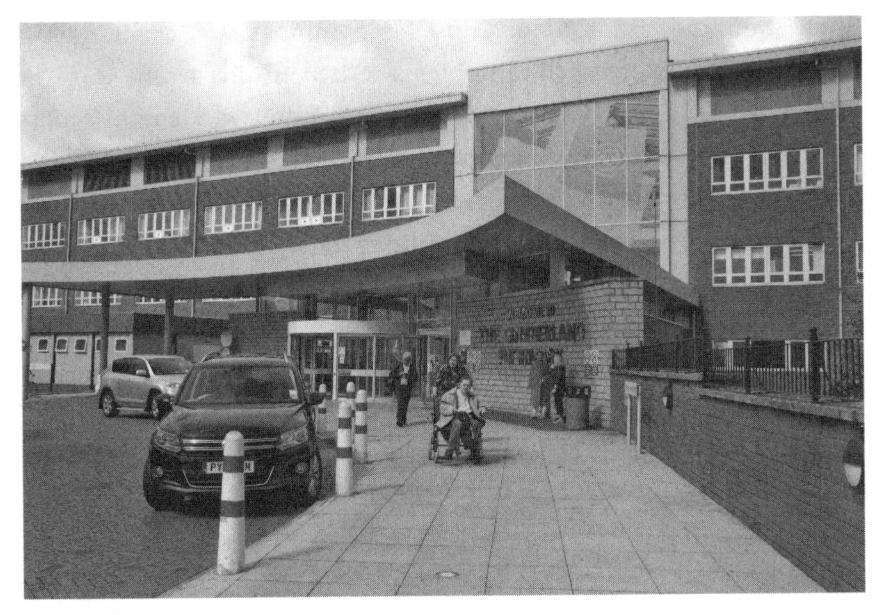

17. The hospitals built under the NHS's second wave of modernisation during the 1990s and 2000s differed from their concrete or prefabricated predecessors. Funded by PFI, they regularly featured red bricks, panel cladding, curved white roofs and tinted glass. Facilities such as the flagship Cumberland Infirmary ran into persistent problems with expense, bed numbers and design failures.

facilities, in 2001 the government invited the then-Prince Charles to become the 'design champion' for PFI hospitals.[101] Placed by *The Times* among 'the annals of ridiculous and empty symbolic gestures', the prince's interventions proved ineffective and PFI hospitals stumbled into persistent controversy.

Poor design caused trouble for NHS patients and staff. In 2000, Blair opened the first PFI hospital, the Cumberland Infirmary in Carlisle (Figure 17). He might have hoped for a better outcome than the leaky pipes and heating issues that soon plagued the facility.[102] At one point, a blocked sewage system flooded an operating theatre with waste. Similarly, a central glass roof brought plenty of light into the hospital, but meant temperatures soared to 33°C (91.4°F) in some parts of the building. Trade unions and NHS campaigners again took a leading role in exposing the problems related to this recent form of marketisation. The health activist John Lister produced a lengthy report for UNISON based on interviews with staff at the Cumberland Infirmary.[103] He uncovered stories of elderly patients who could not hold a handrail because the temperature of the hospital made it too hot to touch. One nurse recalled an emergency where a patient entered cardiac arrest, leaving staff 'running around like headless chickens' searching for a working telephone to call for assistance. The contractor that built the Cumberland Infirmary addressed difficulties at the hospital – compounded later by warnings of a 'major' fire risk – by explaining that on 'a project of this magnitude, there are likely to be a few teething problems, but they are minor'.[104] To be sure, NHS facilities constructed under older, state-centred procurement methods did not escape design difficulties. The local health authority that completed construction of Wonford Hospital near Exeter in 1974 at a cost of £12 million, for instance, discovered a decade later that the building suffered from 'concrete cancer' and needed replacing to the tune of £56 million.[105] Nonetheless, PFI projects frequently fell into scandal, defying the rhetoric of the private sector's comparative efficiency.[106]

PFI hospitals also squeezed bed numbers in the NHS, as they were generally smaller than those they replaced.[107] The average available beds (fully staffed, funded and ready for patients) across the UK fell from 388,000 in 1987/88 to 204,000 when Labour left office in 2009/10.[108] Put another way, across the same period, this decline amounted to a shift from 6.8 beds per 1,000 people to 3.3 per 1,000 people – a stark contrast with Germany or France, which boasted 8.25 beds and 6.43 beds in 2010, respectively.[109] Various longer-term factors contributed to this outcome, ranging from the closure of local hospitals in favour of centralised facilities during the NHS's postwar modernisation to budget restrictions during the 1980s. The end of long-stay institutional care for mental health patients or people with learning disabilities also played a role. However, privately financed and designed NHS hospitals exacerbated this downturn. The contract for the Cumberland Infirmary called for

474 beds, for instance, but the contractors delivered 30 fewer. Soon after it opened, administrators constructed a makeshift cabin in the car park, optimistically called the 'Mulberry Unit', to meet demand.[110] In a familiar occurrence, the new hospital had condensed the total available square footage compared to the two older institutions it replaced. Inspectors found patients complaining about 'the lack of space and privacy' and ward corridors too cramped to walk three abreast.

The costs and scandals that plagued PFI provoked a groundswell of opposition. Veteran NHS campaigners worked with trade unions to produce exposés of the scheme.[111] PFI, in their minds, exemplified a new form of the NHS's 'privatisation'. Activists deployed colourful refrains and imagery to lambast private capital's influence. One Oxford TUC campaign included stickers emblazoned with the slogan: 'PFI No Thanks: Our Health Service and NHS Staff Are NOT FOR SALE'.[112] The focus on the US as the antithesis of the NHS persisted in their illustration of a pig dressed as Uncle Sam, smoking a cigar. National organising groups such as Keep Our NHS Public and The People Versus PFI coordinated grassroots opposition through their websites and mailing lists.

These local campaigns, though, did not always receive unanimous support. Sam Semoff – a US-born health activist and founding member of Keep Our NHS Public, Merseyside – led several legal challenges against the Royal Liverpool University Hospital in the 2010s.[113] Approved by Labour's Secretary of State for Health, Andy Burnham, before his party lost power, this local PFI scheme was viewed by Semoff as further proof of the government's ambition to 'decimate the NHS and turn it into a market-based health care system like in America'. The local press and Liverpool's Labour politicians disagreed. 'My message is "Bog off Semoff"', warned the leader of the City Council, accusing the campaigner of denying new health care facilities to local people. Semoff's two legal challenges against the PFI deal went to the High Court, forcing the local NHS Trust to rerun an earlier public consultation that had not mentioned this form of finance. The matter became settled in an unexpected manner. In 2018, the construction giant behind the

Royal Liverpool University Hospital deal, Carillion, collapsed.[114] The government stepped in and supplied public funds to complete the project, underlining both the volatility of relying on private companies and the continued significance of the state. After these delays, the hospital fully opened in late 2022.

MORE MARKETS, BUT NOT PRIVATISATION

Did the four decades of market-oriented policies in the NHS equate to its privatisation? In fact, the service fared well compared to other nationalised industries, infrastructure or welfare measures first established after the Second World War. As the health policy expert Rudolf Klein also notes, the founding social democratic values of state-administered, universal, free-at-the-point-of-use health care remained more or less intact, regardless of the insistence on market-driven 'modernisation' by New Labour in one direction and warnings about the service being 'sold off' by campaigners in the other.[115] The claims of 'privatisation' sometimes obscured the limits of marketisation in the NHS as well as the continuities and commitments that the service shared with its past. As the abandonment of PFI suggested, marketisation could stall or suffer reversals. There was no triumph for neoliberal politics in British health care. The original goal among free-marketeers to replace the NHS with a system of private health insurance had failed. Even the success of systematically reforming the service in line with market principles – which possessed a much shorter intellectual pedigree as a secondary political objective – proved patchy. Both Conservative and Labour governments marketised the NHS, but these policies did not signal a completed process of transferring resources tantamount to privatisation. By the end of the 2010s, a social democratic health service still existed, albeit now suffering from a diminished degree of funding compared to the prior two decades.

After the 1980s, many communal health care norms and practices that had been embedded in the postwar decades continued. For instance, PFI did not dislodge patients' preference for shared wards, despite the policy's prioritisation of more individualised designs. Many hospitals built under PFI followed the view of private hospitals that patients needed – and desired – separate rooms. This stance contrasted with planners in the postwar period, who brought patients from different backgrounds together in large, communal wards. The South West Acute Hospital at Enniskillen opened in 2012 and provided ensuite rooms for each patient – the first hospital in Northern Ireland to do so.[116] Fitted with televisions and the capacity to speak to a nurse via intercom, their design pursued a different understanding of privacy than the NHS had historically provided. Rather than use curtains and subdivisions on its wards, walls would separate patients from each other. Similarly, the Royal Liverpool University Hospital was constructed as the largest hospital in England providing all single rooms.[117] For PFI's critics, this drive towards individualised rooms formed part of a mission to ripen the NHS for an expansion in private health insurance, whose subscribers expected such a degree of solitude.[118] A growing number of medical experts also contributed to the legitimacy of single rooms by pointing to its health benefits. With rising case numbers of 'superbugs' like MRSA in hospitals during the 2000s, individualised accommodation seemingly offered the chance to reduce the cross-infection that occurred on open wards. US experts – often using US evidence – such as Roger Ulrich advised the NHS to adopt single rooms on these grounds, as well as for other advantages, such as encouraging patients to divulge sensitive information in confidence.[119] The UK and Scottish governments agreed, committing to increasing the numbers of individual rooms within the NHS.[120]

And yet, large sections of the public may have been relieved that policymakers did not come close to accomplishing these ambitions. In an important study, the architectural health researcher Bryan Lawson found that people at two English hospitals on the south coast during the early 2000s did not wholly endorse single rooms.[121] Poole Hospital Trust had recently converted its 1960s-style general wards – divided up with clusters of six or one-bed bays – to sixteen individual bedrooms and three four-bed bays with ensuite bathrooms. When asked at the end of their stay, more patients did give the highest satisfaction rating for the newer, more individualised, rooms. However, overall, 54 per cent of the 473 patients interviewed for the study stated a preference for multiple-bed accommodation, compared to 43 per cent for single rooms. The balance between 'privacy and community', as Lawson described it, did not seem as clear cut as politicians claimed. Age or gender did not indicate patient preference, and instead the reasons for wanting more communal environments usually centred on wanting to avoid loneliness by having others to converse with, as well as wishing to remain in sight of a nurse. Such statements brought these patients close to their forebears in the 1960s and 1970s. Although a higher degree of support for single rooms in the NHS now existed than in prior decades, many patients still seemed to favour more communal designs.[122] Their preferences challenged ideas that the end of the twentieth century witnessed the birth of an atomised and individualistic society. In fact, communalism could live on in the everyday spaces of the health service.

The emphasis on 'privatisation' that framed both activism in support of the NHS and media coverage during the 2000s also obscured developments that came close to achieving some of the service's founding goals. In Hull, the city redeveloped its general practice facilities on more communal lines through a sister initiative of PFI. Emerging in 2001, the Local Improvement Finance Trust (LIFT) enabled the establishment of 'LIFT companies' to build primary care facilities, which would be jointly owned by the Department of Health – through an organisation called Community Health Partnerships (CHP) – and a consortium of private interests.[123] Although not free from controversy, this scheme involved a much higher degree of state ownership and architect-led design than PFI. It channelled £2.2 billion of investment over 10 years, with 90 per cent of the 314 LIFT projects developed in predominantly urban communities with above average health problems.[124] The Hull LIFT projects began with the explicit acknowledgement that they wanted to deliver on the 'clear vision' in 1948 'to have a health centre in every community'. This pursuit of the objectives contained in the original NHS Acts would require substantial transformation, as 75 per cent of GP surgeries in Hull were more than a quarter of a century old. One local resident, Angela Flower, described a scene reminiscent of the early NHS at her local surgery. Based in 'an old terraced house', she described how the 'kitchen was the reception, the living room was the waiting room, and my doctor's office was upstairs'. The Hull LIFT project pitched itself breathlessly as indicative of the 'power of partnership' but still improved on existing provision through thirteen new health centres and a pharmacy. The Wilberforce Centre – named after the Hull-born eighteenth-century anti-slavery campaigner William Wilberforce – opened in 2012, replacing an abandoned office building in the heart of the city. Situated in a large, five-storey structure in a new landscaped public square, it brought together three GP practices, a pharmacy and clinics that included addiction and sexual health services. Serving 100,000 patients a year, this centre symbolised a belated victory in Hull for the coordinated health centre model, which was, after all, first advanced earlier in the twentieth century through documents like the 1920 Dawson Report. In total, LIFT relocated 74 per cent of Hull's GP practices into health centres, underlining how public–private partnerships sometimes delivered objectives close to the original NHS Acts in places where they remained unrealised.

Moreover, although such expansion involved the private sector, the portion of the NHS budget spent on independent providers remained small throughout the 2010s, despite further efforts to open up the service to external competition. To be sure, this decade represented a marked shift in the efforts to marketise the NHS on a comprehensive scale. In 2012, the Conservative–Liberal Democrat coalition government passed the Health and Social Care Act which empowered 'any qualified provider' – whether from the public, private or voluntary sectors – to bid to run NHS-funded services in England.[125] This legislation extended the competitive impulses first brought into the service by the internal market during the 1990s, with Clinical Commissioning Groups (CCGs) – comprised of GPs and other clinicians – now 'buying' services from 'sellers' that included NHS Trusts, the voluntary sector and private companies. These changes therefore also amped up the drive towards a diversity of health providers championed by New

Labour, and campaigners expressed significant anxiety about the imminent – or actual – demise of the NHS.[126]

However, even with this legislation, the share of markets in the provision of UK health care did not expand to the point where it hollowed out the NHS. Although a spike in NHS spending on private health services took place during the first three years following the 2012 Act, this balance remained stable for the rest of the decade.[127] By the start of the 2020s, approximately 22 per cent of NHS funds went to 'independent providers', of which only 7 per cent lay in the private sector. As the political economist Kate Bayliss argues, the transference of resources to the private sector remained 'limited in scope', even if companies had made new inroads into areas such as mental health services.[128] The persistent barriers to firms making a profit in the NHS included uncertainty over rules, less public money to commission their services, and the perceived risks of reputation damage in a policy area where campaigners vigorously exposed failings by private contractors.[129] The role of the NHS's supporters in limiting the footholds secured by private interests once more underlined the historic trend that the service required an active defence. Beyond the formal private sector, the rest of the money spent on independent providers went towards GPs (since 1948, contractors to the NHS), pharmacy services dominated by familiar high street chains such as Boots, national charities including Macmillan Cancer Support and local charities such as hospices. Many of the recipients of NHS funds, then, either did not operate for profit or formed, as the historian Katey Logan describes it, part of a longstanding 'marriage of consumerism and nationalised healthcare'.[130] While the expanded involvement of independent providers followed from the marketisation of the state service's functions, it did not amount to a completed process of privatisation. Nor did it signal an inevitable path to that outcome in the years to come.

The more immediate threat to the NHS's operation came from unprecedented reductions in the funding that any industrialised nation's health budget needed to keep pace with medical developments and growing popular demand for services. Under the Conservatives between 1979 and 1997, the average change in per capita health spending had gone up by 2.03 per cent; under New Labour between 1997 and 2010, it had expanded by approximately 5.67 per cent.[131] However, under the Conservative–Liberal Democrat coalition government between 2010 and 2015, and the period of sole Conservative rule thereafter, this figure actually fell, by 0.07 per cent and 0.03 per cent, respectively. These later years, then, marked an extensive and profound period of reversal for overall NHS finances compared to the New Labour era. A lack of money did not comprise the only problem in the health service, but it did carry longer-term implications, such as an underinvestment in staff recruitment or an inability to continue upgrading medical facilities. This financial tightening also exacerbated unevenness in access to medical services, particularly in England. By the end of the 2010s, for example, more than half of CCGs in England rationed access to cataract surgery – the most common surgical procedure in the NHS – out of a need to save money.[132] The patients left in the wake of these decisions provided a later example of the historic imbalances in the quality of health care that could still exist in Britain. At minimum, addressing such challenges to the NHS's capacities would require expanded health budgets.

***

The NHS bore a closer relationship to markets after the 1980s. Bevan would have struggled to recognise – or contain his disdain for – the internal competition, outsourcing or private capital that now permeated a state institution run by managers in suits with lanyards hanging from their necks. Even the language describing the service and those who relied on it would seem alien. 'Service users', 'stakeholders', 'models of service delivery' – the byzantine language of policy wonks tripping off the tongues of administrators, politicians and journalists alike. Yet the NHS's founders might have taken solace in how its social democratic principles endured. The service remained predominantly funded and managed by the state, universal and free from direct payment. Even its communalism showed signs of survival. Taking a historical view of the tsunami of attempts to marketise the NHS from within ultimately attests to the limits of neoliberal politics in British health care and the surprising resilience of what it sought to change. At the start of the twenty-first century, the service's funding and employee numbers towered over the supposed golden age of the welfare state during the postwar era. The NHS pursued some of its original aspirations with a degree of success and expanded its frontiers into novel areas. To be sure, more money was going into the pockets of unnamed shareholders and their political enablers. Yet, taken as a whole, the depth of markets within the NHS did not match the repeated claims of privatisation. In fact, this term could mischaracterise the pressures facing the service after 2010, more concentrated on budget restrictions that diminished capacity in local areas than a takeover by the private sector. All the same, the fears of privatisation had facilitated a greater identification among workers, campaigners and swathes of the public with the social democratic values behind the NHS. Indeed, the anxiety that surfaced in this period created another cultural tradition that further cemented its place as Britain's best-loved institution – a tradition that strangely involved giving cake, candles and balloons to an arm of the welfare state.

8

BIRTHDAYS AND THE ENDURANCE OF SOCIAL DEMOCRACY

Ellesmere was not a radical place. This small English market town, located near the Welsh border, enjoyed a quiet reputation based on its dairy products and local wetlands. Voters in the surrounding area of North Shropshire had consistently returned Tories and Conservatives to Parliament since 1832. Yet, on 5 July 1988, Ellesmere's residents staged a peculiar sort of protest.[1] Dressed in Victorian clothes, dozens of people attended a tea party outside their local hospital. The children masquerading as street urchins and women wearing bonnets protested the closure of the hospital, one of ten in the region earmarked for such a fate by the Thatcher government. Their decision to assemble on the NHS's anniversary reflected an important transformation in the popular significance of that date. Why did NHS 'birthdays' – as they were known by the end of the twentieth century – become so important? If the health service had survived the 1980s, how did the popular tradition of marking its anniversary that arose in that same moment shape understandings of the institution's history and ideas of 'Our NHS'?

The growth of NHS birthdays as occasions confirmed, and in turn advanced, the endurance of social democratic politics by the end of the twentieth century.[2] From uncertain beginnings, the health service had matured, resisted political opposition and become imbued with welfare nationalism. Though its structures exhibited signs of marketisation, the service had fared better than different parts of the welfare state or public industries. Like these other outcomes, the expanding importance of celebrating NHS anniversaries required deliberate action from the service's supporters. It was not inevitable that a wing of the postwar welfare state would receive public adulation on its 'birthday' (or even that the date would be described in such terms). Activists, campaigners, trade unionists and Labour politicians, as well as members of the public, invented a new popular tradition that championed the social democratic faith in state provision, universalism and communal social services.[3] In the 1990s, the state picked up this practice and made it official.[4] Celebration became the dominant register of these occasions from this point onwards, but they could still expose underlying anxieties about the service's future in the face of marketisation or spending cuts. As the Ellesmere protestors illustrated, NHS birthdays offered the chance to voice both a sense of popular ownership over the institution and opposition to the government's policies.

For all this reflection on what lay ahead for the NHS, as a form of commemoration, the institution's birthdays meant thinking about the past.[5] When anniversaries expanded into a cultural tradition in their own right, they involved 'making history' by advancing a particular narrative of where the service came from, what it replaced and how it had changed since 1948. This account of the institution's past was firmly social democratic. The NHS, it was now widely held, had followed from the determination of Bevan, supplanted the horrors of health care during the 1930s with the benevolence of the state and developed in a more-or-less straight line of progress since. Other interpretations of the service's history, more sympathetic to the charity, mutualism and markets of the interwar period, jostled to be the dominant understanding. To the NHS's critics, the institution's inception in 1948 prevented Britain from taking a different – and in their view, superior – path in funding and organising health care. But these alternative historical narratives were marginalised, deliberately associated by the NHS's supporters with a harsh bygone era in medicine, never to be repeated.

The decision by Ellesmere's residents to dress up in Victorian costume provided a living example of the competition between different historical interpretations encapsulated by NHS anniversaries. In their view, by defending the service they were fighting against a return to the past. To explain her Victorian dress, one woman contended that 'we feel we're getting back to the Victorian era'. 'Here we are in 1988', she added, 'not going forward as we should be with the health service, but going back in time'. As these comments revealed, by using history, NHS birthdays not only brought greater prestige to the service by associating it with progress – and fostered public identification with its social democratic values – but further maligned free-market medicine. The service's anniversaries dovetailed with what the social historian Raphael Samuel called an 'expanding historical culture' during the late twentieth century, defined by interest in historical television documentaries, antiques and memorabilia, as well as an appetite for oral testimonies that unearthed voices from the past.[6] In the case of the NHS, this growing attentiveness to history was marshalled to defend a wing of the welfare state. The endurance of social democracy involved a victory in a battle to frame the public interpretation of the NHS's past.

Popular understandings of the service's history from the turn of the twentieth century onwards were sometimes sanitised or tinged with a romanticised nostalgia. They usually depicted an institution always celebrated by the public since 1948, free from contestation or the discrimination that welfare nationalism had created for its patients and workers hailing from overseas. Moreover, this idea of the NHS as a consensus issue since its inception – rather than the reality of a wing of the welfare state that the left fought for and defended – increased the possibility of the NHS's cultural reputation being co-opted by politicians whose decisions harmed the service. After 2010 in particular, an upbeat, if value-neutral, presentation of the service's origins and significance could act as a smokescreen for unprecedented restrictions on NHS budgets. However, despite these historical erasures and unexpected outcomes, the extensive popular investment in the health service as a form of collective progress further evidenced the endurance of social democratic politics.[7] On the other side of the millennium, the prominence of the service's birthdays reflected a widespread belief in 'Our NHS', a powerful conviction now based on cultural, nationalist and historical foundations.

THE RADICAL BIRTH OF A 'BIRTHDAY'

For the first three decades of the NHS's existence, the anniversaries of its founding were patchily or even hesitantly celebrated. To both Conservative and Labour governments, elaborate festivities seemed an unnecessary use of stretched resources. The service's tenth anniversary in July 1958, for instance, was met with a lack of enthusiasm in Whitehall. One perplexed civil servant drew up a report discussing 'what, if anything, should be done' to mark the date in Scotland.[8] The document insisted that 'there should be no attempt to stimulate a major celebration of the Anniversary', but offered that ministers 'might well refer to it in speeches', albeit only 'where it would fit appropriately into the subject matter'. Conservative Minister of Health Derek Walker-Smith duly completed a short television interview for ITV and issued a statement of thanks to the NHS's staff that avoided extolling any broader values that the service might represent.[9]

Ten years later, in 1968, the Labour Party displayed expanded interest in the NHS's twentieth anniversary. As the welfare nationalism around the service began to swell, Minister of Health Dr Kenneth Robinson organised a conference for medical experts in Westminster to celebrate what he described as a 'notable anniversary' and 'more importantly, to help to shape and fit the Service for the tasks ahead'.[10] The special guest, Jennie Lee – a radical Labour MP and Bevan's widow – delivered an opening address that praised the 'basic philosophy' of the service. She made sure to criticise the US for failing to introduce universal health care and underlined her enduring belief 'in my country being ambitious'. 'I want us to continue to be the trend setters and the pace makers, and I am sure we can do it', Lee added in another assertion of Britain's apparent global leadership in the organisation of medical care. Yet, despite her explicit welfare nationalism, NHS anniversaries remained low-key affairs in the immediate postwar years, observed mostly by medical experts or prominent politicians.[11]

The NHS's thirtieth anniversary on 5 July 1978 occurred in a more challenging environment. In the opulent Lancaster House – a stone's throw from Buckingham Palace – the embattled Labour Prime Minister, Jim Callaghan, delivered a speech at a lunch attended by former health ministers from the two main political parties.[12] The day before, the DHSS had held a conference on the theme of 'Working Together to Reach the Disadvantaged'. However, this bipartisanship and calls for cooperation sat at odds with the industrial action escalating across Britain. Celebrating the NHS did not seem so straightforward on the back of strikes over wages by nurses, junior doctors and ancillary workers, as well as the bruising battle over pay-beds between Barbara Castle and private health interests. Callaghan likely relished the opportunity to lecture free-marketeers in the audience like Enoch Powell that life and health were too precious 'to be abandoned to the test of the market place or the ability to pay'.[13] But he still pleaded with health workers 'to find ways to come to agreement on procedures that will avoid strikes or sudden stoppages that can harm the care and cure of your patients and damage the reputation of the health service itself'. Even as Callaghan spoke, hundreds of employees at six Greenwich hospitals staged a one-hour stoppage in protest at budget cuts and closures.

For all these difficulties, in 1978 the Labour government managed to put forward some central components of what would later become hallmarks of the service's 'birthdays': namely, emphasising its reach across British society and advancing a progressive narrative about its historical origins. Labour urged health authorities to avoid 'significant expense' in marking the day, and the NHS had to share the festivities with social security legislation that had also been enacted in July 1948. Nevertheless, the glossy colour posters produced for the occasion displayed the service as a caring, human institution that supported everyone. Photographs of a cardiac arrest team saving a patient's life, a smiling nurse watching an older man play the piano, and laboratory technicians at work fit into the tradition of presenting the NHS as a humanitarian enterprise, equipped for the future.[14] One poster's depiction of a Black nurse reading a story book to a white child provided a glimpse into the multiracial reality of the service that attendees at most hospitals would be familiar with. Yet such celebration sat uneasily with the protests taking place in those same hospitals. 'How can the unemployed health service staff and the many thousands of sick people on waiting lists celebrate when cuts are destroying our NHS?', asked one campaigning group associated with the strikes in language framed by a tone of crisis.[15]

During the mid-1980s, trade unions largely squared this circle. The Conservative government under Margaret Thatcher was an unlikely candidate to instigate a national jamboree over a state medical system. Combining both celebration and protest, the labour movement stepped up and reinvented the service's anniversaries for their own ends. The NHS's birthdays – and indeed the description of them as such – became established as a regular cultural tradition that involved a wider sweep of the general public. This transition began in response to the Thatcher government's changes to the health service, such as restrictions to the annual growth rate in its budget or outsourcing. In early 1984, the TUC launched a 'Save Your N.H.S. Campaign' and announced that an 'N.H.S. Day' on 5 July would see 'trade unionists around the country' organise 'a series of events to mark the achievements of the Service since 1948 and to highlight the threat to the service posed by the Government's current policies which do not provide sufficient resources to maintain services'.[16] The anniversary provided a window of opportunity to highlight the unions' efforts to, in their own words, 'save' the NHS from cuts and marketisation.

In the summer of 1984, an impressive range of celebrations took place across Britain to mark 'N.H.S. Day'. Most festivities took place in the longstanding strongholds of trade union and Labour Party politics – the North of England, Wales and Scotland – blending political activism and protest with family-centred fun. In the small town of Alva, nestled at the foot of the Ochil Hills in central Scotland, trade unionists and the local council organised speeches, a performance from the town band, a firework display and an under-18s disco.[17] Their petition collected 20,000 signatures from the surrounding Forth Valley for a 'better NHS'. Notably, people from across the constituent nations of the UK marked the occasion in a similar fashion, underlining the NHS's standing as a 'British' institution. Large cities such as Manchester, though, possessed the funds, organisation and population to go further. In the same year, thousands of Mancunians thronged the city centre to join a mass procession towards a carnival in Platt Fields Park that carried on late into the night. Families watched a Punch and Judy puppet show, jumped on a bouncy castle, rode in a hot air balloon and were amazed by the Irish escapologist Blondini ('See him before the N.H.S. take him away').[18] Although comparatively diminished in scale, other initiatives marked the day in the South of England, such as public ballots in Bristol and Taunton calling for higher government spending on the NHS.[19] The presentation of 'Get Well Soon' cards and giant birthday cakes, alongside the organisation of hospital 'open days', cricket matches and relay runs between hospitals threatened with closure, underlined the mix of celebration and protest that distinguished NHS anniversaries during the mid-1980s (Figure 18).

However, not everyone in the labour movement agreed with this balance. Some thought their energies would be better expended elsewhere. When planning 1985's 'N.H.S. Day', the TUC leadership and northern English, Welsh and Scottish trade union branches felt they could build on the successes of the previous year.[20] In Scotland, for instance, the 1984 celebrations had succeeded, they claimed, because of 'the broad based nature of the Campaign'. Similarly, representatives from the North-West boasted that 'NHS Day was treated as a celebration of the service and had been very successful'. Yet some local trade union branches lamented the lack of participation in their area. Representatives from the West Midlands reported a 'very poor response to last year's NHS Day'. Their colleagues from the South-East of England went further, declaring it a 'disaster'. Explanations for this lack of popular support included the assertion that the campaign 'lacked a national focus' and that the Labour Party only half-heartedly cooperated with the TUC. At the heart of the problem, these dissenting voices insisted, lay confusion about whether NHS anniversaries should be joyful occasions of celebration or serious opportunities to display

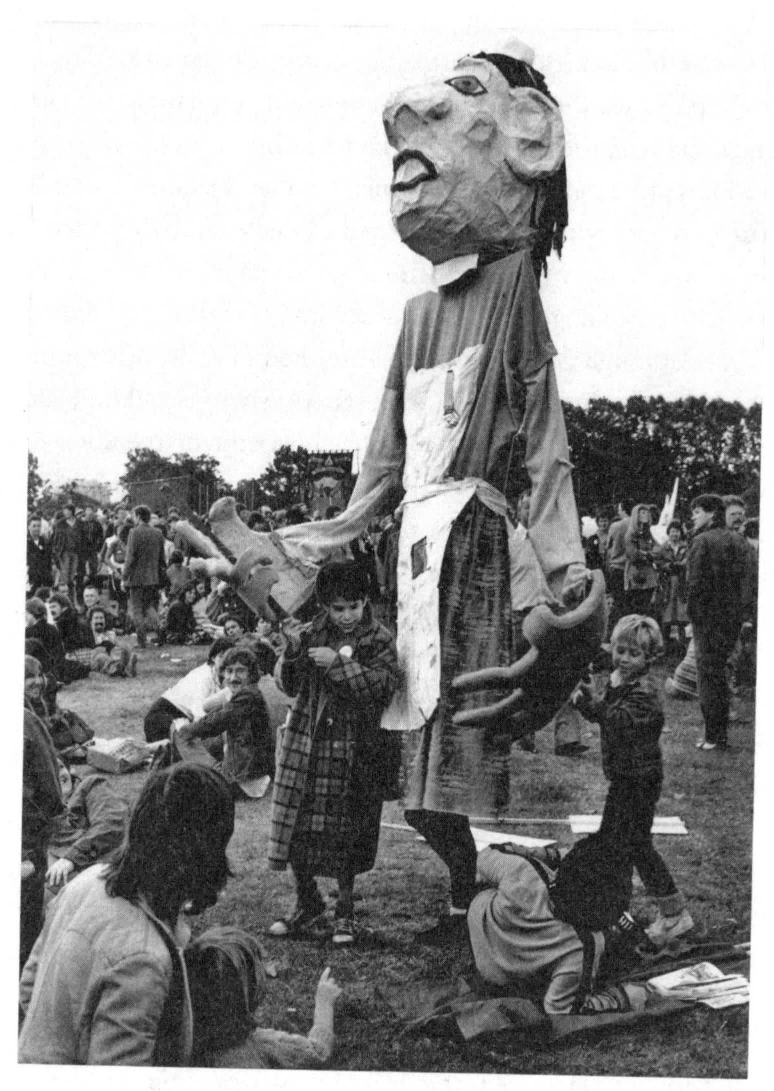

18. In the 1980s, 'N.H.S. Day' emerged as a trade union tradition bringing together community celebration of the health service with protests against the Thatcher government. From the late 1990s, New Labour made the NHS's 'birthdays' national occasions that championed the service's social democratic principles and welfare nationalism. These anniversaries also offered a powerful narrative about the NHS's history that hailed the progress wrought by the state in the field of medicine since 1948.

resistance to the Thatcher government.[21] The later growth of NHS anniversaries, then, was far from inevitable or even agreed upon as a beneficial outcome by all of the service's natural supporters. Nonetheless, the trade unionists sceptical of the advantages of devoting significant time and resources to these occasions continued to support 'N.H.S. Day' as the 1980s advanced. Festivities intensified in 1985 and 1986, with mass rallies and petitions sitting alongside donkey rides and gala evenings.[22] Flyers and posters for these events were emblazoned with bright orange and blue, and the frequent imagery of outstretched hands around a family symbolised the caring qualities of the NHS.[23]

As some trade unionists recognised during their debate over 'N.H.S. Day', future expansion depended on national coordination. The increased interest of the Labour Party provided a step in this direction. After defeat in the 1987 General Election, the party turned to planning a large celebration for the NHS's fortieth anniversary in 1988. Labour cooperated with the trade unions to organise events across the UK and to hold a showcase event in London. Much of their renewed interest in the occasion stemmed from Labour leader Neil Kinnock. Born in the same mining town of Tredegar as his hero, Bevan, Kinnock had earned a reputation as a moderate within the party, taking on the radical left in a bid to make Labour a more attractive proposition for voters.[24] However, the media's focus on these internal battles obscured the cooperation between the Labour leadership and trade unions over the NHS. The red-headed Welshman made important contributions to reshaping the service's cultural meaning in the late 1980s, entrenching its welfare nationalism and popular celebration. A passionate orator, Kinnock centred more of his public appearances on the health service than his predecessors, delivering speeches that combined hard-nosed economic analysis with fiery prose. In one of his first speeches as Leader of the Opposition, he lacerated the Thatcher government for its NHS spending cuts and 'privatisation', which amounted to, in his view, 'social corrosion'.[25] To Kinnock, the government's 'whole philosophy' was 'essentially amoral' because of its insistence 'that most matters of human comfort, convenience and serenity can be best decided by impersonal economic forces'. The NHS took on even greater political and cultural weight for him as the decade wore on. 'Other than liberty itself', professed Kinnock in firmly welfare nationalist terms, 'nothing is more important to the people of this country than the National Health Service'. As 'the strongest citadel of applied socialism', he believed the service needed rigorous defence from the business interests and neoliberal critics aligned against it.

In response to the threat posed by free-marketeers and a squeezed health budget, the NHS's supporters capitalised on the service's fortieth anniversary by stimulating popular celebration that might embarrass the Conservative government. The showpiece event in London took place at Alexandra Palace, a large Victorian entertainment venue that had recently welcomed Led Zeppelin and the Grateful Dead, as well as somewhat less trendy organisations like the Campaign for Real Ale. The event picked up the trade union traditions of 'N.H.S. Day' by providing bands and music, a hot air balloon and a 'Kids' World' play area, and presenting a giant 'birthday card' signed by 1,000 people from Newcastle.[26] In a demonstration of cooperation with the labour movement, Kinnock posed for photos as he conducted the Goldthorpe Colliery Band.[27] The Bakers' Union provided a birthday cake, iced with the name 'Nye Bevan'. As the recipient of baked goods and a greetings card, the NHS was treated almost like a living entity.

Kinnock delivered a lengthy speech, flanked by nurses, balloons and a giant 'NHS Get Well Soon' sign. He recounted a quasi-pilgrimage to visit Jennie Lee, 'an old and very great lady' who had supported Bevan as he shepherded the service into existence.[28] By contrast, he insisted that Thatcher displayed 'full contempt for everything that the NHS is and what it stands for'. Kinnock associated her support for private medicine with the ills of US health care. 'Does anyone other than the highest priests of Thatcherism seriously want any semblance of that system here?', he asked in a pointed reminder of the differences between the two health systems. Kinnock closed his speech in soaring welfare nationalist terms with a call to fight for the NHS's future 'as patriots, people who manifest their love of their country by their commitment to the people of the country and not only to the flag that flies over them'.

The Conservative government delivered no comparable speeches or events for the fortieth anniversary. In fact, the scale of commemoration by the state recalled the muted atmosphere of the late 1950s. The government spent money on a Westminster reception for NHS staff and an exhibition at the Department of Health (DH), which had replaced the DHSS earlier that year.[29] Apart from also funding a video for local health authorities to train health service workers, the government did not promote the occasion on a national scale. In speeches, like one to the Office of Health Economics (OHE) at a special event on 5 July 1988, the Secretary of State presented a qualified picture of the service's successes. The institution's organising framework and lack of direct payment remained, he admitted, 'the jewel in the NHS crown'.[30] But achievements like greater teamwork in general practice, technical developments in surgery like coronary heart bypasses, and greater respect for mentally ill patients, were, he maintained, more the result of 'medical and scientific discoveries of various sorts' than the fruits of any special contribution from the NHS.

Away from the government's measured expressions of congratulations, trade unions persisted with their radical approach to marking the anniversary. In Ebbw Vale, South Wales, a packed schedule began at the Aneurin Bevan Memorial Stones, erected in 1960 on the hillside where the politician once delivered open-air speeches to his constituents.[31] After lunch, attendees marched to the local comprehensive school to hear speeches by the former Labour Leader, Michael Foot MP, the General Secretary of NUPE, Rodney Bickerstaffe, and the Shadow Secretary of State for Wales, Alan Williams. Children's activities and a crèche catered to younger participants. Elsewhere, trade unionists organised four relays of flaming torches, which converged in London on 5 July.[32] One of these torches symbolised 'the eternal flame of the NHS'. In Halifax, Yorkshire – where the documentary *Halifax Laundry Blues* had captured the impacts of outsourcing on laundry employees – workers used fire in a different way. After the local Health Authority refused to accept an NHS birthday cake, they set it ablaze.[33]

NHS birthdays had emerged as a popular – and at times radical – tradition in the 1980s, a period commonly depicted as a barren decade for social democratic politics given the wider difficulties faced by trade unions and the Labour Party. The anxiety provoked by marketisation under the Thatcher government spurred on the creation of this cultural practice which, in turn, furthered the service's prominence in national life. If both celebration and protest shaped the tone of these occasions at first, this mix shifted at the end of the next decade once the state became more invested.

NEW LABOUR AND WELFARE NATIONALISM

The fiftieth anniversary of the NHS in 1998 marked the point when popular interest in the occasion conjoined with extensive state involvement. New Labour, elected a year before, amplified the service's 'birthday' – now commonly understood as such – to an unprecedented degree and entrenched it as a social democratic cultural tradition across the UK. From their perspective, the anniversary provided an opportunity to draw attention to the party's historical achievements and pitch ambitions for the service's 'modernisation'. Through the government's pursuit of these objectives, NHS birthdays became more about celebration than protest, a shift facilitated by the diminished influence of trade unions in national life by the late 1990s. The slick public relations machinery deployed by New Labour to promote the NHS's birthday provided little room for provocative stunts like setting a cake on fire. Indeed, in the government's view, there was no need to protest, even if some members of the public continued to express anxiety about the institution's future. They had a plan to help the service move on from the difficulties it faced when 'N.H.S. Day' emerged during the 1980s. Beyond showcasing their brand of modernisation, New Labour used 'NHS50' to escalate welfare nationalism, tying the service to stamps, currency, the Royal Family and the foremost sites of religious worship in the UK.

New Labour's attitude to the fiftieth anniversary followed their broader policy approach to the NHS. It focused on partnerships with the voluntary and private sectors, with the state taking the predominant role. To ensure overall coherency, the government established a special committee. Based in Leeds, the National Liaison Steering Group brought together the heads of the NHS in England, Wales, Scotland and Northern Ireland, leaders of individual NHS Trusts, the presidents of the Royal Colleges of Medicine, the Patients' Association, voluntary groups and many other figures and organisations besides.[34] New Labour's interest in public relations led them to employ external communications and marketing companies to maximise 'the number of OTS' when promoting the anniversary (in PR-speak, the 'opportunities to see/hear').[35] In a policy document titled 'The Vision Thing', civil servants and political advisors set out the government's plan to use the NHS50 campaign to communicate their aspirations for a service that commanded the full powers of medical science, communications and information technology and administrative flexibility.[36] By emphasising these goals, they hoped to expand 'public confidence' in the institution. 'More than that', they continued in welfare nationalist language, the public needed 'to be excited by what it can achieve, to develop a pride in the service, as a world leader among health services and as a symbol of a modernised Britain'.

NHS50 proved key to rebranding the NHS. By the late 1990s, the administrative mechanisms of the service had become more complex through, for instance, the internal market or the recruitment of external voluntary and private health organisations. However, the imagery around the institution simplified. Officials noted that the fiftieth anniversary heralded 'the first attempt to achieve consistent NHS branding throughout the service' and provided 'the first example of a "one NHS" communications campaign'.[37] These comments referred to the 'NHS50 logo', which did indeed represent the first comprehensive, national branding for the service in its history. The image of a person shaped like the number '50' stepping confidently forward – coloured in blue, white and yellow – provided a stylish and upbeat image to associate with the NHS.[38] The National Liaison Steering Group issued strict guidance on how this logo should be featured on anniversary materials that included 80,000 posters and 35,000 sticker sheets.[39]

At this same moment, the government rolled out the now-famous NHS logo across England, to reinforce 'a consistent visual identity for the NHS' and achieve 'greater public understanding of the totality of NHS services'.[40] Through this branding, New Labour sought to end the proliferation of hundreds of logos in use by individual NHS Trusts since the introduction of the internal market during the early 1990s (described as 'the death of a thousand logos' by one quick-witted civil servant). The 'blue lozenge' in Pantone 300 and Frutiger Bold Italic font became the definitive image of the NHS, and one of the most recognisable brands in the world.[41] The logo confirmed, in the view of the historian Sally Sheard, the NHS as 'bold, in our face, at the centre of our British lives'.[42] Indeed, by this point, the abbreviation 'NHS' was now cemented as the predominant descriptor of the service among the British population, over and above older formulations such as 'the National Health'.

But NHS50 was not just about branding. It transformed the trade union tradition of 'N.H.S. Day' into a national jamboree. The government organised a vast array of events to celebrate the service during the summer of 1998.[43] Roping in Britain's political, religious and civic elite, these proceedings confirmed the significance of the NHS to understandings of national identity by the end of the twentieth century. The Dean of Westminster led a 'National Act of Celebration' at Westminster Abbey and nearly 8,000 people attended a garden party at Buckingham Palace for NHS staff. Over 26,000 people visited a public health exhibition at the Ideal Home Show, also in London. A photo exhibition displaying a typical day in the life of the service (through eight subject areas ranging from cancer treatment to an accident and emergency unit to mental health) toured the country.[44] Corporate sponsors – including HSA Healthcare, Network Photographers, FUJIFILM and GlaxoWellcome – picked up the travel bill. Although the presence of these companies might have marked a change from anniversaries past, the desire to showcase the NHS 'in the round' through such exhibitions – with people at its heart – picked up a cultural practice with origins in the Callaghan government and trade unions. New Labour extended other longstanding symbolism associated with the NHS. The Royal Mint issued commemorative fifty pence coins etched with hands cradling sunbeams, with the number '50' at the bottom. By using an illustration of hands, they harked back to the imagery deployed by the trade unions during 'N.H.S. Day' in the 1980s.[45] These coins jangled around in the purses and wallets of Britons for years to come, providing another example of how NHS50 rewired a social democratic tradition on a national scale. By associating the service with many of the central pillars of civic life, New Labour ramped up welfare nationalism around the NHS.

As in earlier years, a wide assortment of local events took place across the UK, this time inspired by the government. A '50 Ways to Celebrate' pack, issued by the NHS Executive to various parts of the service, sought to get the creative juices flowing by encouraging staff to 'join the rest of the U.K. in celebrating 50 years of our National Health Service in July 1998'.[46] Suggestions ranged from working with local newspapers and voluntary groups, to directly organising the kinds of festivities that now occupied a firm place in the NHS birthday repertoire, such as parades and firework displays. Over 1,000 events took place during the summer of 1998 to mark NHS50.[47] Fun runs, tea parties, church thanksgiving services – a flourishing network of activity spanned the nation in praise of 'Our NHS', spurred on by the government. The question of how to celebrate was left up to local people. Though praising a national institution, such regional variety allowed participants to draw ties to their own communities. The Chief Executive of the NHS in England, Alan Langlands, insisted 'that staff in individual NHS trusts, health authorities and practices celebrate the Anniversary in a way which suits them and the people in their local community'.[48] 'I do not want this to be managed from the centre', he added. But even if not directed in a centralised fashion, through their funding and guidance, the New Labour government facilitated local festivities in a way that their predecessors had not.

The fiftieth anniversary of the NHS attracted a significant degree of participation and most people in the UK were aware of it. Internal reporting by civil servants found that whereas only 8 per cent of people knew about the anniversary at the beginning of 1998, 78 per cent were aware at the end of the birthday week in July.[49] According to surveys, 86 per cent of people had seen something about the anniversary in their local community or in the media, even if some had not immediately known that it related to the occasion. As ever, opinions about the care delivered by the NHS and its wider cultural meaning sometimes diverged. The public feedback about care during the years immediately before New Labour's large budget increases in the early 2000s remained relatively critical. Yet confidence and satisfaction rates in the service still increased by nearly 10 per cent at the end of the anniversary week. NHS birthdays further underlined how public perceptions of the institution reflected cultural and political values, as well as the actual quality of the health care received in hospitals and health centres.

Some members of the public continued to express anxiety about the NHS's future in 1998. A special panel show organised by Channel 4 titled *The Prescription* featured a wave of concern about waiting lists and funding.[50] The belief in NHS crisis, then, could coexist with celebration. Other people complained about the costs involved, or accused staff of wasting time at Buckingham Palace at the expense of their patients.[51] Nevertheless, the scale of celebrations and the depth of participation and awareness among the public underscored the impact of New Labour's interventions. NHS birthdays had become less radical than during the 1980s when trade unions formed their main advocates, and were now subject to corporate partnerships and public relations expertise. Yet many of their traditions and much of their imagery endured, amplified into a national celebration of a state welfare institution like no other. The NHS's supporters – inside and outside government – had placed the service at the heart of British political culture.

MAKING THE HISTORY OF 'OUR NHS'

The growth of NHS birthdays as a mass cultural tradition involved 'making history', with the service's supporters shaping a usable story out of its past. These occasions reflected – and contributed to – the triumph of a historical understanding of the virtues of state-organised and financed health care that fortified the NHS's prestige in the present. This narrative was social democratic, telling a story about the state's contributions, the virtues of collective progress and the perils of free-market medicine. The public did not unthinkingly parrot the now dominant account of the NHS's past, but large numbers of people agreed with it. Trade unions, health activists and eventually the state sourced memories to reinforce this sense of a shared history around the service. These developments challenge the argument, made by the cultural critic Patrick Wright during the 'heritage debates' of the 1980s, that a popular interest in the past only served conservative politics.[52] Instead, the use of history during NHS birthdays provided a welfare institution with further esteem against its neoliberal critics and deepened the notion of 'Our NHS' in the public imagination. As a result, the welfare nationalism surrounding the service acquired historical foundations, deepening its authority.

The strategic deployment of history had been baked into promoting the NHS from the beginning. After all, during the service's foundation, the postwar Labour government had condemned the interwar medical system to justify the need for greater state intervention in medical care. As the NHS's anniversaries grew in prominence, the Labour Party picked up and amplified this tactic.[53] Amidst the rancour of the 1978 anniversary, Jim Callaghan's government released a pamphlet about the history of the health service. *National Health Service: The First Thirty Years* (1978) was authored by Brian Abel-Smith, the left-wing health economist who had battled against free-market opponents to prove the NHS's value for money during the 1950s and 1960s.[54] Now a Labour advisor, Abel-Smith synthesised his academic work for a wider audience. Dedicated to NHS staff, the pamphlet praised Britain as 'the first country in the world to offer free medical care to the whole population', portrayed as a 'bold decision' taken during the Second World War. The NHS improved, he believed, on the earlier system of national health insurance which 'excluded children, wives who did not go out to work, the self-employed, higher paid employees and many old people'. Abel-Smith also highlighted the regional imbalances in the quality of medical care that had existed across the country, as well as the social stigma engendered by customs such as private and 'panel' patients waiting in separate rooms. The NHS had ended this medical inequity, he argued, through the principles of state rationalisation. This 'noble purpose' was built upon by the postwar modernisation of hospital care and general practice, still unfolding when he penned the pamphlet.[55] *National Health Service: The First Thirty Years* provided a critical historical account of what preceded the NHS in 1948 in order to praise what followed.

Subsequent elaborations of this historical narrative went further than Abel-Smith in condemning the medical past. During the 1980s, when NHS anniversaries started to become popular occasions, trade unions often represented their struggles against the Thatcher government's health policies as a fight against a return to the 1930s. For the fortieth anniversary of the NHS, the East Midlands branch of the TUC published a collection of personal testimony titled *Life Before the National Health Service* (1988).[56] In its introduction, this slim pamphlet warned that the Conservatives wanted to create a 'two-tier' health service with charity serving the 'very poor' and private medicine supporting everyone else. 'The best way to illustrate what the future might hold', it suggested, 'is to look back into the past to see what life was like without a National Health Service'. Like Abel-Smith, the TUC pinpointed unevenness and gaps in pre-NHS health care as symptoms of a system 'in turmoil'. The personal testimony included within the volume – procured by writing, they explained, 'hundreds of letters; to newspapers, to Trade Unionists, to old people and to many other Organisations who might be able to tell us' – reinforced such claims. Mrs Semmence, for instance, recalled 'the days when people would walk about half dead because they were sick and unable to afford the 2s 6d to see the doctor'. 'People do not appreciate what they get today', she believed, adding 'God save the NHS'. Mrs Hess recounted that she 'could have wept with joy' when the service began. 'It was a God-send to us', she added. To the trade unions, these memories carried political heft. 'If the public are not concerned about and don't remember the past, if they want jumble sales or flag days, then it will go back to the way it was before 1948', they warned.

Neil Kinnock also advanced the NHS's social democratic historical narrative, as his adulation of Bevan or visits to Jennie Lee showed. Like the trade unions, the Labour leader railed against pre-1948 medical care for its inequity. He frequently praised Bevan – 'a rare man, compelling and visionary' – and quoted his fellow Welshman in speeches: from strictures on the evils of money in medicine to his view that founding the NHS proved that Britain was 'a nation very largely of visionary empiricists'.[57] In doing so, Kinnock reaffirmed Bevan's centrality to the NHS story. To be sure, Bevan's time as Minister of Health in the Attlee government ensured that he would always be associated with the service. But, while alive, he was a somewhat divisive figure. Bevan's hatred for the Conservatives and battles within his own party on behalf of the radical left earned him many enemies. The fond memories later expressed towards the Welshman beyond the Labour Party – and even within it – were far from inevitable.

Indeed, from the 1980s, the rougher edges of Bevan's personality were smoothed out, helping to create a 'founding father' for the NHS as a national inheritance. In 1987, the Welsh sculptor Robert Thomas produced a statue of Bevan that was erected in central Cardiff. Thomas was the son of a miner and member of the 'Rhondda School', a group of artists with a socialist edge to their work that depicted working-class industrial life. His statue of Bevan became a famous symbol of the Welsh capital, facing down Cardiff Castle on a plinth adorned with the phrase 'Founder of the National Health Service'. This focus on Bevan only increased as NHS birthdays expanded in scope and significance. A documentary presented by *Private Eye* editor Ian Hislop about the history of the service on its fiftieth anniversary bore the title *Pennies from Bevan* (1998).[58] Professional historians joined in. The 'official historian' of the NHS, Charles Webster, contributed to a 1998 feature in *Nursing Times* where he answered twenty questions posing as Bevan himself. The hard-nosed queries put to Webster-as-Bevan included, 'What do you do when you're not at work?' and 'When did you last cry?', confirming the softening of the Welshman's historical image decades after his death in 1960.[59]

New Labour picked up this use of history as established by their predecessors within the party and the trade unions. Despite the emphasis on the 'new', the party did not entirely reject its own past as many commentators and academics claimed in the wake of its electoral successes under Blair. To the historian James Cronin, New Labour launched 'a frontal assault on the party's traditions' in order to rebrand itself.[60] Yet as historians such as Emily Robinson have shown, they did not discard Labour's past but widened it to include contributions from Liberals like the politician Lloyd George, the economist John Maynard Keynes and the social reformer William Beveridge.[61] In the New Labour view, the radical tradition belonged to both the Labour Party and the Liberal Party as they attempted to widen their electoral appeal.

However, the NHS stood as the exception. To New Labour, this part of the welfare state was a uniquely Labour achievement. In a speech on its fiftieth anniversary, Blair shared how the service created by the postwar Attlee government had cared for his father after he suffered a stroke and his mother as she died of cancer.[62] Indeed, the expanded use of personal stories by politicians to talk about their attachment to the NHS marked a shift in approach during the New Labour years. 'It is the embodiment of the values I believe in', Blair continued. 'It is the tangible experience of what I mean by "community", working together – and paying taxes together – to create and sustain it in the interests of each individual in the community'. Blair used a phrase regularly deployed by Bevan to describe this ethos, arguing that it lay 'at the heart of any civilised country'. If New Labour baulked at other pillars of 'Old Labour', it expressed few qualms about heightening the welfare nationalism that their predecessors had fostered around the NHS. 'Britain is one of the few countries where they feel your pulse before they feel your wallet if you collapse in the street', boasted Blair in a statement that ignored the reality of health care in nearly all industrialised nations. Gordon Brown regularly praised the NHS for having saved his eyesight after a rugby accident. The Scotsman saw the service as not just 'our party's greatest achievement' but also 'the most-loved institution of our country'.[63] In a direct invocation of its founder, he asserted that millions of Britons 'owe their lives, their health and, in Aneurin Bevan's phrase, their serenity to the existence of the NHS'. For all their embrace of markets in the NHS, New Labour stood alongside their 1970s counterparts in bolstering welfare nationalism.

Nonetheless, as this social democratic historical narrative took hold, the NHS was presented as the harbinger of more-or-less linear medical progress since 1948. Comparisons were usually made between the 1930s and the present and tended to overlook how other countries had made similar advances across the same period with different health systems. The National Liaison Steering Group in charge of NHS50, for instance, distributed a 'Fact Sheet' with graphs that charted improvements in metrics such as infant mortality rates (which fell from 33.9 deaths of infants under one per 1,000 live births in 1948 to 6.1 deaths per 1,000 live births in 1994) and life expectancy (which had risen from 66.4 years for men and 71.2 years for women in 1948 to 74.2 years for men and 79.4 years for women in 1994).[64] The decline of deaths due to contagious diseases such as tuberculosis, meningitis and influenza over the previous fifty years received similar attention. Blue lines cresting upwards or plummeting downwards on Y-axes symbolised an arc of uninterrupted medical advancement, thanks, it was suggested, to nationalised medicine. These statistics were, of course, achievements in their own right. But they did not just take place in the UK. No mention was made of how other industrialised nations had achieved comparable health improvements through systems funded by direct payments or insurance. This 'Fact Sheet' also ignored the stubborn health inequalities – across class, race and region – that Britain still struggled with, despite the calls for greater attention to preventative medicine throughout the service's history. The NHS, it seemed, was a unique blessing.

Hospitals encouraged patients to witness the medical progress secured by the NHS first-hand. In 1998, Liverpool's Alder Hey Children's Hospital invited former patients back to see how things had changed since the 1940s.[65] James Watson recalled treatment for osteomyelitis (a chronic bone condition) in 1946. He shared how a surgeon had nearly amputated his leg but, at the last moment, had tried 'the new wonder drug, penicillin' with success. Watson's story supported the prevalent view that medical care was cruel before the NHS and had only become more humane after its inception. Another patient, Pat Williams, had contracted tuberculosis aged six and spent nearly three years in the hospital with just two hourly visits from her parents each week. 'Times have certainly changed for the better,' she concluded after her visit, 'today children do not lose contact with the outside world and having their parents around can make all the difference'. The NHS, of course, had not immediately ended such restrictions on parents' visiting time in hospitals, and in fact they had continued into at least the 1960s. Yet Williams's statement further supported a social democratic account of the service's compassion and its association with medical advance.

The neoliberal critics of the NHS offered their own histories. To them, the escalation of the institution's anniversaries into ever-more lavish and popular forms posed a serious problem. As the emergence of welfare nationalism showed, private medicine possessed none of the NHS's stature in popular culture or public opinion. Such feeling around the NHS had helped sink plans for the mass take-up of private health insurance. Part of the reputational damage to private alternatives in these years also stemmed from a prevalent historical account that depicted the state system as an escape from a bleak past where income had determined one's health. David Green disagreed with the social democratic interpretation of the NHS's origins in his book *Working-Class Patients and the Medical Establishment* (1985), which provided a history of self-help in Britain from the Victorian period to 1948.[66] Green had served as a Labour councillor in Newcastle upon Tyne during the 1970s but, after an about-turn in his politics, now contributed to the IEA, the neoliberal think tank behind many of the early proposals for a system of private health insurance. In his book, Green provided a celebratory account of the friendly societies that thousands of British workers had paid into to cover the costs of illness before the NHS. Manual workers, he claimed, had created 'organizations for the supply of primary medical care that were not surpassed anywhere in the world'. Yet, for all the friendly societies' achievements, this world, Green argued, was lost to the state – first undermined by the 1911 National Insurance Act and then buried by the NHS. Green therefore retold the NHS's history in less favourable terms, implying that its inception continued to harm health care in the present. It was a mistake, in his view, to have abandoned the mutualism and private payments of the interwar years. The subsequent 'monumental growth of the power of the state', argued Green, had only empowered bureaucrats and the medical profession at the expense of ordinary 'consumers'. 'The story of working-class achievement recounted in these pages', he closed, 'ought not to be ignored by today's public policy makers'.

Nevertheless, being ignored was not the whole problem faced by the advocates of neoliberal alternatives in health care. Rather, the historical arguments advanced by Green and his fellow travellers became the focus of popular derision and ridicule. The social democratic account of the service formed an integral part of the story of 'Our NHS' by the close of the twentieth century. Alternative historical explanations that championed the self-help, financial independence or local charity that underpinned health care before 1948 were successfully maligned by prominent left-wing politicians as the views of a radical minority that fell beyond the pale of mainstream opinion. In Kinnock's assessment, for example, 'their system' – as opposed to 'Our NHS' – represented a past best left behind, never to be repeated.[67] 'It didn't work in all the years up to 1948 and it couldn't work in any of the years from now', charged the Labour leader. This association of private medicine with the past reverberated in popular culture. The comedian Rik Mayall satirised sympathetic interpretations of the pre-NHS era in *The New Statesman* (1987–1994), a sitcom in which he played a sleazy, self-interested Tory MP named Alan B'Stard.[68] In one episode, B'Stard began a speech with his opinion that to solve NHS waiting lists the government should simply 'shut down the health service'. 'In the good old days', he continued, 'you were poor, you got ill, and you died'. 'And these days', he offered by way of comparison, 'people seem to think they have some God-given right to be cured!' In the sketch, B'Stard insisted that today's 'sloppy socialist thinking' only produced 'more poor people', concluding that 'my policies would eradicate poor people, thereby eliminating poverty'. Criticisms of free-market views of the medical past were not just for laughs. The socialist indie rock band The Housemartins climbed up the UK music charts in the mid-1980s with their song 'Flag Day'.[69] This slow-moving track condemned the charitable fundraising that had partly funded hospitals in the pre-NHS era with its depiction of jumble sales and collection boxes as a 'waste of time'. The more sympathetic views of how health care had worked before 1948 enjoyed no comparable cultural output that might allow them to get anywhere near a record player in a teenager's bedroom.

As trade union efforts during the 1980s illustrated, supporters of the service procured public testimony to reinforce their political arguments. Under New Labour, the state began to source popular memories about the NHS's past for the first time. The organisers of NHS50 urged NHS Trusts to find local people born, married or who had qualified as medical professionals on 5 July 1948 and invite them to events.[70] Through being placed in the spotlight, patients and staff became integral participants in constructing the NHS's past. Special history books, the organisers added, which 'remember the most significant events for future generations in pictures, illustrations, facts and personal memories', could be produced for the occasion. Several NHS Trusts took this advice. Lewisham Hospital NHS Trust, for instance, released a slim booklet for local people that encapsulated the social democratic historical narrative around the service.[71] A foreword by the Chief Executive of the Trust quoted Bevan's description of nationalised medicine as lifting a 'shadow from millions of homes'. In a section on 'Fifty Years of Medical Advance', a familiar pattern of health improvements achieved since the service's inception filled the pages. The personal testimony from former NHS staff and patients collected for the pamphlet testified to the caring and communal nature of the institution: from cheery stories of nurses checking surgeons' rubber gloves for holes by blowing them up, to a senior nurse recalling 'the fellowship we shared with each other' on the ward, to a patient praising how staff had made 'my husband and I feel very special' during childbirth. A voluntary group working with elderly patients at Ruskin College, Oxford, collected local memories in another volume, *From Cradle to Grave: 50 Years of the NHS, Memories of Before and After 1948* (1998).[72] In a 'Before the NHS' section, contributors such as Rose Fisher shared how the establishment of the service had brought feelings of security and progress. 'At least if you woke up after 5 July 1948 to find a group of strangers surrounding your bed they would be medical students rather than there to check if you were a deserving recipient of charity', she maintained. Recollections about the NHS's past, now sourced and collated on a systematic basis, reinforced the institution's reputation.[73] Put another way, the service's history was 'made' to provide it with greater esteem in the present.

Not everyone condemned the pre-NHS era of health care – fissures existed at the edges of the dominant interpretation of the institution's history.[74] Asked for her memories in the 1980s as part of the trade union-published *Life Before the National Health Service* volume, D.A. Salisbury recalled the charitable fundraising and workers' insurance schemes of the period with affection.[75] Her husband had served on a medical fund that employees in local factories and businesses in Kettering paid into to cover costs during times of illness. As common in the period, the fund held fundraising events to raise extra money. 'These included', Salisbury remembered, 'flower shows with entertainment to follow, band concerns, whist drives, dances and also each year a carnival where all factories got together and made a day to remember'. Her fond memories of such events challenged the idea that all pre-1948 health care was harsh or merely about determining one's income. The community-centredness of charitable medical fundraising drew close, in her telling, to Green's sympathetic account of the interwar years. Yet such voices were few and far between. In the main, the public did not perceive the earlier world of friendly societies, working-class medical funds and large-scale charitable fundraising with affection. Instead, the state's role in medical care was celebrated as an escape from a harsh past.

'OUR NHS' IN THE TWENTY-FIRST CENTURY

The celebration of the NHS's birthdays confirmed the service's centrality to British life by the twenty-first century. More than just a health system, this was now an institution imbued with a positive image of social democratic universalism, a sense of shared historical progress and the authority of welfare nationalism. However, while this cultural framing may have helped the service build and maintain public support, it carried distinct costs and created unexpected outcomes. The commonplace 'Our NHS' encapsulated the longstanding boundaries that welfare nationalism sometimes fashioned for the service's patients and staff who came from beyond Britain's borders. As a phrase hinged on a possessive word, it sharpened who belonged and who did not. Moreover, the presentation of the institution's history as one of consensus across political lines – rather than as a distinctive legacy of the left that had always been the target of free-market opposition – made it easier for the service's reputation to be co-opted.

As NHS birthdays crystallised into national occasions after the 1990s, they could reveal a popular sense of nostalgia about the institution's past.[76] Romanticised projections of the service's history obscured the political disputes or range of public opinions that had defined the NHS in the postwar decades. The journalist Polly Toynbee was far from the only person declaring that nationalised medicine 'became immediately the most loved and profoundly defended institution in British life' on a special fiftieth anniversary BBC radio broadcast.[77] Such a statement downplayed the mixed opinions about the service and the ideological opposition that existed during and after its commencement. In an effort to distinguish itself, at least partly, from the radicalism of the trade unions in the 1980s, the New Labour government stoked the sentimentalising of the NHS's past to advance its modernisation agenda. 'Setting out a vision for the future of the NHS', explained civil servants and political advisors, 'has always been a key objective of the NHS50 campaign, which has used nostalgia as a "hook" to attract interest before encouraging people to look forward'.[78] One such 'hook' used by NHS Trusts in 1998 was inviting retired staff back to discuss what they cheerfully described as 'the good old days'.[79] At the Bloomfield House Health Centre at Bury St Edmunds, staff participated in a similarly rosy image of the past by dressing up in pressed suits and starched white nurses' uniforms from the 1940s.[80] Their patients could observe a supposed golden era of rigid medical hierarchies and cleanliness performed in front of them. One mile away, at the West Suffolk Hospital, members of the public watched nurses plaster limbs with 'yesteryear's hospital equipment'. Though far from being static or used in a single way, a romanticised nostalgia formed an important part of the historical narrative that permeated NHS anniversaries, and often worked in the institution's favour by animating warm feelings about the past while showcasing medical progress.

However, such presentations of the NHS's past obscured other parts of its history. In 2012, the service featured prominently in the Opening Ceremony of the London Olympic Games.[81] Directed by the film-maker Danny Boyle, this four-hour spectacle painted a picture of British history encompassing the Industrial Revolution, pop music and Commonwealth immigration. In its tone, the ceremony offered an image of a confident and multicultural Britain at ease with itself. To showcase the NHS, hundreds of dancing nurses in matching blue-and-white uniforms pushed trolleys that – when the camera panned over the stadium – spelled out the service's initials. On the one hand, this event confirmed the strength of the welfare nationalism now surrounding the service. The NHS lay at the heart of a projection of national identity and British history to over 400 million people around the world. Indeed, the prominence given to a public welfare institution annoyed some Conservative politicians, including Aidan Burley MP, who dismissed the ceremony as 'leftie multicultural crap'. On the other hand, this event smoothed out some of the less laudable parts of the NHS's history. Burley's dig at 'multicultural crap' referred, in part, to the racial diversity of the nurses featured in the ceremony. Though their presence provided a visual reminder that the institution had always relied on a racially diverse workforce, it could not meaningfully address the discrimination that Black and Asian workers had faced in the past, or indeed continued to endure. The feel-good celebrations of 'Our NHS' at the start of the twenty-first century, then, could encourage a self-satisfied historical narrative about the service that confirmed the heights of welfare nationalism, but rarely offered opportunities to adequately come to terms with its costs.

Moreover, the popular depictions of the institution's past as a matter of consensus, progress and quintessentially 'British' values paradoxically facilitated the NHS's reputation being deployed by politicians working against its interests. The Conservative Party's public embrace of the service in the 2010s illustrated this outcome. Of course, the party had overseen significant parts of the NHS's development since its inception, such as the 1962 Hospital Plan or the first systematic reorganisation of the service's administration in 1973. Nevertheless, throughout the service's history, Conservative politicians had regularly met with groups such as the Fellowship for Freedom in Medicine or think tanks like the IEA who wanted to replace the institution. As Thatcher showed, its leading members sometimes voiced outright hostility towards the social democratic principles behind the NHS.

In the 2010s, this picture changed – the Conservative Party came to publicly embrace the health service, often in welfare nationalist terms, for electoral gain. Before coming to power, future Conservative Prime Minister David Cameron had laid the groundwork with a speech worthy of the Labour Party in its degree of approbation for the institution.[82] For the NHS's sixtieth anniversary in 2008 he symbolically visited Park Hospital where Bevan had 'opened' the service six decades earlier, lavishing praise on the NHS as 'one of the great achievements of our past, it's an institution which embodies, in its very bricks and mortar, in its people, in its services, something which is great about Britain'. 'That something', Cameron explained, 'is equity, the founding value of the NHS: the spirit of fairness for all . . . and the equal right of everyone to care and comfort when they are born, when they are ill, and when they are dying'. Such statements affirmed how the universalism embodied by the NHS, and the cultural identification of the service with Britishness and 'our past', commanded respect. In this regard, the left had achieved a victory by forcing its opponents onto their ground. Cameron also inherited the New Labour approach of discussing his attachment to the institution though personal stories, recounting how its staff had cared for his late son. If Thatcher openly praised her private health insurance plan, Cameron took pains to show how he used the NHS. Yet the social democratic values underpinning the service were expunged from Cameron's historical account through his insistence that nationalised medicine was 'not a dream of socialism'. For anyone listening to his speech, it would seem that the NHS was a common-sense reform, welcomed by all, unchallenged during its inception or in the years since. The historical contributions of activists, campaigners, trade unions, workers, the Labour Party and the service's supporters among the general public were nowhere to be seen.

Once he entered government, Cameron oversaw the largest sustained reduction in NHS spending as a percentage of GDP since the early 1950s.[83] This diminished funding carried consequences for the NHS's capacities, despite the service's overall resilience to the influence of the private sector in this decade. Under Conservative-led governments in the 2010s, the number of people waiting for hospital treatment in England alone rose from 2.5 million to 4.6 million (its highest number to date). The sanitised cultural image of the service's past eased its strategic use by politicians who, through their actions, undermined standards of health care across the country. The fact that Jeremy Hunt was the first Conservative Secretary of State for Health to proudly wear an 'NHS' enamel pin badge on his suit lapel while also being the first to oversee such historic down-turns in key service metrics encapsulated his party's position.

Future Conservative Prime Minister Boris Johnson weaponised the NHS's reputation to much more dramatic effect during the 2016 referendum over the UK's EU membership. The Vote Leave campaign placed the health service at the heart of its message to voters. In one promotional video, Vote Leave presented a fictionalised image of the NHS 'Inside the EU' next to an imagined vision of the service 'Outside the EU'.[84] The footage for the former showed a woman helping a sobbing elderly relative through a hospital swamped with patients and staffed by doctors and nurses visibly under pressure. The footage for the latter showed the pair in the same hospital, with few patients, staffed by smiling doctors and nurses. At the end of the video, Vote Leave told viewers that the taxes spent on EU membership could fund one new hospital every week, encouraging them to 'take back control' so that 'our money' could be spent on 'our priorities, like the NHS'. Johnson amplified this message by travelling around the UK in a large red bus emblazoned with the – later discredited – claim that 'We send the EU £350 million a week, let's fund our NHS instead' (Figure 19).

For Vote Leave, the political power of 'Our NHS' lay not just in fighting faceless bureaucrats based in Brussels, but also in 'taking back control'

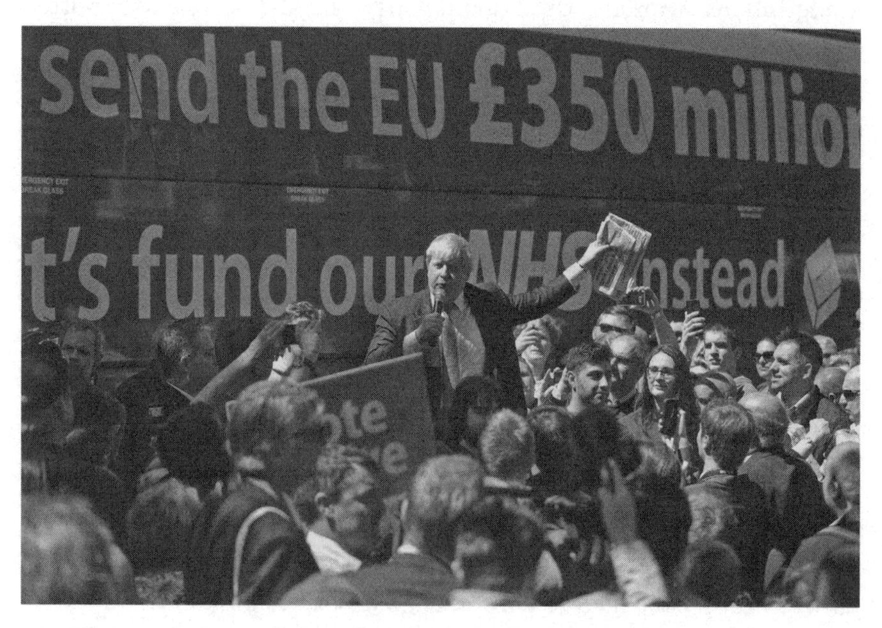

19. The mythology of the NHS as a peculiarly British invention, always adored and consistently supported across the political spectrum, reinforced its standing. However, the sanitising of the service's contested origins as well as the work undertaken by its supporters that had ensured both its survival and iconic status allowed politicians to co-opt its reputation for different political causes. The Vote Leave campaign placed the NHS at the heart of their messaging during the 2016 referendum on Britain's EU membership.

of a service that they implied lay threatened by foreign migrants. These arguments were racialised, as a poster unveiled by the leading Eurosceptic Nigel Farage that depicted a long line of Asian men with the phrase 'Breaking Point' underlined.[85] In this context, the strategic deployment of 'Our NHS' as a form of welfare nationalism echoed the earlier uses of that term against Commonwealth migrants during the postwar decades. It had long been understood as a national inheritance that needed to be protected from foreigners, and it continued to be invoked in this manner. Yet the public's esteem of the NHS was more easily utilised by this type of conservative, xenophobic politics during the 2010s in part because of a sanitised understanding of its past. Even if the NHS remained a social democratic health service, and its universalism and communal principles enjoyed widespread public backing, the figures and organisations who had ensured this outcome – predominantly on the political left – were too often removed from the historical explanation of how these outcomes had come to pass. If their contributions had been recognised as an essential part of the NHS's history, then the institution's reputation might not have been so easily redeployed by those whose decisions placed its services under such strain.

***

Beginning in the postwar years as muted occasions mainly observed by high-ranking politicians and medical experts, in the 1980s NHS birthdays became moments that mixed celebration with protest and brought in a wider swathe of the population. Trade unions motivated much of this transformation. In the following decade, New Labour picked up a flowering cultural tradition, pruning some of its radical roots. Still, NHS birthdays now existed as government-backed, national occasions that celebrated a state-funded and organised universal health system. The growth of welfare nationalism, which had begun in the 1970s, ascended to new heights after the millennium, exemplified by the service's anniversaries.

As an act of commemoration, the expansion of NHS birthdays involved calibrating a positive historical account of the service's origins and achievements. Many members of the public contributed to the growth of a distinctly social democratic narrative about the NHS's past, even if some challenged it. The romanticised understandings of the service's history sometimes advanced by these occasions facilitated its celebration but obscured the challenges the NHS had faced in embedding itself or overcoming political opposition in the past. A cultural image of the NHS as a peculiarly British invention, always adored among the population and consistently supported across the political spectrum, may have buttressed its standing, but defied historical reality. As a result, the service's popular reputation could be more easily co-opted for political gain by those who harmed its operational capacities. The endurance of social democracy through the NHS, then, led to unexpected – and at times ironic – outcomes.

All the same, no other welfare service enjoyed anything comparable to the public and state-backed celebration of the NHS's contribution to British life. People did not bake birthday cakes to mark the point that mothers gained access to child benefit. They did not organise fun runs to celebrate council housing. Nor did they post letters with commemorative stamps that championed unemployment pay. Although this affection could be used opportunistically, and carried costs, the cultural importance of universal health care suffused society, the result of active and deliberate efforts to cement its position as 'Our NHS'.

CONCLUSION

On 5 July 2018, June Rosen returned to the site where Bevan had inaugurated Britain's experiment with nationalised medicine while staying at her family home (Figure 20).[1] The 'first' NHS hospital now occupied a prominent place in commemorations of the service, and, after its fortieth anniversary in 1988, it had acquired a new name: the Trafford General Hospital. It retained an interwar façade that would still be familiar to Bevan, built with red bricks and topped by a clock tower. However, the Welshman would not have recognised more recent additions such as an orthopaedic centre and urgent care unit. Rosen was invited to mark the NHS's seventieth anniversary. Since qualifying in 1958, she had served hospitals in the Manchester area as a physiotherapist. Photographers captured images of Rosen, as well as of a line of staff who showcased nurses' uniforms over the decades. The Mayor of Greater Manchester, Andy Burnham, delivered a speech, and a blue plaque was unveiled to recognise the hospital as the 'birthplace' of the NHS. The day's events underlined the deliberate use of history and the tone of celebration now typical of these occasions, held for a universal health system that remained overwhelmingly funded by taxes, delivered by the public sector and free at the point of use.

In London, amidst the parliamentary rancour around Brexit, embattled Prime Minister Theresa May attended a special ceremony at Westminster Abbey.[2] At the beginning of the event, a nurse placed a copy of the 'House to House' leaflet – which had been used in 1948 to

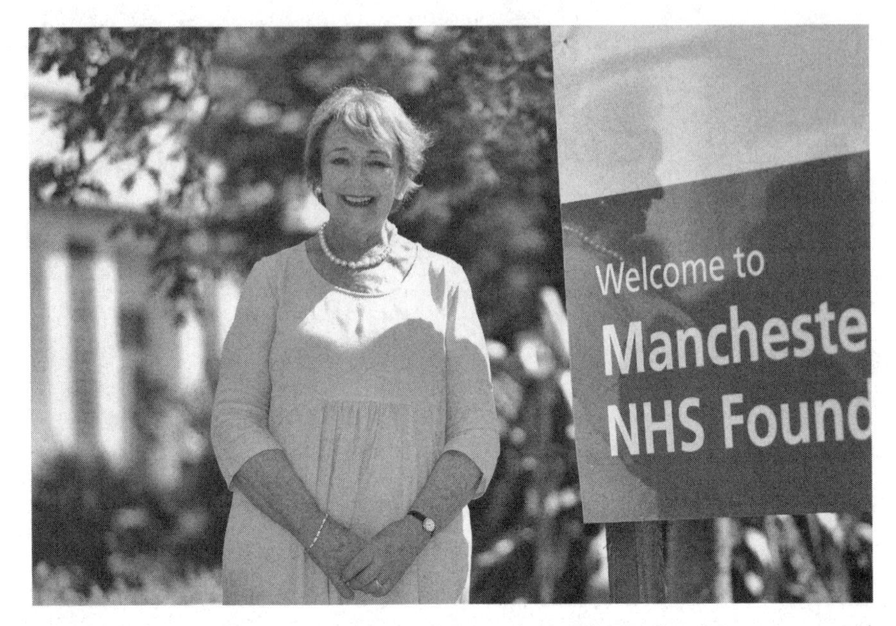

20. June Rosen first met Aneurin Bevan the night before he inaugurated the NHS on 5 July 1948. After qualifying in 1958, Rosen gave decades of service as a physiotherapist to patients in the Manchester area. She was invited to a special ceremony to mark the seventieth anniversary of the NHS in 2018 and only retired two years later during the COVID-19 pandemic.

persuade Britons to sign up to the NHS – on the high altar like a sacred relic. Assorted politicians, members of the royal family, medical professionals and patients sang hymns such as 'Jerusalem Luminosa' and listened to orations honouring the health system's achievements. The Dean of Westminster quoted Bevan's words that the NHS was 'a piece of real socialism; it's a piece of real Christianity too', adding his praise for 'this remarkable, this unique, service to the people of this land'. 'Let us give thanks to God for the National Health Service; for those whose vision and compassion brought it into existence, and those who have served within it these seventy years', intoned one prayer later in the ceremony. The founders of the NHS could not have conceived that one day a Conservative Prime Minister would feel compelled to genuflect to a health system invoked with such reverence in a religious site. Such a venue, which hosted state occasions like coronations and royal weddings, confirmed the welfare nationalism that now surrounded the NHS. It seemed natural – almost to the point where it did not attract comment – that the NHS, as Britain's best-loved institution, would receive the acclaim which lay at the heart of such pomp and ceremony.

Rosen compared her time working in the NHS to being a 'very small cog in an enormous wheel'. Though modestly downplaying her own contributions to the service and its patients, Rosen's words captured something of the vast scale and esteem of the medical system now regularly celebrated on 5 July. The NHS had begun on much less certain ground than its later prestige would suggest. During the Second World War, the public viewed plans for a comprehensive system of 'state medicine' with a mixture of hope, ambivalence, suspicion and sometimes even hostility. The promises by medical reformers to coordinate care and banish direct payment in doctors' surgeries and hospitals did not automatically generate support. The NHS, as a practical reality and a cultural icon, had to be made. At the crucial moment of its foundation, supporters grappled with public perceptions of what greater government intervention in medicine implied. To address their misgivings, they took steps such as safeguarding choice and presenting the service as a protector of the family that would reverse a decline in the nation's birth rate. The foundation of the NHS, then, proved difficult and involved a dialogue with longstanding views among the public about the appropriate role of government that they had inherited from the interwar and Victorian past.

Many such challenges remained as governments modernised the health service across the postwar decades. No golden era of funding, it saw budgets allocated to the welfare state that were low by later standards. Even within the scant spending given to social services, health care stood as the poorer cousin to the likes of education. As a result, no new hospitals opened in 1948 and purpose-built facilities such as health centres remained few and far between. Yet, modernisation also involved changing the everyday practices and routines of the NHS, a social process missed by an exclusive focus on funding and new buildings. Supporters of the institution, from charitable organisations to academics to volunteers, worked to adapt the health service to the wider transformations taking place in Britain. Extending the visiting hours for families and friends in hospitals, welcoming fathers at the birth of a child or building parking spaces near a health centre to reflect swelling car ownership amounted to an institution shifting with the times. The construction of new hospitals and general practice facilities picked up from the 1960s. Indeed, a stroll in most villages, towns and cities in the UK a decade later would reveal the health service to be among the most visible signs of change wrought by the welfare state. Far from perfect, postwar modernisation did not always reach its full potential or banish social divides in the NHS along the lines of class, gender or race, and sometimes even brought these tensions into clear view. The focus of the NHS's supporters at this point on mothers during a 'baby boom' or on working-class families when Britain remained heavily industrialised would later seem less appropriate. Nevertheless, when compared to other parts of the welfare state or public industries that were also founded after the Second World War, the NHS more successfully embedded its communal principles while attending to personal needs. The health service's evolution challenges the argument that a rising tide of individualism in the postwar decades buried social democratic politics, or that its institutions became irrevocably tarnished as bureaucratic and unresponsive.

The 1970s and 1980s represented an important moment in the transformation of the NHS's reputation and its capacity to withstand ideological assault. These years witnessed the rise of welfare nationalism around the service, stoked by its defenders and inflected by its shifting place on the world stage. The NHS's initial supporters offered the service as a model for others in a postwar world where nations sought to extend medical care to a greater sweep of their own populations. While the institution won many admirers, including in key positions in the US, few countries replicated its exact structures or believed British boasts that the NHS stood as the 'envy of the world'. Transatlantic cooperation between medical reformers in the 1940s and 1950s splintered in the face of diverging priorities and persistent attacks on the NHS by US conservatives. In part, welfare nationalism emerged from this rupture, as medical experts, academics, politicians, commentators and cultural figures on the British left moved to differentiate the two nations' health arrangements. These arguments proliferated, helping the NHS to eventually become entrenched in the popular imagination as representative of 'British' values, rather than as a model for pushing forward the frontiers of medical universalism on the world stage. The international aspirations of the NHS's supporters narrowed, even if this development provided the service with greater resilience at home.

As the NHS became understood as reflective of essential 'British' qualities, this framing served to include and exclude certain groups of people. The emphasis on the health service's national distinctiveness was sometimes weaponised against people hailing from beyond Britain who worked in the institution or relied on its care. Critics of the NHS, like the Fellowship for Freedom in Medicine, blended free-market opposition to the service with racialised claims that purportedly inferior foreign doctors replaced their British-born counterparts. Enoch Powell and his supporters deployed the question of access to health services as part of their campaign against Commonwealth immigration. In these ways, another source of welfare nationalism revealed itself, based on who 'belonged' in the service or who had the 'right' to access public health care. The belief in 'Our NHS', then, could involve a sense of superiority over other nations, as well as scapegoats and exclusions directed at marginalised groups within Britain. Statements like the one made in Westminster Abbey in 2018 that the NHS was 'for the people of this land' might be used against the same people who made its services possible. Indeed, Theresa May's participation in the seventieth anniversary celebrations belied her role in creating a 'hostile environment' in immigration policy, which had led to the deportation of a number of former NHS employees who once cleaned hospitals or tended patients.[3]

This swelling support for the NHS hindered neoliberal advances into British health care during the 1980s. The long-held aspirations among free-market intellectuals, think tanks, parts of the medical profession and influential Conservative politicians to replace nationalised medicine with a system of private health insurance ran aground in this decade. These grand ambitions struggled to take off in the face of market instability, the administrative complexity of abolishing a decades-old health service, and an increasing association with the inequities of 'American medicine'. The positive associations with capitalist values that the Conservative Party successfully fostered in areas such as buying a council house or stock market investment became impossible in the field of medicine due to the counterattacks marshalled by the NHS's supporters. In cultural terms, free-market medicine was daubed with the Stars and Stripes, which could not compete with the Union Jack draped over the NHS.

As this disappointment for neoliberal politics unfolded, its proponents shifted position by turning to the introduction of markets within the NHS itself. The spread of outsourcing, and the use of external capital to construct public facilities over the closing decades of the twentieth century, signalled a growing belief among politicians that the private sector knew best. However, the deteriorating conditions for many NHS staff and patients that sometimes – though not always – resulted from the expanded involvement of markets challenged such a rosy view. Indeed, the impact of cuts motivated by efficiency drives or predictions of the institution's imminent capture by private capital escalated feelings of 'crisis' in the health service from the 1980s onwards. In turn, the marketisation unfolding within the NHS motivated trade unions, activists and campaigners to identify with the service's defence even more explicitly, further embedding its prominence in national life. All the same, the spectre of 'privatisation' and crisis raised by these groups may have been politically effective in sharpening public attention, but it could obscure more than it revealed about the history of the NHS. At the start of the new millennium, the service – though changed – received unprecedented levels of government funding, continued to provide the overwhelming majority of medical care and labour, and had expanded into new areas. Policies based on free-market principles, like PFI, could be reversed or abandoned altogether. Marketisation made inroads and reshaped the institution in these years, but the much-proclaimed 'death' of the NHS has yet to pass.

The making of 'Our NHS' as a lived reality and a cultural icon comprised a historical process that took effort by the service's supporters. It was not inevitable. The institution's history illustrates the capacity of social democracy's proponents to win popular backing and defend public institutions from neoliberal assault. Although many individuals and organisations contributed to this outcome, some of the most significant lay on the political left. From activist organisations like the SMA, to welfare experts such as Richard Titmuss, Brian Abel-Smith and Ann Cartwright, to cultural figures like the filmmakers Jack Pizzey, Tony Wardle and Yvette Vanson, to the country's largest public sector trade unions, the survival of social democratic politics in British medicine depended on nimble supporters.

The Labour Party also made decisive contributions, despite being out of power for large periods of the twentieth century – including, most obviously, founding the service along nationalised lines in 1948, as well as less-recognised measures such as addressing the tumult in general practice during the 1960s, the extension of modernisation in the difficult 1970s, and the record levels of funding allocated to the health service after the millennium. New Labour deepened the reach of markets in medical services as part of a recast programme of 'modernisation', but they also brought health spending up to the standards of other industrialised nations, improved waiting lists and times, and expanded the service's frontiers of care. They may have jettisoned older parts of the social democratic approach to the NHS, such as the earlier focus on mothers, families and industrial production, but they also expanded the institution's reach and popular recognition. New Labour made the trade union custom of marking 'N.H.S. Day' a national occasion for celebration. Such actions exemplified how the party boosted welfare nationalism, making later displays like the 2012 Olympic Opening Ceremony possible. The NHS therefore provides evidence of a continuation in social democratic values within the party after the 1980s, and even the invention of new traditions, rather than a total capitulation to neoliberalism.

By contrast, the history of free-market medicine in twentieth-century Britain is riddled with disappointments and disillusionment. Though its most fervent boosters made some gains, they regularly voiced frustration as the Conservative Party neglected to act on their suggestions. Even when the party adopted policy proposals drawn from a wider ecosystem of free-market intellectuals and organisations, it frequently failed to make them a reality. Taken together, the work of the NHS's supporters and the shortcomings of their opponents enabled social democratic politics to endure in Britain. But had the NHS brought the equality of health outcomes that it promised in 1948?

***

It took a global pandemic to make Rosen retire. In early 2020, a novel coronavirus branded 'COVID-19' by the WHO arrived in the UK. As case numbers escalated and her physiotherapy work became too difficult, Rosen ended a career almost as long as the NHS itself. Across the country, the operation and feel of the health service rapidly shifted. To reduce the transmission of infection, hospitals cancelled outpatient appointments, and GP surgeries moved doctors' consultations to mobile phones and videoconferencing platforms. Large waiting rooms in health centres suddenly became a health risk, their plastic chairs covered in tape to ensure social distancing. The same spaces that had embedded communalism within the NHS during the postwar decades were now treated with suspicion and bifurcated with sheets of Plexiglas. Already straining from the low budget increases given by Conservative-led governments in the 2010s, NHS waiting lists and times only worsened.

The author Polly Morland chronicled the everyday ruptures caused by the pandemic while documenting the life of a rural GP. *A Fortunate Woman* (2022) followed the doctor who replaced Dr John Sassall in the same practice that John Berger had studied for *A Fortunate Man* (1967).[4] When compared, the two books revealed many striking transformations in general practice some fifty years later, including a higher proportion of women doctors, the entrenchment of team-based medicine and the extensive use of computers. Nonetheless, several continuities also came to light. General practice remained the subordinate, and often neglected, partner to hospital care. In addition, the doctor in *A Fortunate Woman* showed a similar degree of familiarity with her patients and participation in the life of her village as Berger had encountered with Sassall. It did not seem that the fondness or respect for the local doctor had been entirely lost. COVID-19, though, posed significant challenges to maintaining what Morland described as the 'delicate balancing act of intimacy and friendship' that underpinned the doctor–patient relationship. Garbed in face mask, visor and full protective body equipment, the doctor could complete a full consultation with some of her regular patients without them even realising it was her.

Of course, the impact of the pandemic amounted to more than disruptions to how the service delivered care. It also entailed a tremendous loss of life. By the summer of 2022, over 200,000 people had died from COVID-19 in the UK – a number larger than the population of Portsmouth.[5] These deaths showed the strengths and limits of the NHS, as well as the fractured standing of the political project that it had emerged from. Even if other countries also lost significant numbers of their citizens, the UK fared poorly in comparison. The mortality rate per 100,000 population was more forgiving than in Peru, Slovakia, Brazil, the US and Greece, but worse than in other large European nations such as France and Germany. Much of the immediate damage wreaked by the virus in communities across the country occurred during the first two 'waves' of COVID-19 between March 2020 and May 2021, before effective vaccines became available.

Given the survival of the NHS, and the popular belief in it, why was the UK one of the countries hardest hit by the pandemic? On the one hand, the health service did not collapse, as some feared it might. The large purpose-built 'Nightingale' hospitals, which sprung up in English cities from the West Country to the North-East remained underused, though partly because the NHS still struggled with staff recruitment.[6]

The public mainly heeded Prime Minister Boris Johnson's call to 'Stay at Home, Protect the NHS, Save Lives' – a striking invocation of the health service to mould public behaviour. Britain also fared well with COVID-19 vaccination uptake, again because the public believed in a national service with equality of access that could distribute the vaccinations easily on NHS property or through cooperation with private and voluntary partners. Nonetheless, this engagement with the private sector enriched some supporters of the Conservative government, who profited from the emergency measures put in place during the pandemic. Many of the successful referrals to a special 'VIP Lane' established to speed up the procurement of personal protective equipment (PPE), for instance, came from Conservative politicians.[7] A judge later declared that this process was unlawful. The government may have claimed that it had only acted in Britain's best interests during an emergency, but this justification ignored how multiple companies that had received PPE contracts also donated to the Conservative Party.[8] The beneficiaries of the 'franchise state', which had first emerged in the NHS during the 1980s with the outsourcing of ancillary work to private companies, thrived during the pandemic.

Despite these backdoor dealings, the pre-existing expressions of public support for the health service escalated and took on new forms. 'Clap for Carers' – where Britons stood outside their homes every Thursday evening and participated in a national round of applause for two minutes – formed a prominent illustration of this sentiment. Some commentators dismissed the campaign as a distraction, given the participation of leading politicians, including the Prime Minister, who had overseen failures in PPE procurement.[9] Yet, regardless of the machinations of politicians and private contractors, the engagement of millions of citizens in this ritual confirmed their regard for the NHS, built up in the decades before COVID-19. The children's drawings of rainbows hung in front-room windows or the street art captioned with 'THANK YOU NHS' became an ever-present sign of the public's appreciation.

On the other hand, for all the Herculean efforts of its staff and the depth of popular support, the pandemic revealed the limits of the NHS.

As many experts noted, COVID-19 caused such a high mortality rate in Britain because of a longer-term failure to address economic and social inequality.[10] The pandemic, after all, arrived on the back of a decade of austerity in public spending that ranged beyond the health service. Conservative-led governments cut budgets in nearly every area, with local government funding the hardest hit. The day-to-day spending of local councils in British cities had plummeted by a fifth, leaving scant money for services that included housing and, in England, public health.[11] Northern England suffered the most from austerity, enjoying none of the limited protections that the Welsh, Scottish or Northern Irish governments were able to offer their own councils. With child poverty on the rise, children's centres shuttered, 'zero-hours contracts' spreading in the workplace and wages stagnant, the cuts after 2010 carried serious consequences for health.[12] In some parts of the north of England, life expectancy fell for the first time since the Second World War, particularly among women. COVID-19, then, poured into the chasms of inequality already deepened by austerity. The chance of dying from the virus in the most deprived areas of England for under-65s was 3.7 times higher than in their least deprived counterparts.[13] Similarly, individuals from Black and ethnic minority communities possessed a higher risk of both contracting COVID-19 and dying from it than white Britons.[14]

The pandemic confirmed a truth long known by public health experts: the NHS could only do so much. Figures in the 1960s and 1970s including the epidemiologist Jerry Morris, the social policy academic Richard Titmuss and the GP Julian Tudor Hart had highlighted the problems caused by rising instances of chronic disease and continued inequality in health outcomes. In 1980, an important official committee reported that sharp class divides in standards of health and illness stubbornly persisted, despite over thirty years of the NHS. Named the 'Black Report' (1980) after its chairman, Sir Douglas Black, the document lamented how a failure to address the gap in health improvements between the more affluent social classes and the poorest had, the committee estimated, amounted to a loss of 74,000 lives among those who earned the least.[15] They concluded that 'much of the problem lies outside the scope of the National Health Service'. Factors like 'income, work (or lack of it), environment, education, housing, transport and what are today called "life-styles" all affect health and all favour the better-off', insisted the Black Report. To address health inequality, the committee proposed an anti-poverty strategy that went further than the NHS, 'aimed at radically improving the material conditions of life of poorer groups'. Their solutions included better social housing, cheaper childcare services to aid working parents, new centres for children under five, improved child benefit payments, secure employment and comprehensive disability allowances. Though the Thatcher government released the report quietly on a bank holiday to minimise media attention, it lived on in expert circles as a missed opportunity to tackle what were later called the 'social determinants' of health.[16]

In fact, some areas of government activity that the Black Report recommended for expansion went in the opposite direction. Rather than better social housing being constructed or renovated, local council reserves were sold off. Childcare soared in expense, placing it further out of reach for working families. To be sure, some of the report's recommendations did eventually materialise. New Labour banned tobacco advertising, increased child benefit and introduced a national minimum wage. Yet under the weight of austerity in the 2010s, some of these early twenty-first-century attempts by the state to address social problems were rolled back, including Sure Start Centres, which had proved effective at mitigating health inequality by, for example, driving down children's hospital admissions.[17] The creation of a more equal society that might alleviate longstanding health disparities required the continuation and expansion of such services and initiatives. A building cannot stand on a single pillar.

The NHS survived and even flourished compared to other forms of government intervention aimed at reducing economic and social inequality. However, the fact that social democratic politics endured through the health service only highlighted how its ideals lay unfulfilled or fractured elsewhere. The NHS's comparatively privileged structural integrity and popular standing after the 1980s would not have occurred without the growth of affection for its values and staff. Undoubtedly, the support encapsulated by phrases like 'Our NHS' sometimes contains a great deal of historical erasures and can be weaponised against marginalised groups. Those invested in maintaining the underlying principles of the health service would do well to take a more critical approach to the welfare nationalism that surrounds the institution. Nevertheless, it would be risky to discard such popular attachment entirely. In a century already scarred by a growing distrust of electoral politics and democratic institutions it is not necessarily a bad thing that millions of people believe in a universal and public health service founded to secure a more equal future. It is now regularly voiced from both the right and the left that ending such sentiment would enable substantial 'reform'.[18] However, there has been no shortage of reform to the NHS since the 1970s – the very point when public affection for the institution started to soar. If the link between the swelling popular feeling for the NHS and a lack of reform remains questionable, then the connection between this sentiment and the service's survival is stronger. Campaigners fighting for the expansion of other public services would relish a shred of the approbation that surrounds the NHS, and indeed they often model their proposals on it.[19]

The narratives of 'crisis' that surround the service have long been present. This fact does not diminish the seriousness of the scandals that are sometimes exposed in the NHS, the claims of overwork among staff members, or the complaints by patients about the quality of treatment. Any exhausted employee forced to quit or any patient shunted into the hallway on a trolley due to overcrowding is a cause for concern. Nevertheless, it is important to place the picture of a health service that appears perennially 'in crisis' in a historical perspective and to treat that term with a degree of caution. After all, the NHS's history shows that these narratives appear and intensify at specific moments, such as after the 1980s, when they were tied to budget restrictions and marketisation. They are not preordained. The insistence on crisis can also be exploited for political ends, as in the 1950s, when critics presented the apparent overspending in the NHS as a sign of imminent national ruin (one such iteration of crisis that did not come to pass). In the pandemic's aftermath, familiar claims from the political right that the service is unsustainable and requires replacement have gathered pace in a new atmosphere of crisis.[20] However, history shows that the NHS has been able to work well as a model, to the point where in the late 2000s a leading international health think tank placed it first among all health systems in the world for efficiency and preventing cost barriers to care.[21] Britain is also not the only nation facing difficulties with its health system after the pandemic. According to a 2022 survey of over 23,000 people in 34 countries around the world, 3 out of 5 respondents believed that their health system was overstretched.[22] Moreover, the backlogs in areas like waiting lists that the service faced after the pandemic were largely due, according to an important report undertaken by the King's Fund, to the 'decade of neglect' that preceded it.[23] The history of the NHS shows the importance of asking who is stoking the sense of crisis, and to what ends. It also demonstrates that the service has recovered from serious challenges in the past, and might do so again. In the early 2020s, opinion polls showed that Britons overwhelmingly wanted the existing model to work.[24] Although frustrated with the consequences of existing pressures on the service, the public did not signal any real desire to change direction towards a different system. In 2022, 62 per cent of people in one poll still cited the NHS as the thing that made them 'most proud to be British'. Of course, the NHS – like any health service – should be critiqued and discussion about its future needs to continue, but it is necessary to scrutinise arguments premised on the institution's imminent collapse or claims about widespread public dissatisfaction.

In broader terms, it is possible that social democratic politics could be revived more comprehensively in the future. For those pursuing such a goal, a meaningful first step might be to rethink the declinist narratives that shape how we think about its past. *Our NHS* has shown why a government-organised, universal, free-at-the-point-of-use health service escaped the fate of its counterparts elsewhere in the welfare state and enjoyed popular admiration in a country pivotal to the rise of neoliberalism. It is feasible, then, to see social democracy as capable of adaption and survival, even while recognising its limitations and costs. This vantage point offers lessons – and even hope – for our own moment, when the power of markets can seem unassailable. The pursuit of a better, more equal future through institutions like the NHS might depend on it.

ENDNOTES

INTRODUCTION

1. Author's conversation with June Rosen, 5 September 2022.
2. 'The National Health Service Jigsaw Puzzle', https://www.pdk.co.uk/products/falcon-deluxe-the-national-health-service-jigsaw-puzzle-1000-pieces.
3. Catherine Baker, 'Beyond the Island Story?: The Opening Ceremony of the London 2012 Olympic Games as Public History', *Rethinking History* 19, no. 3 (2015): 409–28.
4. For instance, IPSOS MORI, 'What Makes Us Proud to be British?', 2022, https://www.ipsos.com/en-uk/what-makes-us-proud-be-british.
5. This claim encourages the NHS's supporters and infuriates its critics; see Roger Taylor, *God Bless the NHS* (London: Faber and Faber, 2013); Nigel Cameron, 'Slaying Dragons: Britain's National Religion, the NHS', 2018, https://unherd.com/2018/04/slaying-dragons-britains-national-religion-nhs/.
6. For comparison with other health systems, see Milton Roemer, *National Health Systems of the World, Vol. 1, The Countries* (Oxford: Oxford University Press, 1991), 191–203; Glen O'Hara and George Campbell Gosling, 'Healthcare as Nation-building in the Twentieth Century: The Case of the British National Health Service', in Paul Weindling (ed.), *Healthcare in Private and Public from the Early Modern Period to 2000* (London: Routledge, 2014), 123–41.
7. Rudolf Klein, *The New Politics of the NHS: From Creation to Reinvention* (Boca Raton, FL: CRC Press, 2013), 305.
8. Geoffrey Rivett provides a history of the NHS that closely attends to medical and technological developments; see *From Cradle to Grave: Fifty Years of the NHS* (London: King's Fund, 1998). For selected works that address key twentieth-century health developments in other nations, see Nancy Tomes, *Remaking the American Patient: How Madison Avenue and Modern Medicine Turned Patients into Consumers* (Chapel Hill, NC: University of North Carolina Press, 2016); Julie Livingston, *Improvising Medicine: An African Oncology Ward in an Emerging Cancer Epidemic* (Durham, NC: Duke University Press, 2012); P. Sean Brotherton, *Revolutionary Medicine: Health and the Body in Post-Soviet Cuba* (Durham, NC: Duke University Press, 2012).
9. Keir Waddington, 'Problems of Progress: Modernity and Writing the Social History of Medicine', *Social History of Medicine* 34, no. 4 (2021): 1053–67.
10. Charles Webster, *The Health services Since the War. Volume I. Problems of Health Care: The National Health Service before 1957* (London: HMSO, 1988); Charles Webster, *The Health Services since the War. Volume II. Government and Health Care: The National*

Health Service 1958–1979 (London: HMSO, 1996); Daniel M. Fox, *Health Policies, Health Politics: The British and American Experience, 1911–1965* (Princeton, NJ: Princeton University Press, 1986); Klein, *New Politics of the NHS;* Rivett, *From Cradle to Grave*. For an overview of this work, see Martin Gorsky, 'The National Health Service 1948–2008: A Review of the Historiography', *Social History of Medicine* 21, no. 3 (2008): 437–60. For economists' focus on 'efficiency' and 'value for money', see OECD, *Value for Money in Health Spending* (Paris: OECD, 2010).

11. Recently, scholars have begun to situate the NHS in a wider social and cultural frame; see Alex Mold, *Making the Patient-Consumer: Patient Organisations and Health Consumerism in Britain* (Manchester: Manchester University Press, 2015); Andrew Seaton, ' "Against the Sacred Cow": NHS Opposition and the Fellowship for Freedom in Medicine, 1948–72', *Twentieth Century British History* 26, no. 3 (2015): 424–49; Jack Saunders, 'Emotions, Social Practices and the Changing Composition of Class, Race and Gender in the National Health Service, 1970–79: "Lively Discussion Ensued"', *History Workshop Journal* 88, no. 1 (2019): 204–28; Jennifer Crane, ' "Save Our NHS": Activism, Information-Based Expertise and the "New Times" of the 1980s', *Contemporary British History* 33, no. 1 (2019): 52–74; Agnes Arnold-Forster, 'Racing Pulses: Gender, Professionalism and Health Care in Medical Romance Fiction', *History Workshop Journal* 91, no. 1 (2021): 157–81; Stephanie J. Snow and Angela F. Whitecross, 'Making History Together: The UK's National Health Service and the Story of Our Lives since 1948', *Contemporary British History* 36, no. 3 (2022): 403–29; Jennifer Crane and Jane Hand (eds), *Posters, Protests, and Prescriptions: Cultural Histories of the National Health Service in Britain* (Manchester: Manchester University Press, 2022).
12. For a selection, see Arthur Marwick, *British Society since 1945* (London: Penguin, 2003), 31–5; Brian Harrison, *Seeking a Role: The United Kingdom, 1951–1970* (Oxford: Oxford University Press, 2009), 276; David Kynaston, *Family Britain, 1951–57* (London: Bloomsbury, 2009), 625–6; David Dutton, *British Politics since 1945* (Oxford: Blackwell, 1997), 59–60; Selina Todd, *The People: The Rise and Fall of the Working Class*, 1910–2010 (London: John Murray, 2014), 7, 376.
13. Nick Hayes, 'Did We Really Want a National Health Service? Hospitals, Patients and Public Opinions before 1948', *English Historical Review* 127, no. 526 (2012): 625–61; Seaton, 'Against the "Sacred Cow"'.
14. Alistair Fair, ' "Modernization of Our Hospital System": The National Health Service, the Hospital Plan, and the "Harness" Programme, 1962–77', *Twentieth Century British History* 29, no. 4 (2018): 547–75; Ed DeVane, 'Pilgrim's Progress: The Landscape of the NHS Hospital, 1948–70', *Twentieth Century British History* 32, no. 4 (2021): 534–52.
15. Andrew Seaton, 'The Gospel of Wealth and the National Health: The Rockefeller Foundation and Social Medicine in Britain's NHS, 1945–60', *Bulletin of the History of Medicine* 94, no. 1 (2020): 91–124, especially 117–22; Martin D. Moore, 'Waiting for the Doctor: Managing Time and Emotion in the British National Health Service, 1948–80', *Twentieth Century British History* 33, no. 2 (2022): 203–29.
16. Emily Robinson, Camilla Schofield, Florence Sutcliffe-Braithwaite and Natalie Tomlinson, 'Telling Stories about Post-war Britain: Popular Individualism and the "Crisis" of the 1970s', *Twentieth Century British History* 28, no. 2 (2017): 268–304.
17. Jim Tomlinson, 'A "Failed Experiment"? Public Ownership and the Narratives of Post-War Britain', *Labour History Review* 73, no. 2 (2008): 228–43.
18. 'Welfare nationalism' is a term that has also recently been used in social scientific work on the Scandinavian welfare state when describing opposition to immigrants accessing social services; see chapters in Pauli Kettunen, Saara Pellander and Miika Tervonen (eds),

Nationalism and Democracy in the Welfare State (Cheltenham: Edward Elgar Publishing, 2022). See also Gareth Millward's discussion of 'welfare chauvinism' in *Sick Note: A History of the British Welfare State* (Oxford: Oxford University Press, 2022), 79–89. The use of 'welfare nationalism' in this book builds on this wider scholarship's attention to how social services excluded immigrants and people of colour, but expands the term to include feelings of pride in welfare institutions that could be used as the basis of authority in discussions of international relations.

19. Aneurin Bevan, 'Royal Medico-Psychological Association, 5 September, 1945', in Charles Webster (ed.), *Aneurin Bevan on the National Health Service* (Oxford: Wellcome Unit for the History of Medicine, 1991), 25–9, quote on 28.
20. With apologies to New Zealand, which undertook the world's first attempt to introduce a 'national health service' through the 1938 Social Security Act, see Linda Bryder and John Stewart, '"Some Abstract Socialistic Ideal or Principle": British Reactions to New Zealand's 1938 Social Security Act', *Britain and the World* 8, no. 1 (2015): 51–75.
21. Quoted in W. Taylor Fain, *American Ascendance and British Retreat in the Persian Gulf Region* (Basingstoke: Palgrave Macmillan, 2008), 141–2.
22. Roberta Bivins, *Contagious Communities: Medicine, Migration, and the NHS in Post-War Britain* (Oxford: Oxford University Press, 2015); Julian M. Simpson, *Migrant Architects of the NHS: South Asian Doctors and the Reinvention of British General Practice (1940s–1980s)* (Manchester: Manchester University Press, 2018); Catherine Babikian, '"Partnership Not Prejudice": British Nurses, Colonial Students, and the National Health Service, 1948–1962', *Journal of British Studies* 60, no.1 (2021): 140–68.
23. For Powellism, see Camilla Schofield, *Enoch Powell and the Making of Postcolonial Britain* (Cambridge: Cambridge University Press, 2013); Amy Whipple, 'Revisiting the "Rivers of Blood" Controversy: Letters to Enoch Powell', *Journal of British Studies* 48, no. 3 (2009): 717–35.
24. For decolonisation and British welfare, see Kennetta Hammond Perry, *London is the Place for Me: Black Britons, Citizenship, and the Politics of Race* (Oxford: Oxford University Press, 2015), 70–88; Nicole Longpré, '"An Issue That Could Tear Us Apart": Race, Empire, and Economy in the British (Welfare) State, 1968', *Canadian Journal of History* 46, no. 1 (2011): 63–95, especially 87–9; Jordanna Bailkin, *The Afterlife of Empire* (Berkeley: University of California Press, 2012).
25. For Thatcherism, see Richard Vinen, *Thatcher's Britain: The Politics and Social Upheaval of the Thatcher Era* (London: Simon and Schuster, 2009); Ben Jackson and Robert Saunders (eds), *Making Thatcher's Britain* (Cambridge: Cambridge University Press, 2012).
26. Margaret Thatcher, 'Speech to Conservative Party Conference', October 1982, https://www.margaretthatcher.org/document/105032. When considering the 1980s, historians of the NHS mainly discuss reforms to management structures and internal administration, rather than Conservative engagement with longstanding arguments for private health insurance; see, for instance, Rivett, *From Cradle to Grave*, 291–373.
27. John Boughton, *Municipal Dreams: The Rise and Fall of Council Housing* (London: Verso, 2018).
28. Paul Pierson, *Dismantling the Welfare State?: Reagan, Thatcher, and the Politics of Retrenchment* (Cambridge: Cambridge University Press, 1994), 133–5.
29. Klein, *New Politics of the NHS*, 123–9, 233–5; Alex Mold, 'Making the Patient-Consumer in Margaret Thatcher's Britain', *Historical Journal* 54, no. 2 (2011): 509–28, especially 526–8.
30. This interpretation is particularly strong on the political left: see John Lister (ed.), *Cutting the Lifeline: The Fight for the NHS* (London: Journeyman, 1988); Allyson Pollock, *NHS PLC: The Privatisation of Our Health Care* (London: Verso, 2004).

31. Jennifer Crane also makes this point; see 'Save Our NHS', 57–8.
32. Michael Freeden defines ideologies as clusters of concepts, principles and values arranged in a distinctive way that compete for control over the political arena; see *Ideologies and Political Theory: A Conceptual Approach* (Oxford: Clarendon Press, 1996), 1–9. For definitions of social democracy, see Ben Jackson, 'Social Democracy', in Michael Freeden, Lyman Tower Sargent and Marc Stears (eds), *The Oxford Handbook of Political Ideologies* (Oxford: Oxford University Press, 2013), 348–63; Avner Offer and Gabriel Söderberg, *The Nobel Factor: The Prize in Economics, Social Democracy, and the Market Turn* (Princeton, NJ: Princeton University Press, 2010), 4–7. For its historical origins, see Donald Sassoon, *One Hundred Years of Socialism: The West European Left in the Twentieth Century* (London: I.B. Tauris, 1996); Geoff Eley, *Forging Democracy: The History of the Left in Europe, 1850–2000* (Oxford: Oxford University Press, 2002).
33. Duncan Tanner, *Political Change and the Labour Party, 1900–1918* (Cambridge: Cambridge University Press, 1990).
34. Aneurin Bevan, *In Place of Fear* (London: Heinemann, 1952), 85.
35. For the social and cultural dimensions of social democracy, see Michal Shapira, *The War Inside: Psychoanalysis, Total War, and the Making of the Democratic Self in Postwar Britain* (Cambridge: Cambridge University Press, 2013); Mathew Thomson, *Lost Freedom: The Landscape of the Child and the British Post-War Settlement* (Oxford: Oxford University Press, 2013); Teri Chettiar, '"More than a Contract": The Emergence of a State-Supported Marriage Welfare Service and the Politics of Emotional Life in Post-1945 Britain', *Journal of British Studies* 55, no. 3 (2016): 566–91.
36. Jon Lawrence considers postwar social history through the lens of community and individualism; see *Me, Me, Me? The Search for Community in Post-War England* (Oxford: Oxford University Press, 2019), especially 1–18. For examples of the welfare state seeking to bring people from different backgrounds together in housing and education, see Guy Ortolano, *Thatcher's Progress: From Social Democracy to Market Liberalism Through an English New Town* (Cambridge: Cambridge University Press, 2019), 143–83; Peter Mandler, *The Crisis of the Meritocracy: Britain's Transition to Mass Education since the Second World War* (Oxford: Oxford University Press, 2020), 1–17. In the 1940s, the sociologist T.H. Marshall packaged such ambitions with his idea of 'social citizenship'; see *Citizenship and Social Class and Other Essays* (Cambridge: Cambridge University Press, 1950), 1–85.
37. Bevan, *In Place of Fear*, 82.
38. Many other nations in Europe, for instance, had fewer beds on their wards; see Jeanne Kisacky, *Rise of the Modern Hospital: An Architectural History of Health and Healing, 1870–1940* (Pittsburgh, PA: University of Pittsburgh Press, 2017), 277–91, 304–37.
39. For the 'developmental state', see David Edgerton, *The Rise and Fall of the British Nation: A Twentieth-Century History* (London: Allen Lane, 2018), 307–8; Sam Wetherell, *Foundations: How the Built Environment Made Twentieth-Century Britain* (Princeton, NJ: Princeton University Press, 2020).
40. Including, Edgerton, *Rise and Fall*; Ortolano, *Thatcher's Progress*; Wetherell, *Foundations*; Florence Sutcliffe-Braithwaite, *Class, Politics, and the Decline of Deference in England, 1968–2000* (Oxford: Oxford University Press, 2018); James Vernon, *Modern Britain: 1750 to the Present* (Cambridge: Cambridge University Press, 2017).
41. Jim Tomlinson, *Democratic Socialism and Economic Policy: The Attlee Years, 1945–1951* (Cambridge: Cambridge University Press, 1997); Ina Zweiniger-Bargielowska, *Austerity in Britain: Rationing, Controls, and Consumption, 1939–1955* (Oxford: Oxford University Press, 2000).
42. David Garland, 'The Emergence of the Idea of the "Welfare State" in British Political Discourse', *History of the Human Sciences* 35, no. 1 (2022): 132–57. For histories of the

welfare state, see Peter Baldwin, *The Politics of Social Solidarity: Class Bases of the European Welfare State, 1875–1975* (Cambridge: Cambridge University Press, 1990); Gøsta Esping-Andersen, *The Three Worlds of Welfare Capitalism* (Princeton, NJ: Princeton University Press, 1990); Pat Thane, *Foundations of the Welfare State* (London: Longman, 1996); Susan Pedersen, *Family, Dependence, and the Origins of the Welfare State: Britain and France, 1914–1945* (Cambridge: Cambridge University Press, 1993).

43. James Vernon, *Hunger: A Modern History* (Cambridge, MA: Belknap Press, 2007), 236–71.
44. Edgerton, *Rise and Fall*, 244–5.
45. David Edgerton argues that the postwar period cannot be seen as one of 'social democracy', but acknowledges the NHS's social democratic credentials; see 'What Came Between New Liberalism and Neoliberalism? Rethinking Keynesianism, the Welfare State and Social Democracy', in Aled Davies, Ben Jackson and Florence Sutcliffe-Braithwaite (eds), *The Neoliberal Age?: Britain Since the 1970s* (London: UCL Press, 2021), 30–51, especially 41.
46. This figure is calculated from 1948 to 1973, see Office of National Statistics, 'Gross Domestic Product: Year on Year Growth', https://www.ons.gov.uk/economy/grossdomesticproductgdp/timeseries/ihyp/pn2; Eric Hobsbawm, *Age of Extremes: The Short Twentieth Century, 1914–1991* (London: Michael Joseph, 1994), 257–86, quote on 270. This depiction came to structure most overviews of modern European history; see Tony Judt, *Postwar: A History of Europe Since 1945* (New York: Penguin Books, 2005) and Mark Mazower, *Dark Continent: Europe's Twentieth Century* (New York: A.A. Knopf, 1998).
47. Judt, *Postwar*, 535–58; Mazower, *Dark Continent*, 327–60; John Callaghan, *The Retreat of Social Democracy* (Manchester: Manchester University Press, 2000); Konrad H. Jarausch, *Out of Ashes: A New History of Europe in the Twentieth Century* (Princeton, NJ: Princeton University Press, 2015), 613–38.
48. Philip Mirowski and Dieter Plehwe (eds), *The Road from Mont Pèlerin: The Making of the Neoliberal Thought Collective* (Cambridge, MA: Harvard University Press, 2009); Daniel Stedman Jones, *Masters of the Universe: Hayek, Friedman, and the Birth of Neoliberal Politics* (Princeton, NJ: Princeton University Press, 2012).
49. For definitions of neoliberalism, see Jamie Peck, 'Preface: Naming Neoliberalism', in Damien Cahill, Melinda Cooper, Martijn Konings and David Primrose (eds), *The SAGE Handbook of Neoliberalism* (Los Angeles: SAGE, 2018), xxii–iv; Aled Davies, Ben Jackson and Florence Sutcliffe-Braithwaite, 'Introduction: A Neoliberal Age?', in Davies, Jackson and Sutcliffe-Braithwaite (eds), *The Neoliberal Age?*, 1–29. For competitive individualism, see Florence Sutcliffe-Braithwaite, 'Neo-Liberalism and Morality in the Making of Thatcherite Social Policy', *Historical Journal* 55, no. 2 (2012): 497–520; Aled Davies, James Freeman and Hugh Pemberton, '"Everyman a Capitalist" or "Free to Choose"?: Exploring the Tensions within Thatcherite Individualism', *Historical Journal* 61, no. 2 (2018): 477–501. For criticisms of the term 'neoliberalism', see Daniel T. Rodgers, 'The Uses and Abuses of "Neoliberalism"', *Dissent* 65, no. 1 (2008): 78–87, with replies from Julia Ott, Mike Konczal, N.D.B. Connolly and Timothy Shenk.
50. Quinn Slobodian, *Globalists: The End of Empire and the Birth of Neoliberalism* (Cambridge, MA: Harvard University Press, 2018). For the wider utility of neoliberalism as a concept, see Tehila Sasson, 'Afterword: British Neoliberalism and its Subjects', in Davies, Jackson and Sutcliffe-Braithwaite (eds), *The Neoliberal Age?*, 336–53.
51. Stedman Jones, *Masters of the Universe*, 273–328; David Harvey, *A Brief History of Neoliberalism* (Oxford: Oxford University Press, 2005), 55–63.

52. For social policy, see Pierson, *Dismantling the Welfare State?*; Sutcliffe-Braithwaite, *Class, Politics, and the Decline of Deference*, 163–7.
53. Kim Phillips-Fein, *Invisible Hands: The Making of the Conservative Movement from the New Deal to Reagan* (New York: W.W. Norton, 2009); Fritz Bartel, *The Triumph of Broken Promises: The End of the Cold War and the Rise of Neoliberalism* (Cambridge, MA: Harvard University Press, 2022); Ezra F. Vogel, *Deng Xiaoping and the Transformation of China* (Cambridge, MA: Harvard University Press, 2011).
54. Stephanie L. Mudge, *Leftism Reinvented: Western Parties from Socialism to Neoliberalism* (Cambridge, MA: Harvard University Press, 2018), 43–68. For a challenge to this thesis, see Mark Wickham-Jones, 'Neoliberalism and the Labour Party', in Davies, Jackson and Sutcliffe-Braithwaite (eds), *The Neoliberal Age?*, 226–53.
55. James Vernon, 'The Local, the Imperial and the Global: Repositioning Twentieth-Century Britain and the Brief Life of its Social Democracy', *Twentieth Century British History* 21, no. 2 (2010): 404–18, quote on 418; Alistair Kefford, 'Housing the Citizen-Consumer in Post-war Britain: The Parker Morris Report and the Even Briefer Life of Social Democracy', *Twentieth Century British History* 29, no. 2 (2018): 225–58.
56. William Davies, *The Limits of Neoliberalism: Authority, Sovereignty and the Logic of Competition* (London: SAGE, 2014); Jim Tomlinson, 'The Failures of Neoliberalism in Britain since the 1970s: The Limits on "Market Forces" in a Deindustrialising Economy and a "New Speenhamland"', in Davies, Jackson and Sutcliffe-Braithwaite (eds), *The Neoliberal Age?* 94–111.
57. Edgerton, *Rise and Fall*, 305–6.
58. Aled Davies, *The City of London and Social Democracy: The Political Economy of Finance in Britain, 1959–1979* (Oxford: Oxford University Press, 2017); Ortolano, *Thatcher's Progress*. For other reconsiderations of social democracy, see Sheri Berman, *The Primacy of Politics: Social Democracy and the Making of Europe's Twentieth Century* (Cambridge: Cambridge University Press, 2006); Jeremy Nuttall and Hans Schattle (eds), *Making Social Democrats: Citizens, Mindsets, Realities: Essays for David Marquand* (Manchester: Manchester University Press, 2018).
59. This point of finality is sometimes a result of the case studies that these scholars focus on, rather than a belief that social democracy expired in general; see Davies, *The City of London and Social Democracy*, 181–214; Ortolano, *Thatcher's Progress*, 255–63.
60. Several historians have identified liberalism's permeation of the post-1945 welfare state; see P.F. Clarke, *Liberals and Social Democrats* (Cambridge: Cambridge University Press, 1978); Thane, *Foundations of the Welfare State*. For a long history of liberalism, see Vernon, *Modern Britain*.
61. The health of social democracy is often measured by electoral results; see Tarik Abou-Chadi and Jane Gingrich, 'It's Not Just in Britain – Across Europe, Social Democracy Is Losing Its Way', *The Observer*, 9 May 2021, https://www.theguardian.com/commentisfree/2021/may/09/not-just-britain-across-europe-social-democracy-losing-way.
62. Francis Sejersted, *The Age of Social Democracy: Norway and Sweden in the Twentieth Century* (Princeton, NJ: Princeton University Press, 2011).
63. In this way, the book is informed by the emphasis on 'history from below' in social history and the social history of medicine; see Roy Porter, 'The Patient's View: Doing Medical History from Below', *Theory and Society* 14, no. 2 (1985): 175–98.
64. Nuffield Trust, 'The NHS is One of the World's Largest Employers', 2019, https://www.nuffieldtrust.org.uk/chart/the-nhs-is-one-of-the-world-s-largest-employers.
65. Our World in Data, 'Healthcare Spending', 2017, https://ourworldindata.org/financing-healthcare. The public policy expert Michael Moran suggests that health care politics be considered separately from the welfare state; see *Governing the Health*

Care State: A Comparative Study of the United Kingdom, the United States and Germany (Manchester: Manchester University Press, 1999), 4.

66. Minna Harjula, 'Health Citizenship and Access to Health Services: Finland 1900–2000', *Social History of Medicine* 29, no. 3 (2016): 573–89, especially 586–7.
67. LSE, CPS/12/11, CPS, 'The Reform of the British Medical Services', 1978, 1.
68. For mental health services, see Louise Hide, 'In Plain Sight: Open Doors, Mixed-sex Wards and Sexual Abuse in English Psychiatric Hospitals, 1950s–Early 1990s', *Social History of Medicine* 31, no. 4 (2018): 732–53. For sexual health services, see Robert Irwin, ' "To Try and Find Out What Is Being Done to Whom, by Whom and With What Results": The Creation of Psychosexual Counselling Policy in England, 1972–1979', *Twentieth Century British History* 20, no. 2 (2009): 173–97.

CHAPTER 1 THE NATIONAL HEALTH

1. Edith Summerskill, 'Party Political Broadcast', April 1948, https://www.bbc.co.uk/archive/doctor-edith-summerskill/z7y4scw. Biographical information on Summerskill is drawn from Sally Knapp, *Women Doctors Today* (New York: Thomas Y. Crowell, 1947), 33–46; Edith Summerskill, *A Woman's World* (London: Heinemann, 1967).
2. Richard Titmuss, *Problems of Social Policy* (London: HMSO, 1950).
3. Titmuss's interpretation became a hallmark of scholarship that depicted the conflict as a 'People's War'; see Angus Calder, *The People's War: Britain, 1939–1945* (London: Cape, 1969); Paul Addison, *The Road to 1945: British Politics and the Second World War* (London: Quartet Books, 1977). For a critique, see Sonya O. Rose, *Which People's War?: National Identity and Citizenship in Britain 1939–1945* (Oxford: Oxford University Press, 2003).
4. Fox, *Health Policies, Health Politics*. See also, Harry Eckstein, *The English Health Service: Its Origins, Structure, and Achievements* (Cambridge, MA: Harvard University Press, 1958) and Klein, *New Politics of the NHS*.
5. Charles Webster, 'Conflict and Consensus: Explaining the British Health Service', *Twentieth Century British History* 1, no. 2 (1990): 115–51.
6. John Stewart, *The Battle for Health: A Political History of the Socialist Medical Association, 1930–51* (Aldershot: Ashgate, 1999).
7. BFI, BFI Identifier: N-93123. Rebecca O'Brien, Kate Ogborn, Lisa-Marie Russo. *The Spirit of '45*. Directed by Ken Loach. London: Channel Four Television Corporation, 2013.
8. Hayes, 'Did We Really Want a National Health Service?'
9. Henry Pelling, *Popular Politics and Society in Late Victorian Britain* (London: Palgrave Macmillan, 1979), 1–18. Pat Thane and Jose Harris have argued that opposition to state involvement depended on the particular social policy in question; see Pat Thane, 'The Working Class and State "Welfare" in Britain, 1880–1914', *Historical Journal* 27, no. 4 (1984): 877–900; Jose Harris, 'Did British Workers Want the Welfare State? G. D. H. Cole's Survey of 1942', in Jay Winter (ed.), *The Working Class in Modern British History: Essays in Honour of Henry Pelling* (Cambridge: Cambridge University Press, 1983), 200–14.
10. The Victorian state still regulated individuals and markets; see Patrick Joyce, *The State of Freedom: A Social History of the British State since 1800* (Cambridge: Cambridge University Press, 2013), 1–27; Judith R. Walkowitz, *Prostitution and Victorian Society: Women, Class, and the State* (Cambridge: Cambridge University Press, 1980); Karl Polanyi, *The Great Transformation: The Political and Economic Origins of Our Time* (Boston: Beacon Press, 1944).
11. 'State Medical Service', *New Statesman and Nation*, 6 October 1945, 224.
12. This paragraph's comments on interwar health conditions draw on Charles Webster,

'Healthy or Hungry Thirties?', *History Workshop Journal* 13, no.1 (Spring 1982): 110–29; Anne Hardy, *Health and Medicine in Britain Since 1860* (Basingstoke: Palgrave, 2001); Ray Fitzpatrick and Tarani Chandola, 'Health', in A.H. Halsey and Josephine Webb (eds), *Twentieth-Century British Social Trends* (Basingstoke: Macmillan, 2000), 94–127, especially 101.

13. Geoffrey B.A.M. Finlayson, *Citizen, State, and Social Welfare in Britain 1830–1990* (Oxford: Oxford University Press, 1994), 201–86.
14. Chris Renwick, *Bread for All: The Origins of the Welfare State* (London: Allen Lane, 2017), 72–81; Edgerton, *Rise and Fall*, 224–36.
15. Anne Digby, *The Evolution of British General Practice 1850–1948* (Oxford: Oxford University Press, 1999), 126–53.
16. BL, Oral History of General Practice, Interview with Tom McQuay, Tape 3 (F6631).
17. HMSO, *The National Insurance Act* (London: HMSO, 1911).
18. P.F. Clarke, *Lancashire and the New Liberalism* (Cambridge: Cambridge University Press, 1971).
19. Cited in Derek Fraser, *The Evolution of the British Welfare State: A History of Social Policy since the Industrial Revolution* (London: Palgrave, 2017), 219.
20. BL, Oral History of General Practice, Interview with Kathleen Norton, Tape 3 (F6545).
21. The rest of this paragraph's comments on national health insurance draw from Harris, 'Did British Workers Want the Welfare State?', 203; Ross McKibbin, *Class and Cultures: England, 1918–1951* (Oxford: Oxford University Press, 1998), 44–9, 59–63.
22. Jane Lewis, 'Gender and the Development of Welfare Regimes', *Journal of European Social Policy* 2, no. 3 (1992): 159–73.
23. The following testimony draws on LSE, SUMMERSKILL/1/4, Letter from Laurence Brice, Letter from N. Clarke, Letter from M. Burdon.
24. Cited in Caitríona Beaumont, *Housewives and Citizens: Domesticity and the Women's Movement in England, 1928–64* (Manchester: Manchester University Press, 2013), 102.
25. John Boyd Orr, *Food, Health and Income* (London: Macmillan, 1937), 11–12.
26. Pedersen, *Family, Dependence, and the Origins of the Welfare State*, 320–1.
27. A.J. Cronin, *The Citadel* (London: Victor Gollancz, 1937). Ross McKibbin, 'Politics and the Medical Hero: A. J. Cronin's The Citadel', *English Historical Review* 123, no. 502 (2008): 651–78.
28. Earlier scholars offered an overwhelmingly critical interpretation of interwar hospital provision; see Brian Abel-Smith, *The Hospitals, 1800–1948: A Study in Social Administration in England and Wales* (London: Heinemann, 1964). More recent scholarship revises this view; see John V. Pickstone, *Medicine and Industrial Society: A History of Hospital Development in Manchester and its Region* (Manchester: Manchester University Press, 1985); Steven Cherry, *Medical Services and the Hospitals in Britain, 1860–1939* (Cambridge: Cambridge University Press, 1996); John Mohan, *Planning, Markets and Hospitals* (London: Routledge, 2002); Barry M. Doyle, *The Politics of Hospital Provision in Early Twentieth-Century Britain* (London: Pickering & Chatto, 2014); George Campbell Gosling, *Payment and Philanthropy in British Healthcare, 1918–48* (Manchester: Manchester University Press, 2017).
29. For municipal hospitals, see Alysa Levene, Martin A. Powell, John Stewart and Becky Taylor, *Cradle to Grave: Municipal Medicine in Interwar England and Wales* (Oxford: Peter Lang, 2011), especially 8–28, statistic on 14; John Stewart, '"For a Healthy London": The Socialist Medical Association and the London County Council in the 1930s', *Medical History* 41, no. 4 (1997): 417–36; Clifford Williamson, '"To Remove the Stigma of the Poor Law": The "Comprehensive" Ideal and Patient Access to the Municipal Hospital Service in the City of Glasgow, 1918–1939', *History* 99, no. 334 (2014): 73–99.

30. Nick Hayes and Barry M. Doyle, 'Eggs, Rags and Whist Drives: Popular Munificence and the Development of Provincial Medical Voluntarism Between the Wars', *Historical Research* 86, no. 234 (2013): 712–40.
31. Robert Pinker, *English Hospital Statistics, 1861–1938* (London: Heinemann, 1966), 49.
32. Gosling, *Payment and Philanthropy*, 3–5.
33. Martin Gorsky, John Mohan and Tim Willis, *Mutualism and Health Care: British Hospital Contributory Schemes in the Twentieth Century* (Manchester: Manchester University Press, 2006).
34. Ben Curtis and Steven Thompson, '"A Plentiful Crop of Cripples Made by All This Progress": Disability, Artificial Limbs and Working-Class Mutualism in the South Wales Coalfield, 1890–1948', *Social History of Medicine* 27, no. 4 (2014): 708–27, especially 713.
35. HMSO, *An Interim Report to the Consultative Council on Medical and Allied Services* (London: HMSO, 1920); Esyllt Jones, 'Nothing too Good for the People: Local Labour and London's Interwar Health Centre Movement', *Social History of Medicine* 25, no. 1 (2012): 84–102.
36. 'Finsbury Health Centre', *The Times*, 4 October 1938, 11.
37. Benjamin Moore, *The Dawn of the Health Age* (Edinburgh: Ballantyne Press, 1911), v, 70, 24, 119, 180.
38. Mark Bevir, *The Making of British Socialism* (Princeton, NJ: Princeton University Press, 2011), 131–51.
39. Sidney Webb and Beatrice Webb, *The Break-up of the Poor Law: Being Part One of the Minority Report of the Poor Law Commission* (London: Longman, Green & Co., 1909), 290, 587.
40. Adam Tooze, *The Deluge: The Great War and the Remaking of Global Order, 1916–1931* (London: Penguin, 2015).
41. Somerville Hastings, 'The Future of Medical Practice in England', *The Lancet* 211, no. 5446 (1928): 67–9; PHM, BOX 314 362.4, The Labour Party, Somerville Hastings, 'The People's Health', 1932.
42. Somerville Hastings, 'Can We Afford to Leave the Nation's Health to Private Enterprise?', *Labour Magazine*, April 1931, 543–7.
43. LSE, SUMMERSKILL/7, Michael Summerskill, 'Biography of Edith Summerskill'. The SMA visited again in 1958, see HHC, U DSM/6/36 – 'Notes Prepared for Final Address in the U.S.S.R', 1958.
44. Somerville Hastings, 'The Medical Service of the Future', *The Lancet* 217, no. 5620 (1931), 1115–18, quote on 1115.
45. Cited in Simon Szreter, *Fertility, Class, and Gender in Britain, 1860–1940* (Cambridge: Cambridge University Press, 1996), 1, see 443–532 for explanations; Renwick, *Bread for All*, 88–93. For a European comparison, see Dóra Vargha, *Polio across the Iron Curtain: Hungary's Cold War with an Epidemic* (Cambridge: Cambridge University Press, 2018), 19–51.
46. A.M. Carr-Saunders, *The Population Problem: A Study in Human Evolution* (Oxford: Clarendon Press, 1922); D.V. Glass, *The Struggle for Population* (Oxford: Clarendon Press, 1936).
47. WC, SA/PIC/H/8, 'The Population Investigation Committee: A Concise History to Mark Its Fiftieth Birthday by C. M. Langford', 1988.
48. Glass, *Struggle for Population,* 14–15.
49. Alex Aylward, 'R. A. Fisher, Eugenics, and the Campaign for Family Allowances in Interwar Britain', *British Journal for the History of Science* 54, no. 4 (2021): 485–505.
50. Enid Charles, *The Twilight of Parenthood* (London: Watts & Co., 1934), 192–3, 197, 205, 214.

51. Stewart, *The Battle for Health*, 62–81.
52. Fox, *Health Policies, Health Politics*, 21–36, 52–69.
53. Political and Economic Planning, *Report on the British Health Services: A Survey of the Existing Health Services in Great Britain with Proposals for Future Development* (London: Political and Economic Planning, 1937).
54. Daniel Todman, *Britain's War: Into Battle, 1937–1941* (London: Penguin Books, 2017); Daniel Todman, *Britain's War: A New World, 1942–1947* (London: Penguin Books, 2021).
55. See essays in Harold L. Smith (ed.), *War and Social Change: British Society in the Second World War* (Manchester: Manchester University Press, 1986).
56. Thane, *Foundations of the Welfare State*, 229–38. For Beveridge, see Jose Harris, *William Beveridge: A Biography* (Oxford: Clarendon, 1997).
57. Pedersen, *Family, Dependence, and the Origins of the Welfare State*, 338–41.
58. John Hills, John Ditch and Howard Glennerster (eds.), *Beveridge and Social Security: An International Retrospective* (Oxford: Oxford University Press, 1994).
59. This paragraph's quotes from the Beveridge Report draw from HMSO, *Social Insurance and Allied Services* (London: HMSO, 1942), 5, 158–63.
60. For opposing views of the popularity of the report, see Harris, *William Beveridge*, 415–24; Steven Fielding, Peter Thompson and Nick Tiratsoo, "*England Arise!": The Labour Party and Popular Politics in 1940s Britain* (Manchester: Manchester University Press, 1995), 19–45.
61. Quotes from Labour Party conferences in this paragraph draw from PHM, *The Labour Party Annual Report* (1942), 132; PHM, *The Labour Party Annual Report* (1943), 143–5.
62. PHM, BOX 314 362.4, Labour Party, 'National Service for Health: The Labour Party's Policy', 1943, 1–2.
63. Edith Summerskill, *Wanted – Babies: A Trenchant Examination of a Grave National Problem* (London: Hutchinson, 1943), quotes on 4, 12. For family allowances, see Susan Pedersen, *Eleanor Rathbone and the Politics of Conscience* (New Haven, CT: Yale University Press, 2004).
64. Fox, *Health Policies, Health Politics*, 94–114.
65. David Stark Murray, *The Future of Medicine* (Harmondsworth: Penguin, 1942). The subsequent quote comes from David Stark Murray, *Health for All* (London: Victor Gollancz, 1942), 39.
66. George. H. Gallup, *The Gallup International Public Opinion Polls, Great Britain 1937–1975, Volume One* (New York: Random House, 1976), 43–4.
67. James Hinton, *The Mass Observers: A History, 1937–1949* (Oxford: Oxford University Press, 2013); Penny Summerfield, 'Mass-Observation: Social Research or Social Movement?', *Journal of Contemporary History* 20, no. 3 (1985): 439–52. The rest of this paragraph draws from MOA, SxMOA1/1/8/4/12, File Report 1665 'Feelings About Hospitals' (April, 1943).
68. 'Do We Want a State Medical Service?', *Picture Post*, 12 August 1944, 16–20.
69. In recent years, historians have increasingly used the qualitative material of such surveys while remaining attentive to their challenges; see Lawrence, *Me, Me, Me?*; David Cowan, 'The "Progress of a Slogan": Youth, Culture, and the Shaping of Everyday Political Languages in Late 1940s Britain', *Twentieth Century British History* 29, no. 3 (2018): 435–58.
70. For an overview of the Ministry of Health introducing the EMS, see NA, MH101/1, 'Report by Sir John Hebb on Preparation on Emergency Medical Services, 1923–1939'.
71. Ross McKibbin, *The Ideologies of Class: Social Relations in Britain, 1880–1950* (Oxford: Oxford University Press, 1990), 259–93; Philip Williamson, *Stanley Baldwin: Conservative Leadership and National Values* (Cambridge: Cambridge University Press, 1999).

72. Quotes from members of the public in this paragraph are drawn from MOA, SxMOA1/2/13/1/F/1, '80+ Replies to 5 Questions about Experience of Hospitals and the Way in Which They Are Funded and Organised (1943)', Responses 3, 102, 105.
73. Mass Observation, *Meet Yourself at the Doctor's* (London: Faber and Faber, 2009), 14.
74. Susan R. Grayzel, *At Home and Under Fire: Air Raids and Culture in Britain from the Great War to the Blitz* (Cambridge: Cambridge University Press, 2012), 263–4; James Greenhalgh, 'The Threshold of the State: Civil Defence, the Blackout and the Home in Second World War Britain', *Twentieth Century British History* 28, no. 2 (2017): 186–208.
75. MOA, SxMOA1/2/13/1/F/1, Response 38.
76. MOA, SxMOA1/1/8/10/1 1921, 'Public Attitudes to State Medicine' (1943).
77. MOA, 'Public Attitudes to State Medicine', 44.
78. Cited in 'State Medicine Costs', *Yorkshire Post and Leeds Intelligencer*, 8 March 1948, 2. For other examples, see 'Dictatorship', *Nottingham Journal*, 10 February 1948, 2; 'Health Service', *The Western Morning News*, 23 March 1948, 2.
79. The Labour Party, *Let Us Face the Future: A Declaration of Labour Policy for the Consideration of the Nation* (London: The Labour Party, 1945), 10.
80. Stephen Brooke, *Labour's War: The Labour Party During the Second World War* (Oxford: Oxford University Press, 1992), 231–68; Richard Toye, *The Labour Party and the Planned Economy, 1931–1951* (Cambridge: Cambridge University Press, 2003), 139–55; Jim Tomlinson, 'Managing the Economy, Managing the People: Britain c.1931–70', *Economic History Review* 58, no. 3 (2005): 555–85.
81. Nicklaus Thomas-Symonds, *Nye: The Political Life of Aneurin Bevan* (London: I.B. Tauris, 2014), 135–7.
82. MOA, SxMOA1/1/8/4/12, 'Feelings about Hospitals', 6–7.
83. The following quotes draw from MOA, SxMOA1/2/13/1/F/1, Responses 104, 12, 13, 102, 11, 26.
84. PHM, *The Labour Party Annual Report* (1946), 103.
85. Stewart, '"For a Healthy London"', 417–18.
86. This paragraph draws from House of Commons, 'National Health Service Bill', 30 April 1946, vol. 422, 43–65.
87. HMSO, *National Health Service Act*, (London: HMSO, 1946).
88. Martin Powell, 'The Changing Blueprints of the British NHS: The White Papers of 1944 and 1989', *Health Care Analysis* 2, no. 2 (1994): 111–17, especially 112–14.
89. House of Lords, 'Shortage of Doctors', 29 November 1961, vol. 235, 1131–45. For Beveridge's criticisms of the NHS, see LSE, BEVERIDGE/7/3, William Beveridge, 'The Role of the Individual in the Health Service', 1954.
90. Digby, *The Evolution of British General Practice*, 307–11.
91. 'The Function of the State in Medicine', *Journal of the American Medical Association* 113, no. 1 (1939): 61.
92. For the dispute, see Nicholas Timmins, *The Five Giants: A Biography of the Welfare State* (London: HarperCollins, 2001), 112–26; Webster, *The Health Services since the War. Volume I*, 107–20.
93. 'Is State Medicine Desirable?', *Chester Chronicle*, 1 December 1945, 6.
94. BL, Oral History of General Practice, Interview with Margaret Teuter Samuel, Tape 3 (F4770).
95. Alfred Cox, 'The Health Service Bill', *British Medical Journal* 1, no. 4448 (1946): 541.
96. House of Commons, 'National Health Service', 9 February 1948, vol. 447, 35–160.
97. Gallup, *The Gallup International Public Opinion Polls*, 170.
98. BBCWAC, R41/124 P.C.S., Letter of 13 February 1948.
99. MOA, Diary Number 5296, Entry for May 1946.

100. MOA, Diary Number 5472, Entry for June 1948.
101. CCA, RUSM 1/8, Letters of 23 March 1948 and 28 May 1948.
102. While this line is difficult to source, it was apparently voiced by Bevan to Brian Abel-Smith; see Sally Sheard, 'A Creature of Its Time: The Critical History of the Creation of the British NHS', *Michael Quarterly* 8, no. 4 (2011): 428–41, quote on 435.
103. WC, BBC, 'NHS at 50: Health for a Nation – the Ethical Age' (BBC: Radio 4, 1998).
104. CCA, RUSM 1/8, Letter of 4 March 1948, Letter of 2 July 1948.
105. MOA, File Report 3140, 'A Report on the National Health Service', (1949), 10.
106. The following quotes in this paragraph are drawn from MOA, SxMOA1/2/13/3/1 C File C, 'Questionnaire Drafts and Replies, Survey 02', Interview 02/134, Interview 02/142, Interview 02/004, Interview 02/123.
107. Laura King, *Family Men: Fatherhood and Masculinity in Britain, c. 1914–1960* (Oxford: Oxford University Press, 2015).
108. Individual responses in this paragraph draw on MOA, SxMOA1/2/13/3/1 C File C, Interview 02/001, Interview 02/128.
109. MOA, 'Public Attitudes to State Medicine', viii.
110. MOA, SxMOA1/2/13/1/F/1, '80+ Replies to 5 Questions about Experience of Hospitals'. Percentages collated by the author.
111. Individual responses in this paragraph draw on MOA, SxMOA1/2/13/1/F/1, Responses 50, 6, 19, 20, 11, 37.
112. MOA, SxMOA1/1/12/8/4, File Report 2508, 'Aspects of Charity', August 1947, 14–15.
113. Bevan, *In Place of Fear*, 87.
114. S.F. Marwood, 'Free Choice of Doctor', *British Medical Journal* 1, no. 4193 (1941): 66–8.
115. Tom Wildy, 'The Social and Economic Publicity and Propaganda of the Labour Governments of 1945–51', *Contemporary Record* 6, no. 1 (1992): 45–71; Laura Beers, 'Labour's Britain, Fight for It Now!', *Historical Journal* 52, no. 3 (2009): 667–95.
116. NA, MH55/963, 'House to House': Drafts and Comments, 'Central Publicity Addressed to General Public, Draft Plan'.
117. Gallup, *The Gallup International Public Opinion Polls*, 185.
118. J.M. Lee, 'Clark, Sir Thomas Fife (1907–1985)', *Oxford Dictionary of National Biography*, 2004.
119. NA, MH55/962, Letter from COI, 25 June 1947; NA, MH55/962, Letter from COI, 5 January 1947.
120. NA, MH55/962, 'House to House': Leaflet', Letter to L. Berringer, 16 December 1947.
121. BFI, BFI Identifier: 11586. *Doctor's Dilemma*. London: Central Office of Information, 1948.
122. BFI, BFI Identifier: 62045. Budge Cooper. *Here's Health*. Directed by Donald Alexander. London: Central Office of Information, 1948; BFI, BFI Identifier: 18308. *Children of the City: A Study of Child Delinquency in Scotland*. Directed by Budge Cooper. London: Paul Rotha Productions, 1944.
123. BFI, BFI Identifier: 10992. Central Office of Information. *Your Very Good Health*. Directed by Joy Batchelor and John Halas. London: Halas & Batchelor, 1948.
124. BFI, BFI Identifier: 20691. Central Office of Information. *Charley in New Town*. Directed by Joy Batchelor and John Halas. London: Halas & Batchelor, 1948.
125. BOD, POSTER 1950-21, 'Labour's Health Service Covers Everyone, Tories Voted Against It', 1950.
126. MOA, Diary Number 5043, Entry for 5 January 1949.

127. CCA, ABMS 3/23, J228, 'Survey of Public Opinion on Current Politics', July 1949.
128. See, for instance, 'Genuine Cases?', *Daily Mail*, 20 May 1953, 9.
129. 'Thanks, Nye', *The People*, 10 May 1953, 6.
130. 'Hearing Aid', *Staffordshire Sentinel*, 23 March 1949, 3.
131. The remainder of this paragraph draws from 'Doctor and Patient', *New Statesman and Nation*, 12 February 1949, 148.

CHAPTER 2 ON THE WARD

1. Sarah Campion, *National Baby* (London: Ernest Benn, 1950).
2. My thanks to the 'National Baby' himself, Philip Alpers, for identifying the hospital. Campion discussed writing *National Baby* in a later interview, NARC, New Zealand, NOH-AAA-0183, 'Oral History Interview with Sarah Campion', 1989–1990.
3. Charles Webster, *The National Health Service: A Political History* (Oxford: Oxford University Press, 2002), 29.
4. HMSO, *A Hospital Plan for England and Wales* (London: HMSO, 1962), 1.
5. Office of Health Economics, *Building for Health* (London: OHE, 1970), 6–7.
6. The rise of the modern hospital is often dated to the eighteenth century. For a classic, if contested, work, see Michel Foucault, *The Birth of the Clinic: An Archaeology of Medical Perception* (New York: Vintage Books, 1973). It was not until the twentieth century, however, that hospitals assumed their pre-eminence. See Kisacky, *Rise of the Modern Hospital*; Lindsay Granshaw, 'The Rise of the Modern Hospital in Britain', in Andrew Wear (ed.), *Medicine in Society: Historical Essays* (Cambridge: Cambridge University Press, 1992), 197–218.
7. Office of Health Economics, *Hospital Costs in Perspective* (London: OHE, 1963), 4–6.
8. For the economic crisis in the 1970s and the undoing of other social democratic aspirations, see Davies, *The City of London and Social Democracy*, 127–39.
9. Tony Cutler, 'A Double Irony? The Politics of National Health Service Expenditure in the 1950s', in Martin Gorsky and Sally Sheard (eds), *Financing Medicine: The British Experience since 1750* (London: Routledge, 2006), 201–20; Bank of England, 'A Millennium of Macroeconomic Data', Version 3.1 (2016).
10. For the localised nature of the NHS, see DeVane, 'Pilgrim's Progress'.
11. Robinson et al, 'Telling Stories about Post-war Britain'.
12. Judt, *Postwar*, 535–58. See also, Owen Hatherley, *The Ministry of Nostalgia* (London: Verso, 2016), 11.
13. Webster, *The Health Services since the War. Volume I*, 257–346; Glen O'Hara, *From Dreams to Disillusionment: Economic and Social Planning in 1960s Britain* (Basingstoke: Palgrave Macmillan, 2007), 179–90; Fair, 'Modernization of Our Hospital System'; Tony Cutler, 'Economic Liberal or Arch Planner? Enoch Powell and the Political Economy of the Hospital Plan', *Contemporary British History* 25, no. 4 (2011): 469–89.
14. Jean McFarlane, Kay Richards and C.J. Wells, *Hospitals in the NHS* (London: King's Fund, 1980), 7.
15. For maternity in postwar Britain, see Angela Davis, *Modern Motherhood: Women and Family in England, 1945–2000* (Manchester: Manchester University Press, 2012); Salim Al-Gailani, 'Hospital Birth', in Nick Hopwood, Rebecca Flemming and Lauren Kassell (eds), *Reproduction: Antiquity to the Present Day* (Cambridge: Cambridge University Press, 2018), 553–66.
16. For hospital birth figures, see WC, SA/PIC/H/3/2, National Birthday Trust, *Maternity in Great Britain* (1946), 48–9; HMSO, *Domiciliary Midwifery and Maternity Bed Needs: The Report of the Standing Maternity and Midwifery Advisory Committee* (London: HMSO, 1970).

17. 'Total Fertility Rate in the United Kingdom from 1800 to 2000', 2022, *Statista*, https://www.statista.com/statistics/1033074/fertility-rate-uk-1800-2020/.
18. For lying-in hospitals, see Al-Gailani, 'Hospital Birth', 555–7.
19. The remainder of this paragraph draws on Thomas Ryan, *The History of Queen Charlotte's Lying-in Hospital: From Its Foundation in 1752 to the Present Time, With an Account of Its Objects and Present State* (London: Queen Charlotte's Lying-In Hospital, 1885) and 'Queen Charlotte's Maternity Hospital', https://ezitis.myzen.co.uk/queen-charlottemarylebone.html; LMA, H27/QC/Y/15/001, Photo of Queen Charlotte's Maternity Hospital Exterior, 1930s; Charles Graves, 'Twilight of the Charity Ball', *The Sphere*, 21 May 1949, 280.
20. LMA, H27/QC/A/01/001, Board of Governors Minute Book (1948–1949), Minutes of 28 October 1948.
21. The biographical information on Sarah Campion in this paragraph draws on 'Campion, Sarah', in Roger Robinson and Nelson Wattie (eds), *The Oxford Companion to New Zealand Literature* (Oxford: Oxford University Press, 1998), 88; Rachel Scott (ed.), *I Live Here Now: Sarah Campion in 1950s New Zealand* (Christchurch: Shoal Bay Press, 2000), 9–13.
22. Sarah Campion, *Mo Burdekin* (London: Peter Davies, 1941); Sarah Campion, *Bonanza* (London: Peter Davies, 1942); Sarah Campion, *The Pommy Cow* (London: Peter Davies, 1944).
23. The information on patient numbers in this paragraph is drawn from LMA, H27/QC/A/027/080, 'Annual Report for 1947', 4; LMA, H27/QC/A/027/002, 'Biennial Report 1950–1951', 23. The administrators' quote is from LMA, H27/QC/A/027/081, 'Annual Report for 1949'. The quote from Campion from Campion, *National Baby*, 13.
24. The quotes in this paragraph are from Campion, *National Baby*, 32, 141, 51–2.
25. For conceptions of privacy in the twentieth century, see Deborah Cohen, *Family Secrets: Shame and Privacy in Modern Britain* (Oxford: Oxford University Press, 2013), 4–6; Walter F. Pratt, *Privacy in Britain* (Lewisburg, PA: Bucknell University Press, 1979); David Vincent, *Privacy: A Short History* (Cambridge: Polity Press, 2016).
26. Campion, *National Baby*, 77, 80.
27. Cited in Sally Sheard, 'Getting Better, Faster: Convalescence and Length of Stay in British and US Hospitals', in Laurinda Abreu and Sally Sheard (eds), *Daily Life in Hospital: Theory and Practice from the Medieval to the Modern* (Oxford: Peter Lang, 2013), 299–329, statistic on 318.
28. LMA, H27/QC/Y/15/001, Photo of Maternity Ward, 1930s. For Nightingale wards and their architectural design, see Florence Nightingale, *Notes on Hospitals* (London: Longman, Green, Longman, Roberts, and Green, 1863), 61–4; Julie Willis, Philip Goad and Cameron Logan, *Architecture and the Modern Hospital, Nosokomeion to Hygeia* (Abingdon: Routledge, 2019), 25; Kisacky, *Rise of the Modern Hospital*, 15.
29. Campion, *National Baby*, 77.
30. This paragraph draws from Somerville Hastings, 'Management of Hospitals in Peace and War', *The Lancet* 245, no. 6334 (1945): 71–4.
31. Central Health Services Council, *The Reception and Welfare of In-Patients in Hospitals* (London: HMSO, 1953), 16.
32. Beaumont, *Housewives and Citizens*, 189–214. For their influence among mothers, see Davis, *Modern Motherhood*, 35–40.
33. The comments on gender and privacy in the remainder of this paragraph draw on 'Hospitals Board Asked – Give Women in Wards More Privacy', *Dundee Courier*, 21 January 1952, 3; 'Arbroath Hospital Demands Deputation', *Dundee Courier*, 9 January 1952, 4; 'More Privacy in Hospitals', *Taunton Courier and Western Advertiser*, 5 October 1957, 9.

34. Liverpool offers an illustrative example, see LRO, 920 EVE/7/2/1-19, Letter from Chairman of Everton Women's Helpers League, 12 January 1949.
35. Cited in Frank K. Prochaska, *Philanthropy and the Hospitals of London: The King's Fund, 1897–1990* (Oxford: Oxford University Press, 1992), 165; LRO, 352 PSP/62/58/1-33, Photograph of the League of Friends Shop at the Royal Southern Hospital (1973).
36. H.M. Heafield, 'Hospital Privacy', *The Daily Telegraph*, 3 December 1959, 12.
37. LMA, H27/QC/A/01/001, Board of Governors Minute Book (1948–1949), Minutes of 26 August 1948.
38. Cited in Clifford Williamson, 'The Quiet Time? Pay-beds and Private Practice in the National Health Service: 1948–1970', *Social History of Medicine* 28, no. 3 (2015): 576–95, statistic on 579.
39. Campion, *National Baby*, 14.
40. LMA, H27/QC/A/29/041, Letter of 31 January 1966.
41. Baldwin, *The Politics of Social Solidarity*; Julian Le Grand and David Winter, 'The Middle Classes and the Welfare State Under Conservative and Labour Governments', *Journal of Public Policy* 6, no. 4 (1986): 399–430.
42. Sutcliffe-Braithwaite, *Class, Politics, and the Decline of Deference*, 34–5.
43. Quotes in the remainder of this paragraph are from Campion, *National Baby*, 14, 142.
44. LMA, H27/QC/A/027/081, 'Annual Report for 1949', 22.
45. Jane Lewis and John Welshman, 'The Issue of Never-Married Motherhood in Britain, 1920–70', *Social History of Medicine* 10, no. 3 (1997): 401–18, especially 402.
46. LMA, H27/QC/A/027/080, 'Annual Report for 1947', 23–4; LMA, H27/QC/A/027/081, 'Annual Report for 1949', 24. For almoners, see George Campbell Gosling, 'Gender, Money and Professional Identity: Medical Social Work and the Coming of the British National Health Service', *Women's History Review* 27, no. 2 (2018): 310–28.
47. WC, SA/PIC/H/3/2, National Birthday Trust, *Maternity in Great Britain*, 194.
48. Quotes in this paragraph from Campion, *National Baby*, 99, 100, 97–8, 95.
49. Quotes in this paragraph from Campion, *National Baby*, 138,140, 141, 151.
50. Victoria Bates, '"Humanizing" Healthcare Environments: Architecture, Art and Design in Modern Hospitals', *Design for Health* 2, no. 1 (2018): 5–19.
51. Ayesha Nathoo, *Hearts Exposed: Transplants and the Media in 1960s Britain* (Basingstoke: Palgrave Macmillan, 2009). For postwar medical developments mentioned in this paragraph, see Rivett, *From Cradle to Grave*, 134–62.
52. King, *Family Men*, 174–84.
53. Laura King, 'Hiding in the Pub to Cutting the Cord? Men's Presence at Childbirth in Britain c.1940s–2000s', *Social History of Medicine* 30, no. 2 (2017): 389–407.
54. Campion, *National Baby*, 75.
55. King, 'Hiding in the Pub', 395–6.
56. LMA, H27/QC/A/29/036, Letter of 6 January 1969.
57. LMA, H27/QC/A/29/036, Letter of 14 January 1969.
58. Cited in King, 'Hiding in the Pub', 396–400.
59. Cited in Lewis and Welshman, 'The Issue of Never-Married Motherhood in Britain', 402.
60. LMA, H27/QC/A/29/040, Letter of 3 December 1966; LMA, H27/QC/A/29/040, Letter of 10 January 1967.
61. Margaret Drabble, *The Millstone* (London: Weidenfeld & Nicolson, 1965).
62. Drabble, *The Millstone*, 119–20.
63. BBCWAC, *Woman's Hour*, Films 83/84, Interview with Margaret Drabble, 1 October 1965.

64. Marcus Collins, 'Introduction: The Permissive Society and Its Enemies', in *The Permissive Society and Its Enemies,* ed. Marcus Collins (London: Rivers Oram, 2007), 1–40; Mark Jarvis, *Conservative Governments, Morality and Social Change in Affluent Britain* (Manchester: Manchester University Press, 2005); Stephen Brooke, *Sexual Politics: Sexuality, Family Planning, and the British Left from the 1880s to the Present Day* (Oxford: Oxford University Press, 2011), 146–82; Frank Mort, 'The Permissive Society Revisited', *Twentieth Century British History* 22, no. 2 (2011): 269–98.
65. Brooke, *Sexual Politics,* 174–5.
66. Mold, *Making the Patient-Consumer*, 25.
67. Lise Butler, *Michael Young, Social Science, and the British Left, 1945–1970* (Oxford: Oxford University Press, 2020), 101–57.
68. Ann Cartwright, *Human Relations and Hospital Care* (London: Routledge & Kegan Paul, 1964); subsequent statistic on visitation is on 135.
69. Harry Hendrick, 'Children's Emotional Well-being and Mental Health in Early Post-Second World War Britain: The Case of Unrestricted Hospital Visiting', in Marijke Gijswijt-Hofstra and Hilary Marland (eds), *Cultures of Child Health in Britain and the Netherlands in the Twentieth Century* (Amsterdam: Rodopi, 2003), 213–35.
70. Shapira, *The War Inside*, 198–238; John Bowlby, *Maternal Care and Mental Health* (Geneva, Switzerland: World Health Organization, 1951); Donald Winnicott, *The Child and the Family* (London: Tavistock Publications, 1957).
71. Dolly Smith Wilson, 'A New Look at the Affluent Worker: The Good Working Mother in Post-War Britain', *Twentieth Century British History* 17, no. 2 (2006): 206–29, especially 210–15.
72. HMSO, *The Welfare of Children in Hospital* (London: HMSO, 1959), 4; Mold, *Making the Patient-Consumer*, 25–9.
73. Quotes from Drabble, *The Millstone*, 148–61.
74. BBCWAC, *Woman's Hour*, Films 77/78, 'My Child in Hospital', 23 September 1964.
75. Ruth Davies, 'Marking the 50th Anniversary of the Platt Report: From Exclusion, to Toleration and Parental Participation in the Care of the Hospitalized Child', *Journal of Child Health Care* 14, no. 1 (2010): 6–23, especially 15–18.
76. Victoria Bates, *Making Noise in the Modern Hospital* (Cambridge: Cambridge University Press, 2021).
77. King Edward's Fund for London, *Noise Control in Hospitals* (London: King's Fund, 1958).
78. Prochaska, *Philanthropy and the Hospitals of London*, 164–94.
79. King Edward's Fund for London, *Noise Control in Hospitals*, 9–13.
80. WC, 728038i, King Edward's Fund for London, 'Two Nurses Whispering and Causing a Nuisance to Patients', 1958.
81. This paragraph draws from M. Dorothy Hinks, *'The Most Cruel Absence of Care'* (London: King's Fund, 1974), 6, 21–3.
82. HMSO, *Mental Health Act* (London: HMSO, 1959).
83. Claire Hilton, *Improving Psychiatric Care for Older People: Barbara Robb's Campaign, 1965–1974* (Cham, Switzerland: Palgrave Macmillan, 2017), 57–95.
84. Barbara Robb, *Sans Everything: A Case to Answer* (London: Nelson, 1967).
85. Sally Sheard, *The Passionate Economist: How Brian Abel-Smith Shaped Global Health and Social Welfare* (Bristol: Policy Press, 2014), 233–6.
86. Hilton, *Improving Psychiatric Care for Older People*, 219–22, 225–32.
87. Gerda L. Cohen, 'Hospitals For Patients', *New Statesman*, 8 June 1962, 826–7.
88. HMSO, *A Hospital Plan for England and Wales.*
89. 'The Nation's Hospitals', *The Times*, 24 January 1962, 11.

90. Office of Health Economics, *OHE Guide to UK Health and Health Care Statistics* (London: OHE, 2013), 45.
91. 'General Hospitals', *Architectural Review,* 1 June 1965, 422–46.
92. Jonathan Hughes, 'The "Matchbox on a Muffin": The Design of Hospitals in the Early NHS', *Medical History* 44, no. 1 (2000): 21–56; Fair, 'Modernization of Our Hospital System'.
93. DeVane, 'Pilgrim's Progress', 537–43.
94. Wetherell, *Foundations,* 76–106; Otto Saumarez Smith, *Boom Cities: Architect Planners and the Politics of Radical Urban Renewal in 1960s Britain* (Oxford: Oxford University Press, 2019).
95. Cited in O'Hara, *From Dreams to Disillusionment,* 187.
96. 'Hospital' (1954), *British Pathé,* https://www.youtube.com/watch?v=qygR9TwXHbU.
97. Statistics in this paragraph from Cartwright, *Human Relations and Hospital Care,* 57, 56.
98. Winifred Raphael, *Patients and Their Hospitals* (London: King's Fund, 1969).
99. Winifred Raphael, *Survey of Patients' Opinion Surveys in Hospital* (London: King's Fund, 1974).
100. Raphael, *Patients and Their Hospitals,* 16.
101. Raphael, *Survey of Patients' Opinion Surveys in Hospital,* 19.
102. LRO, 352 PSP/62/39/1-27, Photograph of Mill Road Maternity Ward (1946).
103. LRO, 352 PSP/62/39/82-105, Photograph of Patients in Ward A6 (1977). Placing hospital beds in smaller groups of four was first undertaken in Denmark in 1909. Other countries with large wards gradually copied this style, but it took decades to dislodge the Nightingale pattern of two rows along each wall; see Willis, Goad and Logan, *Architecture and the Modern Hospital,* 45–6.
104. Chris Cordner, '7 Rare Photos as We Look Back at the Ingham Infirmary in South Shields', *Shields Gazette,* 18 April 2021, https://www.shieldsgazette.com/heritage-and-retro/retro/7-rare-photos-as-we-look-back-at-the-ingham-infirmary-in-south-shields-and-the-super-staff-who-worked-there-3203810.
105. The following quotes from Cartwright and patients in this paragraph, as well as the survey statistic, are drawn from Cartwright, *Human Relations and Hospital Care,* 47–9.
106. Perry, *London is the Place for Me*; Ian Sanjay Patel, *We're Here Because You Were There: Immigration and the End of Empire* (London: Verso, 2021).
107. Hinks, *'The Most Cruel Absence of Care',* 22.
108. Clair Wills, *Lovers and Strangers: An Immigrant History of Post-War Britain* (London: Allen Lane, 2017), 247–63.
109. Buchi Emecheta, *Second-Class Citizen* (London: Allison & Busby, 1974), quotes in this paragraph on 60, 124. Emecheta also emigrated from Nigeria, endured a similarly abusive relationship with her husband and worked in the same jobs as her protagonist; see her autobiography, Buchi Emecheta, *Head Above Water* (London: Ogwugwu Afor, 1984).
110. Mathew Thomson, 'Representation of the National Health Service in the Arts and Popular Culture', in Crane and Hand (eds), *Posters, Protests, and Prescriptions,* 231–54, especially 239–44.
111. Quotes in the rest of this paragraph from Emecheta, *Second-Class Citizen,* 110, 126.
112. Sutcliffe-Braithwaite, *Class, Politics, and the Decline of Deference,* 34–55.
113. This paragraph draws from E.J.R. Burrough, 'Hospitals – A Plea for Privacy', *The Listener,* 12 May 1977, 605–6.
114. NA, MH 123/243, 'Hospital Building Notes No. 4 – Ward Units', 1961. For Tatton-Brown's thinking on hospitals, see W. Paul James and William Tatton-Brown, *Hospitals: Design and Development* (London: Architectural Press, 1986).

115. NA, MH 123/243, 'Hospital Building Notes No. 4 – Ward Units', 1961.
116. NA, MH 123/268, 'Hospital Building Notes No. 27 – Maternity Units', 1961.
117. Kisacky, *Rise of the Modern Hospital,* 154–6.
118. Willis, Goad and Logan, *Architecture and the Modern Hospital*, 48–50.
119. NA, MH 123/243, 'Hospital Building Notes No. 4 – Ward Units', 1.
120. Burrough, 'Hospitals – A Plea for Privacy', 606.
121. Dorothy Milton, 'Hospital Privacy', *Daily Telegraph*, 25 November 1959, 10; K. Vickers, 'Communal Life in Hospital,' *Daily Telegraph*, 30 November 1959, 10; Etheldred Browning, 'Hospital Privacy', *Daily Telegraph*, 10 December 1959, 10.
122. The statistics and quote in the rest of this paragraph are from Cartwright, *Human Relations and Hospital Care*, 63, 47, 67–8.
123. Cited in David Owen, *In Sickness and in Health: The Politics of Medicine* (London: Quartet Books, 1976), 33.
124. Susan Francis, Rosemary Glanville, Ann Noble and Peter Scher, *50 Years of Ideas in Health Care Buildings* (London: Nuffield Trust, 1999), 49.
125. The rest of this paragraph draws from WC, Tony Highfield, *Memories of the NHS: 50 Years of the NHS 1948–1998* (Walsall: Walsall Hospitals NHS Trust, 1998), 40–3.

CHAPTER 3 AT THE HEALTH CENTRE

1. This depiction of a typical visit to the doctors in the 1940s draws on Joseph S. Collings, 'General Practice in England Today: A Reconnaissance', *The Lancet* 255, no. 6604 (1950): 555–85; Stephen J. Hadfield, 'A Field Survey of General Practice, 1951–2', *British Medical Journal* 2, no. 4838 (1953): 683–706; Stephen Taylor, *Good General Practice* (Oxford: Oxford University Press, 1955); BFI, BFI Identifier: 13716, Richard Cawston. *On Call to a Nation*. London: BBC, 1958; Nick Bosanquet and Chris Salisbury, 'The Practice', in Irvine Loudon, John Horder and Charles Webster (eds), *General Practice Under the National Health Service, 1948–1997: The First Fifty Years* (Oxford: Oxford University Press, 1998), 45–64; Lucinda McCray Beier, *For Their Own Good: The Transformation of English Working-Class Health Culture, 1880–1970* (Columbus, OH: Ohio State University Press, 2008).
2. This paragraph draws on Medical Practitioners' Union, *Report on Health Centres* (London: Medical Practitioners' Union, 1960); 'Impressions of Health Centres, Urban and Rural – Stranraer', *British Medical Journal* 1, no. 5447 (1965): 1429–30; 'Hythe Health Centre', *British Medical Journal* 2, no. 5452 (1965): 42–3; Ann Cartwright, *Patients and Their Doctors: A Study of General Practice* (New York: Atherton Press, 1967); Ann Cartwright and Robert Anderson, *General Practice Revisited: A Second Study of Patients and Their Doctors* (London: Tavistock Publications, 1981); Ruth Cammock, *Health Centres Handbook* (London: Borough of Newham Medical Architecture Research Unit, 1973); BFI, BFI Identifier: 1379. *Health at the Centre*. London: London Television Service, 1974.
3. Historians tend to agree on the improvements in general practice; see Charles Webster, 'The Politics of General Practice', in Loudon, Horder and Webster (eds), *General Practice Under the National Health Service*, 26–34; Simpson, *Migrant Architects of the NHS*, 45–50; Shaul Bar-Haim, '"The Drug Doctor": Michael Balint and the Revival of General Practice in Postwar Britain', *History Workshop Journal* 86, no. 1 (2018): 114–32.
4. Michael Ryan, 'Health Centre Policy in England and Wales', *British Journal of Sociology* 19, no. 1 (1968): 34–46; Phoebe Hall, Hilary Land, Roy Parker and Adrian Webb, *Change, Choice, and Conflict in Social Policy* (London: Heinemann, 1975), 277–310.
5. Marcos Cueto, 'The Origins of Primary Health Care and Selective Primary Health Care', *American Journal of Public Health* 94, no. 11 (2004): 1864–74; Catherine Mas, *Culture in the Clinic: Miami and the Making of Modern Medicine* (Chapel Hill, NC: University of North Carolina Press, 2022), 103–39.

6. In 1979, 16 per cent of GPs performed all of their work in a health centre, and a further 6 per cent undertook part of their work in such settings; WC, Ann Cartwright and Robert Anderson, 'Patients and Their Doctors: Report on Some Changes in General Practice Between 1964 and 1977 for the Royal Commission on the National Health Service', March 1979, 6.
7. The dichotomy between GPs working in health centres and those opting for group practice is not as stark as historians suggest; see John Fry, *General Practice and Primary Health Care, 1940s–1980s* (London: Nuffield Provincial Hospitals Trust, 1988), 42. Officials and experts often referred to both as part of the same movement towards more communal methods.
8. Christine Hogg, *Patients, Power and Politics: From Patients to Citizens* (London: SAGE, 1999), 42–5; Bruce Wood, *Patient Power?: The Politics of Patients' Associations in Britain and America* (Buckingham: Open University Press, 2000); Charlotte Williamson, *Towards the Emancipation of Patients: Patients' Experience and the Patient Movement* (Bristol: Policy Press, 2010).
9. Collings, 'General Practice in England Today'.
10. Taylor, *Good General Practice*, 202.
11. Bosanquet and Salisbury, 'The Practice', 46–7.
12. 'Payment of Wives', *British Medical Journal,* 24 July 1976, 239.
13. For deference to doctors, see Sutcliffe-Braithwaite, *Class, Politics, and the Decline of Deference*, 89. For 'training' patients, see Taylor, *Good General Practice*, 179.
14. Philip Auld, *Honour a Physician* (London: Hollis & Carter, 1959).
15. NA, MH 134/48, Medical Advisory Committee Sub-Committee on Health Centres, 'M.A.C. (H.C.) 6', 1947, 1.
16. HMSO, *National Health Service Act*, 21–2. In Scotland, the Department of Health held responsibility for building health centres; NA, MH 134/62, Failed Projects: Review of Causes, 1960–1961, 'Review of Health Centre Projects Which Failed to Mature in Early Stages'.
17. NA, MH 52/644, Health Centres: Administrative Scheme, 1947–1953, City of Manchester Public Health Committee, 'Report of the Medical Officer of Health on the Provision of Health Centres', 1943.
18. NYAM, Library of Social and Economic Aspects of Medicine of Michael M. Davis, Box 64, Legislation & Regulations, Ministry of Health, 'Circular 3/48', February 1948.
19. NA, MH 52/644, Letter from Ministry of Health to Town Clerk, Manchester, 22 March 1950.
20. 'Six Doctors Boycott Bevan Clinic', *Daily Mail,* 5 July 1950, 3.
21. This paragraph's comments on doctors' attitudes to health centres draws on 'A Field Survey of General Practice, 1951–2', *British Medical Journal,* 683–706. For single-doctored practices, see Bosanquet and Salisbury, 'The Practice', 48.
22. NA, MH 134/49, 'Draft of Circular 3/47'. For this paragraph's discussion of the TUC and MPU, see NA, MH 134/51, General Secretary to H.A. Marquand, 18 January 1951; 'Health Centres', *Medical World* 81, no. 12 (1950).
23. Charles Webster called them a 'catastrophic failure'; see *The Health Services since the War. Volume I*, 387. This stance replicated prior critical interpretations of health centre development; Eckstein, *The English Health Service*, 247–52.
24. There is no definitive list of health centre openings. This estimate is produced by the author and includes health centres in all four nations of the UK, both 'official' centres opened under the terms of NHS Acts and 'unofficial' centres opened outside of the Acts by philanthropic organisations.

25. 'London AKA Around Britain', 1949, *British Pathé*, https://www.britishpathe.com/video/london-aka-around-britain/query/bevan.
26. Ortolano, *Thatcher's Progress*, 112–25.
27. NA, MH 134/51, D.J. Mitchell to A.J.F. Danielli from, 17 April 1953.
28. Charles F. Stott, 'Three Years in a Health Centre', *Medical World*, April 1957, found within NA, MH 134/64.
29. This paragraph's comments on Sighthill Health Centre draw on NA, MH 134/51, Department of Health for Scotland, 'Sighthill Health Centre, Opening Brochure' (1953); 'Scotland's First Health Centre', *The Lancet* 261, no. 6769 (1953): 1038–41; 'Health Centre', *Architects' Journal* 118, no. 3049 (1953): 169–76.
30. NA, MH 134/51, Letter to Mr Emery, 20 May 1953.
31. LMA, SC/PHL/02/604, Photograph of Entrance Hall, AA1337 (1954). The following information on attitudes to Woodberry Down is drawn from NA, MH 134/64, 'Report on Woodberry Down'; Ronald Gibson, 'Organization and Management of Health Centres', *British Medical Journal* 2, no. 5705 (1970): 353–6.
32. MOA, SxMOA1/1/8/10/1 1921, 'Public Attitudes to State Medicine', 1943, 28.
33. W.S. Parker, 'Administration of Health Centres', *The Lancet* 253, no. 6565 (1949): 1119–20.
34. MOA, 'Public Attitudes to State Medicine', 34.
35. Cartwright, *Patients and Their Doctors,* 165–7.
36. This paragraph's comments on the William Budd Health Centre draw on R.H. Parry, J. Sluglett and R.C. Wofinden, 'The William Budd Health Centre, The First Year', *British Medical Journal* 1, no. 4858 (1954): 388–92; 'Impressions of Health Centres, 5. Oldest and Newest – Bristol', *British Medical Journal* 1, no. 5451 (1965): 1662–4.
37. BA, 40826/PUB/71 'William Budd Health Centre, Knowle, Bristol – Knowle Nurses' Rest Room', 1952.
38. NA, MH 134/63, 'Report on William Budd Health Centre'.
39. R.C. Wofinden, 'Health Centres and the General Medical Practitioner', *British Medical Journal* 2, no. 5551 (1967): 565–7.
40. This paragraph's descriptions of William Budd Health Centre's physical environment are informed by photographs, see BA, 40826/PUB/39, 'Health Centre, Leinster Avenue, Knowle – Main Building', 1950s; BA, 40826/PUB/64, 'William Budd Health Centre, Knowle, Bristol – Private Waiting Room', 1952.
41. NA, MH 134/63, 'Report on William Budd Health Centre', 8.
42. ERO, D/DU 943/21, 'Three New "Health Centres" for Harlow', 7 May 1954; H.E. Bach et al, 'The Health Centres of Harlow, The Second Phase', *British Medical Journal* 2, no. 7055 (1958): 1055–60. The Nuffield Trust pursued 'the improvement of a great publicly provided service'; see Gordon McLachlan, *A History of the Nuffield Provincial Hospitals Trust, 1940–1990* (London: Nuffield Provincial Hospitals Trust, 1992), 69–71. For Taylor's support, see *Good General Practice*, 120–1.
43. S. Taylor, 'Haygarth House, Harlow, Building a Health Centre', *The Lancet* 259, no. 6701 (1952): 253–7.
44. The remainder of this paragraph draws on ERO, D/DU 943/21, 'Three New "Health Centres" for Harlow', 5; 'Russian Doctors at New Town', *The Times*, 10 December 1954, 4.
45. For the Rockefeller Foundation, see John Farley, *To Cast Out Disease: A History of the International Health Division of the Rockefeller Foundation (1913–1951)* (Oxford: Oxford University Press, 2004). For its interest in the NHS, see Seaton, 'The Gospel of Wealth and the National Health'.
46. Dorothy Porter, 'Introduction', in Dorothy Porter (ed.), *Social Medicine and Medical Sociology in the Twentieth-Century* (Amsterdam, GA: Rodopi, 1997), 1–31; John

Stewart, 'John Ryle, the Institute of Social Medicine and the Health of Oxford Students', *Family & Community History* 7, no. 1 (2004): 59–71.

47. For this paragraph's discussion of the centre's beginnings, see UMA, MMC/5/7/18/3/2, H.W. Ashworth, 'History of Darbishire House'. For Rockefeller funding, see RAC, RF, RG 1.2. (FA387), Series 401: England, Box 7, Folder 51, 'Grant to Manchester Health Centre', 1954. For patient numbers, see RAC, RF, RG6, SG 1 Series 2: Postwar, Box 23, Folder 205, University of Manchester, 'Annual Report, 1954–55', 'Annual Report, 1955–56', 'Annual Report, 1956–57'.
48. Medical Practitioners' Union, *Report on Health Centres*, 7; RAC, University of Manchester, 'Annual Report, 1956–57'.
49. RAC, RF, Officers' Diaries, RG 12, M-R (FA393), Box 277, Maier, John (1954), Entry for 18 February 1954.
50. See Bruce Cardew, 'An Appointment System Service for General Practitioners: Its Growth and Present Usage', *British Medical Journal* 4, no. 5578 (1967): 542–3. See also, Moore, 'Waiting for the Doctor'.
51. 'Appointment Systems in General Practice', *British Medical Journal* 1, no. 5427 (1965): 125.
52. RAC, University of Manchester, 'Annual Report, 1955–56'.
53. 'A Field Survey of General Practice, 1951–2', 701.
54. Medical Practitioners' Union, *Report on Health Centres*, 18.
55. This paragraph's comments on expanded interest in health centres draws from The King's Fund, *Health Centres: Papers Delivered at a Conference at the Hospital Centre* (London: King's Fund, 1966); Medical Practitioners' Union, *Report on Health Centres*, 26, 37–8; NA, MH 134/63, 'Summary of Health Centres and Group Practices, Interim Report', 1959.
56. The number of health centres in this paragraph draws from 'Health Centres: Facts and Figures', *The Lancet* 294, no. 7627 (1969): 945–8; Cartwright and Anderson, *General Practice Revisited*, 62; MMI Publications, *The Directory of Health Centres* (London: MMI Publications, 1984), 421.
57. 'Health Centre Explosion', *British Medical Journal* 4, no. 5582 (1967): 759–60.
58. Webster, *The Health Services since the War. Volume II*, 264–83.
59. Simpson, *Migrant Architects of the NHS*, 251.
60. This paragraph draws on, HMSO, *Health Centres: A Design Guide* (London: HMSO, 1970). The document was first issued to local authorities in the late 1960s.
61. GA, DX107/26, Souvenir Booklet for Official Opening of Dowlais Health Centre and Hollies Health Centre, April 1972.
62. John Berger, *A Fortunate Man, : The Story of a Country Doctor* (New York: Pantheon Books, 1967); quotes from the book in the following two paragraphs can be found on 94, 97.
63. Chelsea Saxby, 'Nostalgia and the NHS', *The Polyphony* (April 2020), https://thepolyphony.org/2020/04/07/nostalgia-and-the-nhs/.
64. BFI, BFI Identifier: N-968060. *Towards a Better Life – Community Health* London: FCO, 1986.
65. Statistics on women doctors drawn from Taylor, *Good General Practice*, 50; Laura Jefferson, Karen Bloor, and Alan Maynard, 'Women in Medicine: Historical Perspectives and Recent Trends', *British Medical Bulletin* 114, no. 1 (2015): 5–15.
66. DHC, 5579M/0/7 – Devon Area Health Authority, 'Health Centres in Devon', Exeter, 1982, 1–2.
67. DHC, 5579M/0/7, 'Health Centres in Devon', 4–8.
68. DHC, 8003H – National Health Service, Devon, 1960s–1990s, 'Photograph of Okehampton Health Centre', 1960s, 'Photograph of Seaton Health Centre', 1960s.
69. DHC, 8003H, 'Photograph of Ilfracombe Health Centre', 1960s.

70. This paragraph draws on George Weisz, *Chronic Disease in the Twentieth Century: A History* (Baltimore, MD: Johns Hopkins University Press, 2014); Abdel R. Omran, 'The Epidemiologic Transition: A Theory of the Epidemiology of Population Change', *The Milbank Quarterly* 83, no. 4 (2005): 731–57; Randall M. Packard, *A History of Global Health: Interventions into the Lives of Other Peoples* (Baltimore, MD: Johns Hopkins University Press, 2016), 249–66.
71. This paragraph draws on Jane Lewis, *What Price Community Medicine?: The Philosophy, Practice and Politics of Public Health since 1919* (Brighton: Wheatsheaf Books, 1986), 100–24; Virginia Berridge, *Marketing Health: Smoking and the Discourse of Public Health in Britain 1945–2000* (Oxford: Oxford University Press, 2007); Dorothy Porter, *Health, Civilization, and the State: A History of Public Health from Ancient to Modern Times* (London: Routledge, 1999).
72. The comments in this paragraph on Morris, Doll and Hill draw on J.N. Morris et al, 'Coronary Heart-Disease and Physical Activity of Work', *The Lancet* 262, no. 6796 (1953): 1111–20; Richard Doll and Austin Bradford Hill, 'Smoking and Carcinoma of the Lung', *British Medical Journal* 2, no. 4682 (1950): 739–48; J.N. Morris, 'Tomorrow's Community Physician', *The Lancet* 294, no. 7625 (1969): 811–16.
73. HMSO, *National Health Service Reorganisation Act* (London: HMSO, 1973).
74. DHC, 5579M/0/7, 'Health Centres in Devon', 28–9.
75. MMI Publications, *The Directory of Health Centres*, 25–6. For other 1980s health centres, see 'Building Study: An Angle on Health Centres, Trevor Denton Wayland Tunley', *Architects' Journal* 182, no. 31 (1985): 19–31.
76. Granada Television, *The Practice*. Directed by Sarah Harding, David Richards, Pedr James, Charles Kitchen and Matthew Robinson. Manchester: Granada Television, 1985.
77. Matthew Hilton, *Consumerism in Twentieth-Century Britain: The Search for a Historical Movement* (Cambridge: Cambridge University Press, 2003), 243–67.
78. Tomes, *Remaking the American Patient*, 257–67.
79. WC, SA/PAT/A/1/1: Box 1 Patients Association Committee Minutes, 'Minutes of the First Meeting of the Committee of the Patients Association', 24 January 1963; Mold, *Making the Patient-Consumer*, 29–34.
80. WC, SA/PAT/C/12 Consumers' Association.
81. Such as 'Spectacles', *Which?*, February 1969, 42–5. For *Which?*, see Hilton, *Consumerism in Twentieth-Century Britain*, 205–18.
82. Gordon Thomas and Ian D. Hudson, *The National Health Service and You* (London: Panther Books, 1965), 1.
83. Richard Titmuss, *Commitment to Welfare* (London: Allen & Unwin, 1968), 212.
84. Thomas and Hudson, *The National Health Service and You*, 21.
85. Glen O'Hara, 'The Complexities of "Consumerism": Choice, Collectivism and Participation within Britain's National Health Service, c.1961–c.1979', *Social History of Medicine* 26, no. 2 (2013): 288–304; Hilton, *Consumerism in Twentieth-Century Britain*, 268–97; Robinson et al, 'Telling Stories about Post-war Britain', 276–8.
86. This paragraph draws on Lesley Doyal, 'Women, Health and the Sexual Division of Labour: A Case Study of the Women's Health Movement in Britain', *Critical Social Policy* 3, no. 7 (1983): 21–32; Jesse Olszynko-Gryn, 'The Feminist Appropriation of Pregnancy Testing in 1970s Britain', *Women's History Review* 28, no. 6 (2019): 869–94.
87. The comments on Lin Layram's experience are drawn from 'To Lose a Breast Seemed More Terrible Than Dying', *Spare Rib*, no. 37 (July 1975): 12–14.
88. Bar-Haim, 'The Drug Doctor', 114–15; Thomas Osborne, 'Mobilizing Psychoanalysis: Michael Balint and the General Practitioners', *Social Studies of Science* 23, no. 1 (1993): 175–200.

89. Michael Balint, *The Doctor, His Patient and the Illness* (New York: International Universities Press, 1957).
90. Bar-Haim, 'The Drug Doctor', 123–5.
91. Kevin Browne and Paul Freeling, *The Doctor–Patient Relationship* (Edinburgh: E. & S. Livingstone, 1967), 13–21.
92. For the development of CHCs, see Mold, *Making the Patient-Consumer*, 43–9.
93. BFI, BFI Identifier: 90393, Association of Welsh Community Health Councils. *You and Your Health*. Directed by Harley Jones. Harley Jones Films, 1979.
94. Mold, *Making the Patient-Consumer*, 53–61.
95. NA, BS 6/3540 Health Centres, Kensington, Chelsea and Westminster (South) CHC, 'The Family Doctor in Central London', October 1977, 8.
96. NA, BS 6/3540, 'Patient Attitudes to Health Centres in Northern Ireland' (1978), 3. The following statistics in this paragraph are found on 2, 24.
97. WC, Cartwright and Anderson, 'Patients and Their Doctors: Report on Some Changes in General Practice Between 1964 and 1977', 2.
98. Margot Jefferys and Hessie Sachs, *Rethinking General Practice: Dilemmas in Primary Medical Care* (London: Tavistock Publications, 1983), 158.
99. Cartwright and Anderson, 'Patients and Their Doctors', 17.
100. Quoted from Jefferys and Sachs, *Rethinking General Practice*, 164.
101. Jefferys and Sachs, *Rethinking General Practice*, 167–8.
102. Cartwright and Robert Anderson, *General Practice Revisited*, 65.
103. The comments in this paragraph on the CHGEM draw on BCA, RC/RF/14/05/B, 'Community Health and the NHS Response' and 'HELP Maternity Language Course'.
104. 'Patient Participation in Running a Primary-Care Service', *The Lancet* 306, no. 7933 (1975): 497.
105. 'Consumer Representation in Health-Centre Management', *The Lancet* 305, no.7917 (1975), 1187.
106. Ruth Cammock, *Primary Health Care Buildings: Building and Design Guide for Architects and their Clients* (London: Architectural Press, 1981).
107. Cammock, *Health Centres Handbook*, quote on 47.
108. NA, MH 160/1071, Ruth Cammock, 'Confidentiality in Health Centres and Group Practices', 1974.
109. NA, MH 160/1071, Letter to C. Alderman, 14 January 1975.

CHAPTER 4 THE ENVY OF THE WORLD

1. This paragraph draws from NYAM, Box 62, Bibliography: England: 2, Michael M. Davis, 'My Observations Last Summer of the British National Health Service', 1960.
2. Packard, *A History of Global Health*, 91–104; Anne-Emanuelle Birn, Yogan Pillay and Timothy H. Holtz, *Textbook of Global Health* (Oxford: Oxford University Press, 2017), 477–528.
3. Julie Livingston, *Debility and the Moral Imagination in Botswana: Disability, Chronic Illness and Aging* (Bloomington: Indiana University Press, 2005), 196–233; John Manton and Martin Gorsky, 'Health Planning in 1960s Africa: International Health Organisations and the Post-Colonial State', *Medical History* 62, no. 4 (2018): 425–48.
4. International Labour Organization, 'ILO Declaration of Philadelphia', 1944, http://www.ilo.org/legacy/english/inwork/cb-policy-guide/declarationofPhiladelphia1944.pdf; Martin Gorsky and Christopher Sirrs, 'The Rise and Fall of "Universal Health Coverage" as a Goal of International Health Politics, 1925–1952', *American Journal of Public Health* 108, no. 3 (2018): 334–42.

5. For the UN, human rights and the WHO, see Lynn Hunt, *Inventing Human Rights: A History* (New York: Norton, 2007), 200–8; Samuel Moyn, *The Last Utopia: Human Rights in History* (Cambridge, MA: Harvard University Press, 2010), 44–83; 'Universal Declaration of Human Rights', 1948, http://www.un.org/en/universal-declaration-human-rights/; Amy L. Sayward, *The Birth of Development: How the World Bank, Food and Agriculture Organization, and World Health Organization Changed the World* (Kent, OH: Ohio University Press, 2006); Nitsan Chorev, *The World Health Organization between North and South* (Ithaca, NY: Cornell University Press, 2012); Marcos Cueto, Theodore M. Brown and Elizabeth Fee, *The World Health Organization: A History* (Cambridge: Cambridge University Press, 2019).
6. For the NHS and decolonisation, see Bivins, *Contagious Communities*; Simpson, *Migrant Architects of the NHS.*
7. Caroline Elkins, *Britain's Gulag: The Brutal End of Empire in Kenya* (London: Pimlico, 2005); Ortolano, *Thatcher's Progress*, 184–211; Laura Quinton, 'Britain's Royal Ballet in Apartheid South Africa, 1960', *Historical Journal* 64, no. 3 (2021): 750–73.
8. Aneurin Bevan, 'Manchester, 4 July 1948' in *Aneurin Bevan on the National Health Service*, ed. Webster, 123–6, quote on 123.
9. Seaton, 'The Gospel of Wealth and the National Health'. The progressive New York health reformer Ernst P. Boas reflected this approach; see APS, Ernst P. Boas Papers, Series V, British Health System – Notes', 1950.
10. Roberta Bivins, '"A Spawning of the Nether Pit"? Welfare, Warfare, and American Visions of Britain's National Health Service, 1948–58', in Crane and Hand (eds), *Posters, Protests, and Prescriptions*, 283–322.
11. James T. Kloppenberg, *Uncertain Victory: Social Democracy and Progressivism in European and American Thought, 1870–1920* (Oxford: Oxford University Press, 1986). Daniel T. Rodgers, *Atlantic Crossings: Social Politics in a Progressive Age* (Cambridge, MA: Harvard University Press, 1998), 502–8. For challenges to a pessimistic view of postwar US liberalism, see Jonathan Bell and Timothy Stanley (eds), *Making Sense of American Liberalism* (Urbana, IL: University of Illinois Press, 2012).
12. The historiography on why the US does not possess universal health care is vast; see Monte M. Poen, *Harry S. Truman versus the Medical Lobby: The Genesis of Medicare* (Columbia, MO: University of Missouri Press, 1979); Lawrence R. Jacobs, *The Health of Nations: Public Opinion and the Making of American and British Health Policy* (Ithaca, NY: Cornell University Press, 1993); Beatrix Hoffman, *The Wages of Sickness: The Politics of Health Insurance in Progressive America* (Chapel Hill, NC: University of North Carolina Press, 2001); Colin Gordon, *Dead on Arrival: The Politics of Health Care in Twentieth-Century America* (Princeton, NJ: Princeton University Press, 2003); Jill S. Quadagno, *One Nation, Uninsured: Why the U.S. Has No National Health Insurance* (Oxford: Oxford University Press, 2005).
13. Bevan, 'Royal Medico-Psychological Association', in Webster (ed.), *Aneurin Bevan on the National Health Service*, 25–9, quote on 28.
14. Beatrix Hoffman, *Health Care for Some: Rights and Rationing in the United States Since 1930* (Chicago: University of Chicago Press, 2012), 39–40; Alan Derickson, *Health Security for All: Dreams of Universal Health Care in America* (Baltimore, MD: Johns Hopkins University Press, 2005), 97–100.
15. NYAM, Box 61, Beveridge Report 1942, Social Insurance and Allied Services, 'Luncheon in Honor of Sir William Beveridge & Lady Beveridge', June 1943.
16. NYAM, Box 95–8, Medical Society of the County of New York, Health Insurance Plan, 'Text of Mayor's Speech on Health Insurance Plan', 30 April 1944, 4.
17. The classic one-volume overview of developments in modern US medicine is Paul Starr, *The Social Transformation of American Medicine: The Rise of a Sovereign Profession*

and the Making of a Vast Industry (New York: Basic Books, 1982). For hospital care, see Charles E. Rosenberg, *The Care of Strangers: The Rise of America's Hospital System* (New York: Basic Books, 1987). For bacteriology, see Nancy Tomes, *The Gospel of Germs: Men, Women, and the Microbe in American Life* (Cambridge, MA: Harvard University Press, 1998).

18. For selected works, see Deirdre Benia Cooper Owens, *Medical Bondage: Race, Gender, and the Origins of American Gynecology* (Athens, GA: University of Georgia Press, 2017); Susan Lynn Smith, *Sick and Tired of Being Sick and Tired: Black Women's Health Activism in America, 1890–1950* (Philadelphia: University of Pennsylvania Press, 1995); Keith Wailoo, *Dying in the City of the Blues: Sickle Cell Anemia and the Politics of Race and Health* (Chapel Hill, NC: University of North Carolina Press, 2001).
19. For a biography of Davis, see Alice Taylor Davis, *Michael M. Davis: A Tribute* (Chicago: Center for Health Administration Studies, 1972); George Rosen, 'Michael M. Davis', *American Journal of Public Health* 62, no. 3 (1972): 321–3. For the settlement movement and 'slumming', see Seth Koven, *Slumming: Sexual and Social Politics in Victorian London* (Princeton, NJ: Princeton University Press, 2004).
20. Jonathan Engel, *Doctors and Reformers: Discussion and Debate over Health Policy, 1925–1950* (Columbia, SC: University of South Carolina Press, 2002), 17–19.
21. Including: Michael M. Davis, *National Health Insurance: What Is It? How Would It Work? Why Is It? Needed? Alternatives?* (New York: League for Industrial Democracy, 1956).
22. NYAM, Box 62, Pamphlets: 1, Medical Administration Service, '". . . On the Move.": A Distinguished Report on a Proposed Reorganization of Medical Practice in Great Britain', 1943.
23. NYAM, Box 53, C.N.H. – Articles and Speeches, 'Why I Believe in National Health Insurance', 26 October 1948. Davis set out his appeal to the US South in publications such as *How a National Health Program Would Serve the South* (New York: Committee on Research in Medical Economics, 1949).
24. Harry S. Truman Presidential Library, Independence, 'Special Message to the Congress Recommending a Comprehensive Health Program', 19 November 1945, https://www.trumanlibrary.gov/library/public-papers/192/special-message-congress-recommending-comprehensive-health-program.
25. This paragraph's comments on US public opinion draw from Poen, *Harry S. Truman Versus the Medical Lobby*, 66–7; Eric Schickler and Devin Caughey, 'Public Opinion, Organized Labor, and the Limits of New Deal Liberalism, 1936–1945', *Studies in American Political Development* 25, no. 2 (2011): 162–89, especially 185–6; Tomes, *Remaking the American Patient*, 139; 'Playing Politics with the Health Issue', *New Republic*, 3 May 1948, 19.
26. Carl Malmberg, *140 Million Patients* (New York: Reynal and Hitchcock, 1947), quotes in the remainder of this paragraph on 22, 29–31, 230.
27. Hoffman, *Health Care for Some*, 24–6; FDRL, Eleanor Roosevelt Papers, Box 1391, 'National Health', 'Toward Better National Health' and 'The Need for a National Health Program'.
28. Davis quotes in this paragraph are from NYAM, 'Why I Believe in National Health Insurance', 15–16.
29. If mentioned by historians, the CNH is usually depicted as ineffectual and divided; see Starr, *Social Transformation of American Medicine*, 280, 286; Derickson, *Health Security for All*, 103–10; Engel, *Doctors and Reformers*, 258.
30. This paragraph's comments on Eleanor Roosevelt draw on FDRL, Eleanor Roosevelt Papers, Box 1545, Committee for the Nation's Health, 1946–1952, 'Committee for the Nation's Health Appeal', 21 September 1946; BFI, BFI Identifier: 17739. Crown

Film Unit. *His Fighting Chance*. Directed by Geoffrey Innes. London: Central Office of Information, 1949.

31. Poen, *Harry S. Truman Versus the Medical Lobby*, 83; NYAM, Box 53, C.N.H. – Statement of Purpose; NYAM, Box 61, NPC – Counter Attack Material, 'Contributions by Large Drug Companies to the National Physicians Committee'.
32. Gordon, *Dead on Arrival*, 21; Quadagno, *One Nation, Uninsured*, 36–43; Poen, *Harry S. Truman Versus the Medical Lobby*, 45–7. For 'free enterprise', see Lawrence Glickman, *Free Enterprise: An American History* (New Haven, CT: Yale University Press, 2019).
33. NA, MH 55/967, 'Speech by Clem Whitaker to the Public Relations Society of America', 6 December 1949, 5.
34. NYAM, Michael M. Davis Papers, Box 61, NPC – Ads, Pamphlets, Mailing, 'The Rebellion of British Doctors', *Editor and Publisher*, 6 March 1948.
35. NYAM, Michael M. Davis Papers, Box 61, NPC – Ads, Pamphlets, Mailing, 'America's Vital Issue', 1949.
36. Bivins, 'A Spawning of the Nether Pit', 300–5; Michael Holm, *The Marshall Plan: A New Deal for Europe* (New York: Routledge, 2016), 87–8. For US involvement in postwar Europe, see Charles S. Maier, *In Search of Stability: Explorations in Historical Political Economy* (Cambridge: Cambridge University Press, 1987), 153–84.
37. Daniel M. Fox, 'The Administration of the Marshall Plan and British Health Policy', *Journal of Policy History* 16, no. 3 (2004): 191–211.
38. NYAM, Box 64, A.M.A. on British N.H.S., AMA, '100 Questions and Answers on the British National Health Service', 1949.
39. 'British Socialism Leveling Classes', *New York Times*, 27 November 1947, 8.
40. A. Lawrence Abel, 'Where Britain's Planners Went Wrong', *Medical Economics* 29, no. 219 (1951): 219–33.
41. NYAM, Box 64, Comments and Articles on British N.H.S. 2, 1948–1950, *American Druggist* (July 1949).
42. NYAM, Box 64, Comments and Articles on British N.H.S. 1, 1948–1950, 'C.N.H. Newsletter to "Labor Editors and Editorial Writers"', 19 November 1948.
43. NYAM, Box 62, Costs of British Plan, 'Phony A.M.A. Figures/On British Health Costs/Exposed'; NYAM, Box 62, Bibliography – England: 1, C.N.H. Document, 'The National Health Service'.
44. NYAM, Box 64, C.N.H. Releases on the British N.H.S., Channing Frothingham to Editors and Editorial Writers, 23 November 1948.
45. NYAM, Box 64, C.N.H. Releases on the British N.H.S., Frederick E. Robin to Arthur Box.
46. NYAM, Box 64, C.N.H. Releases on the British N.H.S., Michael Mark Davis to David Stark Murray, 15 October 1948. Murray also corresponded with Ernst P. Boas; see APS, Ernst. P. Boas Papers, Series I, The Physicians Forum Inc, Ernst P. Boas to David Stark Murray, 16 September 1954.
47. For wartime British propaganda in the US, see Angus Calder, *The Myth of the Blitz* (London: Jonathan Cape, 1991), 209–27.
48. See NYAM, Box 64, British Information Services 1948–1951.
49. NA, MH 55/967, 'Interviews with American Journalists'.
50. *Time*, 21 March 1949.
51. NYAM, Box 64, Comments and Articles on British N.H.S. 2, 1948–1950, *American Druggist*, (July 1949), 94.
52. Thomas-Symonds, *Nye*, 207, 213. For anti-American sentiment on the British left, see John F. Lyons, *America in the British Imagination: 1945 to the Present* (New York: Palgrave Macmillan, 2013), 41–7.
53. Aneurin Bevan, 'Speech to Institute of Hospital Administrators, 5 May, 1950', in Webster (ed.), *Aneurin Bevan on the National Health Service*, 165.

54. House of Commons, 'Mr. Aneurin Bevan (Statement)', 23 April 1951, vol. 487, 34–43.
55. This paragraph draws from LSE, TITMUSS/2/121, 'Speech to Civil Servants in the Ministry of Health', 1950.
56. Martin Francis, 'The Labour Party: Modernisation and the Politics of Restraint', in Becky Conekin, Frank Mort and Chris Waters (eds), *Moments of Modernity: Reconstructing Britain, 1945–1964* (New York: New York University Press, 1999), 152–70.
57. David Stark Murray and L.C.J. McNae, *Now for Health: The What, Why + How of the National Health Service* (London: St. Botolph Publishing, 1949), 4.
58. *Medicine Today & Tomorrow* 6, no. 6 (June 1948), 1.
59. NYAM, Box 64, C.N.H. Releases on British N.H.S., 'English Physician Praises Working of National Health Plan', 5 May 1950.
60. 'Granny Is Gone!', *Reader's Digest*, March 1950, 35–8. Harold Stassen outlined his contempt for the NHS in his platform for the presidency; see *Where I Stand* (Garden City, NY: Doubleday, 1947), 187–95.
61. Quotes by Ogilvie in this paragraph are drawn from 'The Granny Racket', *British Medical Journal*, 1, no. 4655 (1950), 683–5; 'Mr. Stassen's Granny', *The Spectator*, 17 March 1950, 9.
62. NYAM, Box 63, British Doctors' Opinions, 'CNH Newsletter – The Granny Racket'.
63. NA, MH 55/967, Claude Pepper to Aneurin Bevan, 19 January 1950.
64. The rest of this paragraph's comments on responses to the Stassen controversy draw from NA, MH 55/967, M.A. Hamilton to Stephen Heald, 16 May 1950; NA, MH 55/967, Note by Mr. Pater, April 1950; NA, MH 55/967, 'Notes on Mr. Stassen's Article on Health Service'; NA, MH 55/967, Geoffrey de Freitas to Arthur Blenkinsop, 7 June 1950; NA, MH 55/967, Gilbert McAllister to Aneurin Bevan, 27 March 1950; NA, MH 55/967, Professor Edmond Privat to Aneurin Bevan, 9 August 1950; NA, MH 55/967, A. Howard Scrase to Aneurin Bevan, 10 March 1950.
65. NA, MH 55/967, A. Howard Scrase to Aneurin Bevan, 10 March 1950.
66. Engel, *Doctors and Reformers*, 305.
67. Derickson, *Health Security for All*, 110–13.
68. Christy Ford Chapin, *Ensuring America's Health: The Public Creation of the Corporate Health Care System* (Cambridge: Cambridge University Press, 2015), 196–9.
69. Chapin, *Ensuring America's Health*, 194–232; Tomes, *Remaking the American Patient*, 256.
70. Paul F. Gemmill, *Britain's Search for Health: The First Decade of the National Health Service* (Philadelphia: University of Pennsylvania Press, 1960); Almont Lindsey, *Socialized Medicine in England and Wales: The National Health Service, 1948–1961* (Chapel Hill, NC: University of North Carolina Press, 1962).
71. Titmuss and Abel-Smith regularly appeared in the acknowledgements of US studies of the NHS; see, for instance, Eckstein, *The English Health Service*. For Davis's correspondence, see LSE, ABEL-SMITH/8/12, Michael M. Davis to Brian Abel-Smith, 3 March 1960; NYAM, Box 62, National Health Service: Popular Pamphlets, Michael M. Davis to Richard Titmuss, 3 March 1960.
72. This paragraph draws on The Beatles. *Revolver*. Capitol Records X 42576, 1966, LP; *Monty Python's Flying Circus*. 'Royal Episode 13'. Directed by Ian MacNaughton. Written by Graham Chapman, John Cleese, Michael Palin, Terry Jones, Eric Idle. BBC, 22 December 1970.
73. NYAM, Box 64, US Press on British N.H.S. Favorable, 'How the British Feel About the National Health Plan', *The Machinist*, 12 October 1961.
74. NYAM, Box 62, British Information Service, 'The British Health Service Delivers a Baby', *AFL-CIO News*, 8 February 1958.

75. W.E.B. Du Bois, 'Socialism and the American Negro', 9 April 1960, http://credo.library.umass.edu/view/full/mums312-b206-i053.
76. TL, Julius Bernstein Papers, Box 21, Folder 15, David Stark Murray to Julius Bernstein, 28 December 1962.
77. 'Can Sanders' Civil Rights Experience at U. of C. Translate on Campaign Trail?', *Chicago Tribune* (2015), https://www.chicagotribune.com/politics/ct-bernie-sanders-university-of-chicago-met-20150826-story.html.
78. 'Now British Doctors Tell You What Government Medicine Is Really Like', *Medical Economics* 38, no. 51 (1961): 51–63.
79. NYAM, Box 62, Experience with National Health Service, Horace Cotton, 'Britain's Hospitals Are Years Behind'.
80. Quotes in this paragraph are drawn from House of Commons, 'National Health Service', 30 July 1958, vol. 592, 1382–506; House of Commons, 'National Health Service', 8 May 1963, vol. 677, 439–559.
81. Lord Stephen Taylor, 'Dynamics of American Medicine', *The Lancet* 273, 7069 (1959): 405–6.
82. Quintin Hogg, 'Britain Looks Forward,' *Foreign Affairs* 43, no. 3 (1965): 409–25.
83. This paragraph draws from LSE, TITMUSS/5/650, AMA, 'A Case Against Socialized Medicine', 1962.
84. Jewkes was a prominent critic of the NHS; see John Jewkes and Sylvia Jewkes, *The Genesis of the British National Health Service* (Oxford: Blackwell, 1961). For the Mont Pelerin Society, see Mirowski and Plehwe (eds), *The Road from Mont Pèlerin.*
85. 'Cet Animal Est Méchant', *British Medical Journal* 2, no. 5147 (1959): 294.
86. R.A.B. Rorie, 'General Practice Outmoded?', *British Medical Journal* 1, no. 5345 (1963): 1612; 'Pay As You Go', *The Times,* 15 September 1958, 11. For an earlier instance, see 'All Robbers?', *New Statesman and Nation,* 22 August 1953, 202–3.
87. 'Distorted Comparisons', *The Times,* 2 July 1962, 13.
88. TL, PAM 2362, R.W. Tucker, 'The Case for Socialized Medicine', 1961, 26–7.
89. NYAM, Box 64, Dr J.R. Seale – St. Mary's Hospital London, John Seale to Michael Davis, 10 January 1959.
90. NA, MH 55/967, S.A. Heald to C. Bellairs at the Conservative Research Department, November 1953.
91. NA, MH 55/967, 'Request for Interview with Minister', 1953.
92. BFI, BFI Identifier: 10065. Frank Gardner. *Health Services in Britain.* Directed by Frank Gardner. London: The Foreign Office, 1962.
93. 'The Case for Britain's Health Service', *New York Times,* 18 November 1962, 42, 47, 49, 50.
94. BFI, BFI Identifier: 753086. London Television Service. *The British Way of Health.* Directed by Richard Marquand. London: London Television Service, 1973.
95. UCB, Helen E. Nelson Papers, BANC MSS 86/178 c, Carton 23, Folder 6, AFL-CIO, 'The Case for National Health Insurance', 1970.
96. BOD, MS. Castle. 309, Edward Kennedy to Barbara Castle, 14 May 1975.
97. Barbara Castle, *The Castle Diaries 1974–76* (London: Weidenfeld & Nicolson, 1980), 358–9.
98. WC, GC/201/A/1/30, George Godber, 'The British Health System: Can We Learn From It, Pro or Con?', 1978.
99. LSE, ABEL-SMITH/10/75, 'Secretary of State's Lecture at Harvard Medical School', 1979.
100. CCA, PJAY 5/3/3, 'Speech by Mrs Margaret Jay to the Woman's National Democratic Club', March 1978.

101. This paragraph draws from Mildred Blaxter, Sheila Murray Bethel and Elizabeth Paterson, *Mothers and Daughters: A Three-Generational Study of Health Attitudes and Behaviour* (London: Heinemann, 1982); UK Data Service, SN4943, 'Mothers and Daughters: Accounts of Health in the Grandmother Generation, 1945–1978', Interview G30, Interview GG9.

CHAPTER 5 IMMIGRATION AND EMIGRATION

1. Author's conversation with Ossie Fernando, 4 May 2022.
2. Simpson, *Migrant Architects of the NHS*; Babikian, "Partnership Not Prejudice".
3. Laurence Monnais-Rousselot and David Wright (eds), *Doctors Beyond Borders: The Transnational Migration of Physicians in the Twentieth Century* (Toronto: University of Toronto Press, 2016); David Wright, Sasha Mullally and Mary Colleen Cordukes, '"Worse than Being Married": The Exodus of British Doctors from the National Health Service to Canada, c.1955–75', *Journal of the History of Medicine and Allied Sciences* 65, no. 4 (2010): 546–75; Fallon Mody, 'Revisiting Post-War British Medical Migration: A Case Study of Bristol Medical Graduates in Australia', *Social History of Medicine* 31, no. 3 (2018): 485–509.
4. British imperial administrators laid the groundwork for these legacies by spreading medical customs and schools throughout the empire. See Margaret Anne Crowther and Marguerite Dupree, *Medical Lives in the Age of Surgical Revolution* (Cambridge: Cambridge University Press, 2007); Douglas M. Haynes, *Fit to Practice: Empire, Race, Gender, and the Making of British Medicine, 1850–1980* (Rochester, NY: University of Rochester Press, 2017).
5. See, for example, NA, MH 149/2351, 'Summary Report of the Career Experiences of Hospital Doctors in the North West & Merseyside Regions' (1981).
6. Robbie Shilliam, *Race and the Undeserving Poor: From Abolition to Brexit* (Newcastle upon Tyne: Agenda Publishing, 2018), 91–3; Grace Redhead, '"A British Problem Affecting British People": Sickle Cell Anaemia, Medical Activism and Race in the National Health Service, 1975–1993', *Twentieth Century British History* 32, no. 2 (2021): 189–211.
7. Schofield, *Enoch Powell and the Making of Postcolonial Britain*; Elizabeth Buettner, '"This Is Staffordshire Not Alabama": Racial Geographies of Commonwealth Immigration in Early 1960s Britain', *Journal of Imperial and Commonwealth History* 42, no. 4 (2014): 710–40, especially 716–17.
8. Seaton, 'Against the "Sacred Cow"'.
9. The FFM are generally ignored. Marvin Rintala, *Aneurin Bevan and the Medical Lords* (Portland, OR: Frank Cass, 2003) discusses the organisation, but dismisses them as playing 'no significant role in British politics', quote on 123.
10. Nigel Lawson, *The View from No. 11: Memoirs of a Tory Radical* (London: Bantam Press, 1992), 613.
11. David Wright, Nathan Flis and Mona Gupta, 'The 'Brain Drain' of Physicians: Historical Antecedents to an Ethical Debate, c. 1960–79', *Philosophy, Ethics, and Humanities in Medicine* 3, no. 24 (2008): 1–8.
12. Alec Cairncross, *Years of Recovery: British Economic Policy 1945–51* (London: Methuen, 1985), 385–408.
13. Babikian, '"Partnership Not Prejudice"', especially 141–2.
14. NA, FCO 50/31, Letters to Heads of Chancery, 25 August 1967.
15. The comments in this paragraph on Nola Ishmael are drawn from Ann Kramer and Abigail Bernard, *Many Rivers to Cross: The History of the Caribbean Contribution to the NHS* (London: Sugar Media Limited, 2006), 34, quotes on 48, 73.
16. This paragraph's statistics of overseas medical practitioners in the NHS draw from Stephanie J. Snow and Emma Jones, 'Immigration and the National Health Service:

Putting History to the Forefront', *History and Policy* (March 2011), http://www.historyandpolicy.org/policy-papers/papers/immigration-and-the-national-health-service-putting-history-to-the-forefront.

17. Aneez Esmail, 'Asian Doctors in the NHS: Service and Betrayal', *British Journal of General Practice* 57, no. 543 (2007): 827–34.
18. This paragraph's comments on the WHO draw from WHO, 'Health Manpower Development: Progress Report' (1975), 11, https://apps.who.int/iris/handle/10665/152510; Oscar Gish and Iain Guest, 'The Immigrant Doctor', *New Internationalist* (March 1974): 13–18.
19. 'India to "Hold" Doctors', *Sunday Times*, 28 February 1965, 2.
20. 'SOS – for Commonwealth Doctors', *Daily Mirror*, 14 October 1965, 2.
21. 'Loss of Skilled Worrying India', *New York Times*, 24 March 1974, 5.
22. NA, MH 149/1007, 'Immigration of Doctors from Overseas: Effect upon the Staffing of the NHS'.
23. This paragraph draws from NA, MH 149/352, M. Hardie to I.R. Murray, March 1965; NA, MH 149/353, 'Notes for Supplementaries'; NA, MH 149/353, Note of 16 September 1965.
24. House of Lords, 'Shortage of Doctors', 29 November 1961, vol. 235, 1131–45.
25. Roberta Bivins, 'Picturing Race in the British National Health Service, 1949–1988', *Twentieth Century British History* 28, no. 1 (2017): 83–109, especially 97–8.
26. Biographical information on Horder is drawn from Mervyn Horder, *The Little Genius: A Memoir of the First Lord Horder* (London: Duckworth, 1966); L.J. Witts, 'Horder, Thomas Jeeves, first Baron Horder (1871–1955)', *Oxford Dictionary of National Biography* 2011.
27. RCP, BOX MS.3128, FFM, *Bulletin No. 19* (December 1952), 2. For membership, see RCP, BOX MS.3128, FFM, *Bulletin No. 1* (November 1948); RCP, BOX MS.3124, 'FFM Members on Staffs of Teaching Hospitals', 1959.
28. RCP, BOX MS.3128, FFM, *Bulletin No. 67* (April 1968), 31–2.
29. Jim Tomlinson, '"Inventing 'Decline": The Falling Behind of the British Economy in the Postwar Years', *Economic History Review* 49, no. 4 (1996): 731–57; David Edgerton, *Science, Technology and British Industrial 'Decline'* (Cambridge: Cambridge University Press, 1996); Guy Ortolano, *The Two Cultures Controversy: Science, Literature and Cultural Politics in Postwar Britain* (Cambridge: Cambridge University Press, 2009), 161–93.
30. For early disputes over spending, see Klein, *New Politics of the NHS*, 24–30; Tony Cutler, 'Dangerous Yardstick? Early Cost Estimates and the Politics of Financial Management in the First Decade of the National Health Service', *Medical History* 47, no. 2 (2003): 217–38.
31. Jim Tomlinson, 'Welfare and the Economy: The Economic Impact of the Welfare State, 1945–1951', *Twentieth Century British History* 6, no. 2 (1995): 194–219, especially 203–6.
32. Ffrangcon Roberts, 'The Cost of the National Health Service', *British Medical Journal*, 1, no. 4598 (1949): 293–7, quote on 297. See also Ffrangcon Roberts, *The Cost of Health* (London: Turnstile Press, 1952).
33. Friedrich Hayek, *The Constitution of Liberty: The Definitive Edition* (Chicago: University of Chicago Press, 2011), 421–4.
34. 'King's Physician a Visitor', *New York Times*, 30 May 1949, 15.
35. Horder's remarks are drawn from NA, MH 55/967, Lord Horder, 'Freedom in Medicine' (September 1952).
36. RCP, MS-HALER/3121/6, 'Harrogate Meeting' (December 1953).
37. NVHK, 'National News'.
38. RCP, BOX MS.3128, FFM, *Bulletin No. 18* (October 1952), 21–4.

39. RCP, BOX MS.3128, FFM, *Bulletin No. 18* (October 1952), 5; RCP, BOX MS.3128, FFM, *Bulletin No. 20* (April 1953), 4; CPA, CRD 2/27/9, Health Sub-Committee Minutes, 1946–54.
40. The quotes in the rest of this paragraph draw from Roy Lewis and Angus Maude, *Professional People* (London: Phoenix House, 1952), 1–12, 186; RCP, BOX MS.3128, FFM, *Bulletin No. 28* (March 1955), 9–15.
41. This paragraph's comments on the Fellowship's views towards the Guillebaud Committee draw from RCP, BOX MS.3128, FFM, *Bulletin No. 21* (July 1953), 5; RCP, MS.3131, FFM, *Memorandum of Evidence Submitted to the Committee of Inquiry into the Costs of the National Health Service* (February 1954).
42. Richard Titmuss and Brian Abel-Smith, *The Cost of the National Health Service in England and Wales* (Cambridge: Cambridge University Press, 1956), 60–1; Rivett, *From Cradle to Grave,* 112–15. For Titmuss, see Ann Oakley, *Father and Daughter: Patriarchy, Gender, and Social Science* (Bristol: Policy Press, 2014).
43. NA, PREM 11/1492, 'Report of Committee of Enquiry into Cost of Running the National Health Service', 9.
44. House of Commons, 'National Health Service (Cost)', 7 May 1956, vol. 552, 845–960. For this paragraph's subsequent discussion of FFM reaction to the Guillebaud Report, see RCP, BOX MS.3131, FFM, *A Critical Examination of The Guillebaud Report on the Cost of the National Health Service* (London: FFM, 1957), quote on 1.
45. For GP disillusionment, see Digby, *The Evolution of British General Practice*, 336–8; R.M.C. Welldon, 'The Crisis in General Practice: A Trainee Assistant's Viewpoint', *Medical Care* 3, no. 4 (1965): 249–56; Rosemary Stevens, *Medical Practice in Modern England: The Impact of Specialization and State Medicine* (New Brunswick, NJ: Transaction, 2003), 153–68.
46. '"Lord Moran's Ladder": A Study of Motivation in the Choice of General Practice as a Career', *Journal of the College of General Practitioners* 7, no. 1 (1964): 38–65, quote on 38.
47. Audra J. Wolfe, *Freedom's Laboratory: The Cold War Struggle for the Soul of Science* (Baltimore, MD: Johns Hopkins University Press, 2018).
48. RCP, FFM, *Bulletin No. 1*, 5.
49. Donald McIntosh Johnson, *A Doctor Regrets . . . Being the First Part of 'A Publisher Presents Himself'* (London: Christopher Johnson, 1949); Donald McIntosh Johnson, *A Doctor Returns. Being the Third Part of 'A Publisher Presents Himself'* (London: Christopher Johnson, 1956), quotes in this paragraph drawn from 235, 239, 242, 83.
50. Donald McIntosh Johnson, *The British National Health Service: Friend or Frankenstein?* (London: Christopher Johnson, 1962), quotes in this paragraph drawn from 9, 103, 113.
51. LSE, JOHNSON/3/3, Donald McIntosh Johnson to Miss. Georgina B. Eteson, 2 August 1963.
52. Eli Rubin, *Nationalisation* (London: De Vero Books, 1961); LSE, JOHNSON/3/3, Letter from Eli Rubin, 16 July 1962.
53. 'The Birmingham Action Group', *British Medical Journal* 1, no. 5433 (1965): 518.
54. Samuel Mencher, *Private Practice in Britain: The Relationship of Private Medical Care to the National Health Service* (London: G. Bell & Sons, 1967), 82–6.
55. RCP, BOX MS.3128, FFM, *Bulletin No. 62* (November 1965), 2–5.
56. RCP, FFM, *Bulletin No. 62*, 4.
57. Exact figures are impossible to reach, but for an overview, see Wright, Flis and Gupta, 'The 'Brain Drain' of Physicians'.

58. This paragraph draws on 'Doctors Emigrating at Rate of 700 a Year', *The Times,* 16 March 1962, 6; 'The Disappearing Doctor', *Punch*, 22 August 1962, 262; *Daily Express,* 23 August 1966, 6.
59. Nevil Shute, *The Far Country* (London: Heinemann, 1952).
60. Shute, *The Far Country,* 314. For a typical depiction of 'abuse' of NHS services, see 'Genuine Demand for Spectacles', *The Times*, 29 October 1949, 2.
61. J.R. Seale, 'Supply of Doctors', *British Medical Journal* 2, no. 5266 (1961): 1554–5.
62. J.R. Seale, 'A General Theory of National Expenditure on Medical Care', *The Lancet* 274, no. 7102 (1959): 555–9.
63. HMSO, *Report of the Committee to Consider the Future Numbers of Medical Practitioners and the Appropriate Intake of Medical Students* (HMSO: London, 1957).
64. RCP, FFM, *Bulletin No. 50*, 7.
65. This paragraph's comments draw from BL, FFM, *The Supply of Doctors and the Future of the British Medical Profession* (London: FFM, 1962), quote on 4.
66. 'Emigration of Doctors', *The Times,* 9 April 1962, 11.
67. LSE, JOHNSON/3/3, Letter from Associated Re-Diffusion Ltd., 5 March 1962.
68. BFI, BFI Identifier: 751031. Bernard Braden. 'Richard Rossdale'. *Then and Now.* Directed by Bernard Braden. London: Adanac Productions, 1967.
69. The comments by Enoch Powell and Kenneth Robinson on the emigration debate in this paragraph are drawn from 'Mr. Powell's Denial of Mass Emigration of Doctors', *The Times,* 7 June 1962, 8; 'Medical Emigration from Great Britain and Ireland', *British Medical Journal,* 1, no. 5391 (1964): 1173–8; 'B.M.A. Birmingham Meeting', *British Medical Journal,* 2, no. 5516 (1966): 715–16; House of Commons, 'National Health Service (Nursing, Medical and Other Professional Staffs)', 27 March 1962, vol. 656, 1081–320, especially 1082–3.
70. John Enoch Powell, *A New Look at Medicine and Politics* (London: Pitman Medical, 1966), 36.
71. Brian Abel-Smith and Kathleen Gales, *British Doctors at Home and Abroad* (London: Codicote Press, 1964), quotes in this paragraph are from 43, 49, 57–8.
72. Abel-Smith and Gales, *British Doctors*, 13.
73. 'Address at a New York Rally in Support of the President's Program of Medical Care for the Aged', 20 May 1962. The American Presidency Project, https://www.presidency.ucsb.edu/documents/address-new-york-rally-support-the-presidents-program-medical-care-for-the-aged.
74. BL, FFM, *The Supply of Doctors and the Future of the British Medical Profession* (London: FFM, 1962), 7.
75. FFM, *Supply of Doctors*, 8.
76. 'Letter from H. Chatterjee', *British Medical Journal*, 2, no. 5402 (1964): 186.
77. NA, MH 149/2351, 'Summary Report of the Career Experiences of Hospital Doctors in the North West & Merseyside Regions', 7.
78. RCP, FFM, *Bulletin No. 51*, 6.
79. This paragraph draws from NA, MH 149/1007, H. Vincent Corbett to John Biggs Davidson, 27 August 1970; NA, MH 149/1007, Note to Mr S.I. Smith, 21 September 1970.
80. NA, MH 149/2351, 'Summary Report of the Career Experiences of Hospital Doctors in the North West & Merseyside Regions', 19.
81. WC, Ruskin College Agewell Group, *From Cradle to Grave: 50 Years of the NHS. Memories of Before and After 1948* (1998), 22–3.
82. Quotes from this speech are drawn from John Enoch Powell, *Freedom and Reality* (London: Batsford, 1969), 213–19.
83. Wetherell, *Foundations*, 98–106.

84. Reynolds, *When I Came to England*, 89–93, quote on 90.
85. Schofield, *Enoch Powell*, 237–61; Whipple, 'Revisiting the "Rivers of Blood" Controversy'.
86. CCA, POLL 3/2/1/15, S.J. Turner to Enoch Powell, 12 November 1973.
87. For Irish workers, see Wills, *Lovers and Strangers*, 87–106.
88. Details of this exchange draw from CCA, POLL 3/2/1/15, D. Pardoe to Enoch Powell, 3 February 1972; CCA, POLL 3/2/1/15, Enoch Powell to D. Pardoe, 1 February 1972.
89. This paragraph draws from CCA, POLL 3/2/1/15, G.D. Shepherd to Enoch Powell, 24 March 1972; CCA, POLL 3/2/1/15, James Johnson to Enoch Powell, 18 March 1972.
90. Longpré, '"An Issue That Could Tear Us Apart"'.
91. This paragraph draws from CCA, POLL 3/2/1/15, Baine Milnes to Enoch Powell, 7 June 1973; CCA, POLL 3/2/1/15, Mrs. Robinson to Enoch Powell, 11 December 1972.
92. This paragraph draws from Simpson, *Migrant Architects*, 80–2, and Christopher Kyriakides and Satnam Virdee, 'Migrant Labour, Racism and the British National Health Service', *Ethnicity & Health* 8, no. 4 (2003): 283–305, especially 288–93.
93. NA, BS 6/7, A.F.A. Sayeed to Harold Wilson, 17 October 1975.
94. Perry, *London Is the Place for Me*, 48–88.

CHAPTER 6 THE LIMITS OF FREE-MARKET MEDICINE

1. Details of this meeting and the Charing Cross dispute are drawn from Castle, *The Castle Diaries 1974–76*, 130–8; 'Give In. . . Or We Will Starve Patients Out', *Daily Mail*, 12 July 1974, 2. For Castle, see Anthony Howard, 'Castle, Barbara Anne, Baroness Castle of Blackburn (1910–2002)', Oxford Dictionary of National Biography, 2006.
2. Historians rarely now see the postwar period as a time of 'consensus'; see Harriet Jones and Michael Kandiah (eds), *The Myth of Consensus: New Views on British History, 1945–64* (Basingstoke: Macmillan, 1996).
3. LSE, TITMUSS/2/121, 'Joint Meeting on the Cost of the Health Service', 1954.
4. Tony Butcher and Ed Randall, 'The Politics of Pay-beds: Labour Policy and Legislation', *Policy and Politics* 9, no. 3 (1981): 273–93; Williamson, 'The Quiet Time?'.
5. For Britain in the 1970s, see Lawrence Black and Hugh Pemberton, 'Introduction: The Benighted Decade? Reassessing the 1970s', in Lawrence Black, Hugh Pemberton and Pat Thane (eds), *Reassessing 1970s Britain* (Manchester: Manchester University Press, 2013), 1–24, especially 14–15; John Shepherd, *Crisis? What Crisis?: The Callaghan Government and the British 'Winter of Discontent'* (Manchester: Manchester University Press, 2013).
6. Robert Saunders, 'Crisis? What Crisis? Thatcherism and the Seventies', in Jackson and Saunders (eds), *Making Thatcher's Britain* (Cambridge: Cambridge University Press, 2012), 25–42.
7. Castle, *The Castle Diaries, 1974–76*, 309.
8. Stuart Hall, among many others, depicted Thatcher's politics as motivated by a desire to roll back the state; see 'Thatcherism – Rolling Back the Welfare State', *Thesis Eleven* 7, no. 1 (1983): 6–19. For a contrasting view, see Slobodian, *Globalists*.
9. See, for instance, Rudolf Klein, 'Why Britain's Conservatives Support a Socialist Health Care System', *Health Affairs* 4, no. 1 (1985): 41–58. An exception – notably also published in the 1980s – is Ben Griffith, Steve Iliffe and Geof Rayner, *Banking on Sickness: Commercial Medicine in Britain and the USA* (London: Lawrence and Wishart, 1987).

10. WC, PP/AWD/H.11/5/2, P.G. Gray and Ann Cartwright, 'General Practice Under the National Health Service', 1952.
11. 'The Beveridge Plan', *British Medical Journal*, 2, no. 4275 (1942): 700.
12. Arthur Bryant, *BUPA, 1947–1968: A History of the British United Provident Association* (London: BUPA, 1968); Douglas Robb, *BUPA 1968–1983: A Continuing History* (London: BUPA, 1984).
13. Industry statistics in this paragraph draw from Bryant, *BUPA, 1947–1968*, 40; NA, MH170/343, Lee Donaldson Associates, 'Provident Scheme Statistics', 1979.
14. LSE, TITMUSS 2/197, BUPA, 'Private Treatment in Illness', 1962.
15. Information on companies and group schemes in this paragraph draws on Ralph Harris and Michael Solly, *A Survey of Large Companies* (London: IEA, 1959), 22; WC, EPH428 Medical Insurance Ephemera: Box 1, BUPA, 'Why Private Treatment?', 1971; WC, SA/DAT/D/43, Private Patients Plan, 'Private Medical Insurance: Facts and Figures', 1984.
16. For an exploration of waiting times and elective procedures, see Luigi Siciliani and Jeremy Hurst, 'Tackling Excessive Waiting Times for Elective Surgery: A Comparative Analysis of Policies in 12 OECD Countries', *Health Policy* 72, no. 2 (2005): 201–15.
17. Julie Anderson, Francis Neary, John. V. Pickstone and John Raftery, *Surgeons, Manufacturers and Patients: A Transatlantic History of Total Hip Replacement* (Basingstoke: Macmillan, 2007), 108.
18. Mencher, *Private Practice in Britain*, 29.
19. NUAA, SL279 Sun Life, Branch Manager Conference Notes, 'Marketing Permanent Health Insurance', 1972.
20. Quotes from BUPA and PPP in this paragraph draw on WC, EPH428, BUPA, 'Why Private Treatment?'; LSE, TITMUSS 2/197 BUPA and Sickness Insurance Schemes, PPP, 'The Hospital Service Plan', 1962, 1.
21. Horace Cotton, 'Why Do Britons Buy Health Insurance?,' *Medical Economics*, 1960s, found in NYAM, Box 62, Experience with National Health Service.
22. The individual comments about privacy at the end of this paragraph are drawn from NA, BS6/23, Letter from Ann R. Fowler; CCA, POLL 3/2/1/15, Angela Waddington to Enoch Powell, 3 March 1972.
23. Economists such as Kenneth Arrow laid the intellectual groundwork for medical economics in the early 1960s. See his influential article, 'Uncertainty and the Welfare Economics of Medical Care', *American Economic Review* 53, no. 5 (1963): 941–73. For its historical background, see Eleanor MacKillop, Sally Sheard and Michael Lambert (eds), *The Development of Health Economics and the Role of the University of York* (Liverpool: Department of Public Health and Policy, University of Liverpool, 2018), 6–8.
24. Office of Health Economics, *Health Services in Western Europe* (London: Office of Health Economics, 1963); Brian Abel-Smith, *An International Study of Health Expenditure and Its Relevance for Health Planning* (Geneva: WHO, 1967).
25. For the IEA, see Richard Cockett, *Thinking the Unthinkable: Think-Tanks and the Economic Counter-Revolution, 1931–1983* (London: HarperCollins, 1995); Ben Jackson, 'The Think-Tank Archipelago: Thatcherism and Neo-liberalism', in Jackson and Saunders (eds), *Making Thatcher's Britain*, 43–61.
26. IEA, *Monopoly or Choice in Health Services?: A Symposium of Contrasting Approaches* (London: IEA, 1964).
27. D.S. Lees, *Health through Choice: An Economic Study of the British National Health Service* (London: IEA, 1961), quotes in this paragraph from 7, 20, 61–2.
28. For Buchanan, see Nancy MacLean, *Democracy in Chains: The Deep History of the Radical Right's Stealth Plan for America* (New York: Viking, 2017).

29. Arthur Seldon, *After the N.H.S.* (London: IEA, 1968).
30. IEA, *Choice in Welfare* (London: IEA, 1963); IEA, *Choice in Welfare* (London: IEA, 1965), quote in this paragraph from 21, survey percentages from 36–7.
31. Melinda Cooper, *Family Values: Between Neoliberalism and the New Social Conservatism* (New York: Zone Books, 2017), 67–117; Ben Jackson, 'Free Markets and Feminism: The Neo-Liberal Defence of the Male Breadwinner Model in Britain, c. 1980–1997', *Women's History Review* 28, no. 2 (2019): 297–316.
32. This paragraph's comments on affluence draw from John Kenneth Galbraith, *The Affluent Society* (Boston, MA: Houghton Mifflin, 1958); Ian Gazeley, 'Manual Work and Pay, 1900–70', in Nicholas Crafts, Ian Gazeley and Andrew Newell (eds), *Work and Pay in Twentieth-Century Britain* (Oxford: Oxford University Press, 2007), 55–79. For the limits to affluence, see Brian Abel-Smith and Peter Townsend, *The Poor and the Poorest* (London: G. Bell & Sons, 1965).
33. Ian Gazeley, 'Income and Living Standards, 1970–2010', in Roderick Floud, Jane Humphries and Paul Johnson (eds), *The Cambridge Economic History of Modern Britain: Volume II. 1870 to the Present* (Cambridge: Cambridge University Press, 2014), 155–6.
34. Daniel T. Rodgers, *Age of Fracture* (Cambridge, MA: Belknap Press, 2011), 64–6.
35. Rodney Lowe, 'Modernizing Britain's Welfare State: The Influence of Affluence, 1957–1964', in Lawrence Black and Hugh Pemberton (eds), *An Affluent Society? Britain's Postwar 'Golden Age' Revisited* (Aldershot: Ashgate, 2004), 35–52. For this paragraph's discussion of Wyndham Davies and Paul Dean, see Wyndham Davies, *Health or Health Service?: Reform of the British National Health Service* (London: Charles Knight & Co. Ltd, 1972), quote on 107; BFI, 'Paul Dean' (1968), https://player.bfi.org.uk/free/film/watch-paul-dean-1968-online.
36. BMA, *Health Services Financing* (London: BMA, 1970), 149–51.
37. This paragraph's comments on the meetings of the Conservative Party Research Department draw from BOD, CPA, CRD 4/7/15 'British United Provident Association', 26 January 1966; BOD, CPA, CRD 4/7/16, Note of 13 March 1968; BOD, CPA, CRD 4/7/16, 'Private Provision', 1968.
38. Conservative Central Office, *A Better Tomorrow: The Conservative Programme for the Next Five Years* (London: Conservative Party, 1970).
39. John Appleby, '70 Years of NHS Spending', 2018, https://www.nuffieldtrust.org.uk/news- item/70-years-of-nhs-spending#then-and-now.
40. Lawrence Black and Hugh Pemberton, 'Introduction: The Benighted Decade? Reassessing the 1970s', in Black, Pemberton and Thane (eds), *Reassessing 1970s Britain*, 14–15.
41. Griffith, Iliffe and Rayner, *Banking on Sickness*, 78–103.
42. Saunders, 'Emotions, Social Practices', 216–21.
43. Cal Flyn, 'NHS Strikes and the Decade of Discontent', 2018, https://wellcomecollection.org/articles/WyjRuCcAACvGno__.
44. 'The Year the Health Service Caught the Militancy Bug', *Financial Times*, 1 August 1974, 16.
45. MRC, MSS.292B/847.3/1, J. Ripley to TUC General Secretary, 5 May 1961.
46. The Labour Party, *Let Us Work Together: Labour's Way Out of the Crisis* (London: The Labour Party, 1974); The Labour Party, *Britain Will Win with Labour* (London: The Labour Party, 1974).
47. Duncan Gallie, 'The Labour Force', in Halsey and Webb (eds), *Twentieth-Century British Social Trends*, 282–323, statistic on 309.
48. Joan Higgins, *The Business of Medicine: Private Health Care in Britain* (Basingstoke: Macmillan, 1988), 125–30.

49. MRC, MSS.292B/847.3/4, 'National Health Service: Private Patients' Facilities' (1973).
50. Philip Begley and Sally Sheard, 'McKinsey and the "Tripartite Monster": The Role of Management Consultants in the 1974 NHS Reorganisation', *Medical History* 63, no. 4 (2019): 390–410.
51. The remainder of this paragraph draws from MRC, MSS.292D/847.306/1, '1973 Congress Resolution: NHS Hospital Services and Pay Beds', 1973; MRC, MSS.292D/847.306/1, E.C. Moore to General Secretary of TUC, 6 February 1973.
52. This paragraph draws from Gloria Levin, 'Arthur Levin', *British Medical Journal,* 318, no. 7199 (1999): 318; BUA, DM977, Box 2, *Labour Research* (June 1978).
53. 'Dr. Arthur Levin's Hospital Offers Sick Arabs T.I.E.C. – Tender, Loving, and Expensive', *People*, 16 January 1978.
54. Private hospitals outside of London had fewer overseas patients. See BUA, DM977, Box 2, 'Note on Visits to Three Private Hospitals', February 1978.
55. BUA, DM977, Box 2, 'Transcript of *Tonight* interview', 18 April 1978.
56. 'The Mecca of the West', *Guardian*, 27 September 1976.
57. BOD, MS. Castle 311, 'Private Practice in NHS Hospitals and Other Matters', 26 July 1974.
58. Lindsay Anderson, *Britannia Hospital,* directed by Lindsay Anderson, London: Film & General Productions Ltd, 1982.
59. BOD, MS. Castle 311, 'Private Practice in the National Health Service', 13 August 1974.
60. ULA, D709 2/6/1/10, David Owen, 'Private Practice and Private Hospitals', 1974.
61. ULA, D709 2/6/1/11, David Owen to Barbara Castle, 24 October 1975.
62. This paragraph's discussion of Richard Titmuss and Julian Tudor Hart draws from Titmuss, *Commitment to Welfare*, 188–99, quote on 196; Julian Tudor Hart, 'The Inverse Care Law', *The Lancet* 297, no. 7696 (1971): 405–12.
63. For RAWP, see Martin Gorsky and Virginia Preston (eds), *The Resource Allocation Working Party: Origins, Implementation and Development, 1974–1990* (London: Institute of Contemporary British History and London School of Hygiene and Tropical Medicine, 2014).
64. BOD, MS. Castle 320, Independence in Medicine, 'The Case for Independence in Medicine', 1976.
65. Robb, *BUPA 1968–1983*, 26.
66. The remainder of this paragraph's comments on the 'Independence in Medicine' campaign draws from BOD, MS. Castle 315, 'A Memorandum by Organisations Representing the Medical and Dental Professions and by the Independent Hospital Group', September 1975, 5; 'The Week', *British Medical Journal* 1, no. 6011 (1976): 722; BOD, MS. Castle 320, BMA, 'A Message From the General Medical Services Committee', 18 March 1976.
67. George H. Gallup, *The Gallup International Public Opinion Polls, Great Britain 1965–1975, Volume Two* (New York: Random House, 1976), 1376; BOD, MS. Castle 320, 'The Case for Independence in Medicine', 5.
68. Cited in Klein, *New Politics of the NHS*, 89.
69. For 'Thatcherism', see Jackson and Saunders (eds), *Making Thatcher's Britain*; Vinen, *Thatcher's Britain.*
70. Sutcliffe-Braithwaite, 'Neo-Liberalism and Morality in the Making of Thatcherite Social Policy'.
71. Pierson, *Dismantling the Welfare State?*; Sutcliffe-Braithwaite, *Class, Politics, and the Decline of Deference*, 163–7.

72. Ben Jackson, 'Richard Titmuss versus the IEA: The Transition from Idealism to Neo-Liberalism in British Social Policy', in Lawrence Goldman (ed.), *Welfare and Social Policy in Britain Since 1870: Essays in Honour of Jose Harris* (Oxford: Oxford University Press, 2019) 147–61, especially, 150–4.
73. Boughton, *Municipal Dreams*, 169–95; Bernhard Rieger, 'Making Britain Work Again: Unemployment and the Remaking of British Social Policy in the Eighties', *English Historical Review* 133, no. 562 (2018): 634–66.
74. NA, MH 170/346, Conservative Health Study Group, 'Final Report Draft Document on Health Care', January 1979, 2.
75. Conservative Central Office, *Conservative Manifesto 1979* (London: The Conservative Party, 1979).
76. This paragraph's comments on Thatcher's views on the NHS draw from House of Commons, 'Debate on the Address', 15 May 1979, vol. 967, 52–198; Ken Clarke, *Kind of Blue: A Political Memoir* (London: Macmillan, 2016), 192; 'Politician Patients', People's History of the NHS, https://peopleshistorynhs.org/encyclopaedia/politician-patients/; Margaret Thatcher, *The Downing Street Years* (New York: HarperCollins, 1993), 607.
77. Appleby, '70 Years of NHS Spending'.
78. This paragraph's statistics on insurance subscribers and private hospitals draws from Michael Calnan, Sarah Cant and Jonathan Gabe, *Going Private: Why People Pay for Their Health Care* (Buckingham: Open University Press, 1993), 2; Higgins, *The Business of Medicine*, 1.
79. The rest of this paragraph's comments on US medical insurance companies draw from Higgins, *The Business of Medicine*, 124; 'Provident Associations Put Up Capital', *Financial Times,* 7 January 1981, 15; NA, MH 170/348, 'Note of a Meeting with the British Insurance Association', 21 May 1981.
80. Slobodian, *Globalists*. The remainder of this paragraph draws from John Mohan, *A National Health Service? The Restructuring of Health Care in Britain since 1979* (Basingstoke: Macmillan, 1995), 155–8.
81. NA, MH 170/350, 'Progress Report', 22 October 1981.
82. NA, MH 170/351, 'Alternative Finance for Health Care: Report of the Working Party', 1982.
83. 'Tories to Unveil New Health Care', *Daily Mail,* 2 December 1981, 9; 'Thatcher Backs Shake-up for NHS Finance', *The Times*, 12 December 1981, 26.
84. Clarke, *Kind of Blue*, 192.
85. The remainder of this paragraph draws on NA, MH 170/349, G.G. Hulme to Sir Kenneth Stowe, 31 July 1981; NA, MH170/349, Charles Hall, 'The US Health Care System – A Briefing Note', 1981; NA, MH170/346, 'Social Security in France', 23 July 1979; NA, MH170/347, Gerald Vaughan Speech to Conservative Medical Society Symposium, 21 November 1980.
86. LSE, CPS/12/2, Health Study Group Meeting Minutes, 5 November 1979.
87. NA, MH 170/344, Lee Donaldson Associates, 'The Private Sector of Health Care', 1981.
88. NA, T 639/130, 'Public Expenditure in the Longer Term', 1982; 'Thatcher's Think-Tank Takes Aim at the Welfare State', *The Economist*, 18 September 1982, 25–6.
89. 'Storm Over Secret Think Tank Report', *The Observer*, 19 September 1982, 2.
90. Thatcher, *Downing Street Years*, 276–7.
91. Margaret Thatcher, 'Speech to Conservative Party Conference', October 1982.
92. LSE, CPS/12/5, Minutes of a Meeting of the Health Group, 21 October 1982.
93. Conservative Central Office, *The Conservative Manifesto, 1983* (London: The Conservative Party, 1983).

94. LSE, CPS/12/5, Minutes of a Meeting of the Health Group, 21 October 1982.
95. NA, MH 170/343, 'Research into Unit Costs in Health Care', 1980.
96. For path dependence, see Pierson, *Dismantling the Welfare State?*, 47–50.
97. This paragraph draws on Peder Clark, '"Problems of Today and Tomorrow": Prevention and the National Health Service in the 1970s', *Social History of Medicine* 33, no. 3 (2020): 981–1000; Alex Mold, Peder Clark, Gareth Millward and Daisy Payling, *Placing the Public in Public Health in Post-War Britain, 1948–2012* (Cham, Switzerland: Palgrave Macmillan, 2019), 100–6.
98. WC, SA/HEC/B/4/20, Health Education Authority, 'Look After Your Heart Publicity Campaign', 1989.
99. The financial information on the private health insurance market in this paragraph draws on 'Why the Insurers Were the First to Put the Brakes on Costs', *The Times*, 14 June 1984, 17; 'Spectre of Overbedding' *Financial Times*, 13 February 1985, 18; 'Companies' Health Benefit Costs Spiral', *Financial Times*, 8 June 1982, 10; Calnan, Cant and Gabe, *Going Private*, 12–13.
100. Amy Edwards, '"Financial Consumerism": Citizenship, Consumerism and Capital Ownership in the 1980s', *Contemporary British History* 31, no. 2 (2017): 210–29.
101. NA, MH 170/346, Conservative Health Study Group, 'Final Report Draft Document on Health Care', 1979, 3.
102. This paragraph draws on LSE, CPS/12/2, Minutes of a Meeting of the Health Group, 17 October 1979; LSE, CPS/12/2, Minutes of a Meeting of the Health Group, 12 September 1979; LSE, CPS/12/6, Minutes of a Meeting of the Health Group, 12 November 1981.
103. Calnan, Cant and Gabe, *Going Private*, 42.
104. For an overview of these changes, see David Coleman, 'Population and Family', in Halsey and Webb (eds), *Twentieth-Century British Social Trends*, 27–93.
105. This paragraph's comments on private insurance advertisements draw on WC, EPH430 Medical Insurance Ephemera: Box 3, BUPA, 'When you're building a career the last thing you want to go wrong . . . is you', 1991; WC, EPH429 Medical Insurance Ephemera: Box 2, BUPA, 'I'm Fit, I'm Healthy. What Do I Need Private Health Care For?', 1980s.
106. Calnan, Cant and Gabe, *Going Private*, 28.
107. For the relationship between television and the NHS in this period, see Patricia Holland, Hugh Chignell and Sherryl Wilson, *Broadcasting and the NHS in the Thatcherite 1980s: The Challenge to Public Service* (London: Palgrave Macmillan, 2013).
108. This paragraph's comments on the documentary draw on Paul Hamann. *I Call It Murder*. London: BBC, 27 November 1979 (This programme was broadcast again on 8 May 1982); Author's conversation with Jack Pizzey, 20 November 2017; Hoffman, *Health Care for Some*, 169–87.
109. The rest of this paragraph draws from Kennetta Hammond Perry, '"U.S. Negroes, Your Fight is Our Fight": Black Britons and the 1963 March on Washington', in Robin D.G. Kelley and Stephen Tuck (eds), *The Other Special Relationship: Race, Rights and Riots in Britain and the United States* (London: Palgrave, 2015), 7–24; Lyons, *America in the British Imagination*, 114–17; Kieran Connell, *Black Handsworth: Race in 1980s Britain* (Berkeley: University of California Press, 2019).
110. NA, MH 170/343, 'Discussion of "I Call It Murder" on "Man Alive"'.
111. BFI, BFI Identifier: 645336. Duncan Dallas. *Sick in Sheffield, Broke in Beverly Hills*. Directed by John Willis. Leeds: Yorkshire Television, 2 August 1982.
112. BFI, BFI Identifier: 344106. Thames Television. 'Right Wing Medicine'. *The Week*. London: Thames Television, 28 January 1988.

113. BFI, BFI Identifier: 340332. Yvette Vanson and Tom Hayes. *Kentucky Fried Medicine*. Directed by Yvette Vanson. London: Vanson Wardle Productions, 23 May 1988.
114. Calnan, Cant and Gabe, *Going Private*, quotes in this paragraph from 55, 52.
115. 'Unhealthy System of Caring', *Liverpool Echo*, 5 April 1990, 8.
116. 'Health Care International', *The Economist*, 28 April 1984, 25.
117. Social and Community Planning Research, *British Social Attitudes Cumulative Sourcebook: The First Six Surveys* (Brookfield, VT: Gower, 1992), A–10.
118. Social and Community Planning Research, *British Social Attitudes*, F–11.
119. 'BUPA: Sir Bryan Nicholson and Peter Jacobs, Prescribing a Run of Healthy Profits', *The Times*, 2 April 1994, 23.
120. Ray Whitney, *National Health Crisis: A Modern Solution* (London: Shepheard-Walwyn, 1988), 8, 109.
121. Lawson, *The View from No. 11*, 613.
122. Martin Gorsky, "Searching for the People in Charge': Appraising the 1983 Griffiths NHS Management Inquiry', *Medical History* 57, no. 1 (2013): 87–107.
123. HMSO, *The National Health Service and Community Care Act* (London: HMSO, 1990); Eleanor MacKillop, Sally Sheard, Philip Begley and Michael Lambert (eds), *The NHS Internal Market* (Liverpool: Department of Public Health and Policy, University of Liverpool, 2018).
124. IEA, *The NHS Reforms: Whatever Happened to Consumer Choice?* (London: IEA, 1990).

CHAPTER 7 PUBLIC SERVICE, PRIVATE CONTRACTS

1. 'Hospital Cleaners Settle in for a Lengthy Strike', *Guardian*, 18 June 1984, 2; Kate Ascher, *The Politics of Privatisation: Contracting Out Public Services* (Basingstoke: Macmillan, 1987), 192–7.
2. Charles Webster describes this period as one of 'continuous revolution', in *The National Health Service: A Political History*, 140–8.
3. Anne-Emanuelle Birn, Laura Nervi and Eduardo Siqueira, 'Neoliberalism Redux: The Global Health Policy Agenda and the Politics of Cooptation in Latin America and Beyond', *Development and Change* 47, no. 4 (2016): 734–59; John Lister (ed.), *Europe's Health for Sale: The Heavy Cost of Privatisation* (Faringdon: Libri Publishing, 2011).
4. Our World in Data, 'Healthcare Spending'.
5. Ascher, *Politics of Privatisation*, 46–7.
6. For the 'franchise state', see Andrew Bowman et al, *What a Waste: Outsourcing and How It Goes Wrong* (Manchester: Manchester University Press, 2015), particularly 1–20. Other scholars have identified a similar cluster of interests by a different name. For the 'shadow state', see Alan White, *Who Really Runs Britain?: The Private Companies Taking Control of Benefits, Prisons, Asylum, Deportation, Security, Social Care and the NHS*, updated edn (London: Oneworld, 2017).
7. This is a point also made by Jack Saunders; see 'The Making of "NHS staff" as a Worker Identity, 1948–85', in Crane and Hand (eds), *Posters, Protests, and Prescriptions*, 25–53, especially 42–7.
8. Lister (ed.), *Cutting the Lifeline*; Pollock, *NHS PLC*.
9. Jane Gingrich, 'Marketization', in Mark Bevir (ed.), *Encyclopedia of Governance II* (Thousand Oaks, CA: SAGE, 2007), 547–8; Jane Gingrich, *Making Markets in the Welfare State: The Politics of Varying Market Reforms* (Cambridge: Cambridge University Press, 2011), 1–23.
10. Michael B. Forsyth, *Reservicing Health* (London: Adam Smith Institute, 1982).
11. Office of Health Economics, *OHE Guide to UK Health and Health Care Statistics*, 81.

12. Office of Health Economics, *Hospital Costs in Perspective* (London: OHE, 1963), 15; Department of Health and Social Security, *Health Care and Its Costs* (London: HMSO, 1983), 5.
13. Ascher, *Politics of Privatisation*, 54–96.
14. This paragraph's comments on deindustrialisation draw on Jim Tomlinson, 'De-industrialization: Strengths and Weaknesses as a Key Concept for Understanding Post-war British History', *Urban History* 47, no. 2 (2020): 199–219, statistics on 203.
15. See James Vernon, 'Heathrow and the Making of Neoliberal Britain', *Past & Present* 252, no. 1 (2021): 213–47.
16. Ascher, *Politics of Privatisation*, 74; House of Commons, *Register of Members' Interests* (London: House of Commons, 1986).
17. MRC, 864/135, Photo of Margaret Thatcher at the 1983 Conservative Conference.
18. Mark Hollingsworth, *MPs for Hire: The Secret World of Political Lobbying* (London: Bloomsbury, 1991), 70–6.
19. DHSS, 'Circular HC (83) 18, Competitive Tendering in the Provision of Domestic, Catering and Laundry Services', September 1983.
20. Angela Coyle, 'Going Private: The Implications of Privatization for Women's Work', *Feminist Review* 21 (1985): 5–23.
21. Cited in Margaret Halsey, *Invisible Hands – Contract Cleaning: A Theological Reflection* (Manchester: The William Temple Foundation, 1996), 12.
22. Office of Health Economics, *OHE Guide to UK Health and Health Care Statistics*, 81.
23. MRC, MSS.229/CO/P/2/11, Joint NHS Privatisation Research Unit, *The NHS Privatisation Experience: Competitive Tendering for NHS Services* (1990), 14.
24. For the impact of outsourcing on women, see Coyle, 'Going Private'; Halsey, *Invisible Hands*.
25. Equal Opportunities Commission for Northern Ireland, *Report on Formal Investigation into Competitive Tendering in Health and Education Services in Northern Ireland* (Belfast: Equal Opportunities Commission for Northern Ireland, 1996), 2–3.
26. Angela Coyle, *Dirty Business: Women's Work and Trade Union Organisation in Contract Cleaning* (Birmingham: West Midlands Low Pay Unit, 1986), 10.
27. Sarah Fielder, Gareth Rees and Teresa Rees, *The New Services: Contract Cleaning and Catering* (Cardiff: University of Wales Social Research Unit, 1991), 17.
28. Gabriel Winant, *The Next Shift: The Fall of Industry and the Rise of Health Care in Rust Belt America* (Cambridge, MA: Harvard University Press, 2021), especially 218–58.
29. BFI, BFI Identifier: 188175. Judith Weymont. *Halifax Laundry Blues*. Directed by Marilyn Gaunt. Leeds: Yorkshire Television, 1985.
30. For the health unions' recruitment of women workers, see Saunders, 'Emotions, Social Practices'.
31. MRC, MSS.292D/847/5, TUC Health Services Committee, 'Privatisation of NHS Services', 26 May 1983.
32. Information-collecting played an increasingly important role in pro-NHS campaigns after the 1980s; see Crane, 'Save Our NHS', 63–5.
33. For the alleged failures of contractors, see MRC, MSS.229/CO/P/2/11, Joint NHS Privatisation Research Unit, *The NHS Privatisation Experience*, 16, 19–31.
34. MRC, MSS.389/PUB/85, NHS Privatisation Research Unit, *Tender Tactics: A Negotiators' Guide to Privatisation in the NHS* (1991).
35. MRC, MSS.229/CO/P/2/11, Joint NHS Privatisation Research Unit, *The NHS Privatisation Experience*, 4.
36. This paragraph's comments on Barking Hospital are drawn from Coyle, *Dirty Business*, 7–8; Steve Vines, 'Cleaners Celebrate Second Year of Strike', *Guardian*, 17 March 1985, 2.

37. Thames News, 'Barking Hospital Cleaners Strike', 13 June 1984, https://www.youtube.com/watch?v=iigGOy3mTG4&list=PLrAOKtLlXAn-jF_bTvmQB-a7xmW7_8GQA&index=2.
38. MRC, 864/18, 'Photograph of Barking Strikers with Meet the Boss Leaflets', 1984.
39. 'Barking Hospital Contract Renewed', *Guardian*, 3 April 1985, 2.
40. Gallie, 'The Labour Force', in Halsey and Webb (eds), *Twentieth-Century British Social Trends*, 309.
41. Coyle, *Dirty Business*, quote on 25.
42. For a critical assessment of union strategy in these years, see Lister (ed.), *Cutting the Lifeline*, 103–5.
43. MRC, MSS.229/CO/P/2/11, Joint NHS Privatisation Research Unit, *The NHS Privatisation Experience*, 5.
44. Tory Reform Group, *High Noon in the National Health Service* (London: Tory Reform Group, 1984), quotes on 6, 21.
45. 'Contracted In', *The Economist*, 18 January 1986, 24.
46. Key Note Report, *Contract Cleaning: An Industry Sector Overview* (Key Note Publications, 1988), 18.
47. 'Monopoly Is Dead, Long Live Cartel?', *The Economist*, 26 May 1984, 24.
48. MRC, MSS.229/CO/P/2/11, Joint NHS Privatisation Research Unit, *The NHS Privatisation Experience*, 6.
49. Jane Griffiths, *Contract Cleaning: 2000 Market Report* (Key Note Publications, 2000), 1.
50. This paragraph draws on 'The NI Interview: The Health Workers of Hillingdon', *The New Internationalist*, October 1997, 31; 'Striking Cleaner Goes Back to Work After Five Years Waiting', *This Is Local London*, 1 November 2000, https://www.thisislocal-london.co.uk/news/120552.striking-cleaner-goes-back-to-work-after-five-years-waiting/.
51. This stance caused tensions between the Hillingdon strikers and UNISON; see MRC, 601/D/2/4/10, 'A Special Appeal to All Our Supporters!', 9 March 1998.
52. For '24 hours to save the NHS', see Nigel Crisp, *24 Hours to Save the NHS: The Chief Executive's Account of Reform 2000 to 2006* (Oxford: Oxford University Press, 2011).
53. Tony Blair, *Let Us Face the Future – the 1945 Anniversary Lecture* (London: Fabian Society, 1995), 4. For histories of New Labour, see Steven Fielding, *The Labour Party: Continuity and Change in the Making of 'New Labour'* (Basingstoke: Palgrave Macmillan, 2003); Richard Carr, *March of the Moderates: Bill Clinton, Tony Blair, and the Rebirth of Progressive Politics* (London: I.B. Tauris, 2019).
54. Anthony Giddens, *The Third Way: The Renewal of Social Democracy* (Cambridge: Polity Press, 1998).
55. Philip G. Cerny and Mark Evans, 'Globalisation and Public Policy Under New Labour', *Policy Studies* 25, no. 1 (2004): 51–65; Helen McCarthy, *Double Lives: A History of Working Motherhood* (London: Bloomsbury, 2020), 323–54.
56. Stuart Hall, 'New Labour's Double-Shuffle', *Soundings* 2003, no. 24 (2003): 10–24.
57. For New Labour and the NHS, see Nick Bosanquet, 'The Health and Welfare Legacy', in Anthony Seldon (ed.), *Blair's Britain, 1997–2007* (Cambridge: Cambridge University Press, 2007), 385–407; Carol Propper and Mary-Anne Venables, 'An Assessment of Labour's Record on Health and Healthcare', *Oxford Review of Economic Policy* 29, no. 1 (2013): 203–26.
58. Mark Bevir, *New Labour: A Critique* (London: Routledge, 2005), especially 29–53. Sutcliffe-Braithwaite, *Class, Politics, and the Decline of Deference*, 173–202.
59. Gordon Brown, 'Speech at Social Market Foundation', 20 March 2002, https://www.ukpol.co.uk/gordon-brown-2002-speech-at-social-market-foundation/.

60. This paragraph's comments on NHS spending draw on King's Fund, 'How Much Has Been Spent on the NHS Since 2005?', 2010, https://www.kingsfund.org.uk/projects/general-election-2010/money-spent-nhs; Nicholas Timmins, *The Most Expensive Breakfast in History: Revisiting the Wanless Review 20 Years On* (London: Health Foundation, 2021); Office of Health Economics, *OHE Guide to UK Health and Health Care Statistics*, 45; Bank of England, 'A Millennium of Macroeconomic Data'.
61. This paragraph's comments on NHS employment numbers draw from Office of Health Economics, *OHE Guide to UK Health and Health Care Statistics*, 81; Nuffield Trust, 'The NHS Is One of the World's Largest Employers'.
62. This paragraph draws on Robert Steinbrook, 'Saying No Isn't NICE – The Travails of Britain's National Institute for Health and Clinical Excellence', *New England Journal of Medicine* 359, no. 19 (2008): 1977–81, quotes on 1979, 1977.
63. King's Fund, *A High-Performing NHS?: A Review of Progress 1997–2010* (2010), https://www.kingsfund.org.uk/sites/default/files/high-performing-nhs-progress-review-1997-2010-ruth-thorlby-jo-maybin-kings-fund-april-2010_0.pdf, 15.
64. NHS Direct, 'History of NHS Direct' https://web.archive.org/web/20081217040304/http://www.nhsdirect.nhs.uk/article.aspx?name=HistoryOfNHSDirect.
65. BBC News, 'Public Given Say on NHS Reforms', 28 October 2005, https://www.bbc.co.uk/news/1/hi/health/4385034.stm.
66. National Centre for Social Research, *British Social Attitudes: The 27th Report: Exploring Labour's Legacy* (London: SAGE, 2010), 73–102.
67. Tony Blair, *A Journey* (London: Arrow, 2011), 283.
68. Klein, *New Politics of the NHS*, 210.
69. David Osborne and Ted Gaebler, *Reinventing Government: How the Entrepreneurial Spirit Is Transforming the Public Sector* (New York: Plume, 1992).
70. Christopher Hood, 'Gaming in Targetworld: The Targets Approach to Managing British Public Services', *Public Administration Review* 66, no. 4 (2006): 515–21.
71. Eve Worth, *The Welfare State Generation: Women, Agency and Class in Britain since 1945* (London: Bloomsbury, 2022), 111–35, statistic on 112. See also Gingrich, *Making Markets in the Welfare State*, 79–130.
72. For continuities between the Conservatives and New Labour in administering the NHS, see Carol Propper, 'Competition in Health Care: Lessons from the English Experience', *Health Economics, Policy and Law* 13, no. 3/4 (2018): 492–508.
73. From the 1970s, feminists critiqued the patriarchal assumptions of the postwar welfare state; see, for instance, Elizabeth Wilson, *Women and the Welfare State* (London: Tavistock Publications, 1977). For women and New Labour, see essays in Claire Annesley, Francesca Gains and Kirstein Rummery (eds), *Women and New Labour: Engendering Politics and Policy?* (Bristol: Policy Press, 2007).
74. Colm Murphy, *Futures of Socialism: 'Modernisation', the Labour Party and the British Left, 1973–1997* (Cambridge: Cambridge University Press, 2023), 123–51.
75. Webster, *The National Health Service: A Political History*, 240–4.
76. Department of Health, *The NHS Plan. A Plan for Investment. A Plan for Reform* (London: HMSO, 2000), quotes on 10, 26.
77. Department of Health, *Delivering the NHS Plan: Next Steps on Investment, Next Steps on Reform* (London: TSO, 2002); Nicholas Mays, Anna Dixon and Lorelei Jones (eds), *Understanding New Labour's Market Reforms of the English NHS* (London: The King's Fund, 2011), especially 6–9.
78. 'How Firebrand Milburn Became a Model Manager', *Guardian*, 7 May 2001, https://www.theguardian.com/society/2001/may/07/nhsstaff.health.
79. Department of Health, *For the Benefit of Patients: A Concordat with the Private and Voluntary Health Care Provider Sector* (London: HMSO, 2000).

80. Mays, Dixon and Jones (eds), *Understanding New Labour's Market Reforms*, 16–29; Mold, *Making the Patient-Consumer*, 169–91.
81. Angela Coulter, 'What Do Patients and the Public Want from Primary Care?', *British Medical Journal* 331, no. 7526 (2005): 1119–201.
82. Will Bartlett et al, 'Provider Diversity in the NHS: Impact on Quality and Innovation', 2011, https://centaur.reading.ac.uk/24490/, statistic on 102.
83. Stephen Williams and R.H. Fryer, *Leadership and Democracy: The History of The National Union of Public Employees. Volume 2, 1928–1993* (London: Lawrence & Wishart, 2011), 544–6.
84. Coyle, *Dirty Business*, 30.
85. Griffiths, *Contract Cleaning: 2000 Market Report*, 51.
86. Jane Broadbent, Jas Gill and Richard Laughlin, *The Private Finance Initiative in the National Health Service: Nature, Emergence and the Role of Management Accounting in Decision Making and Post-Decision Project Evaluation* (London: CIMA, 2004), 17–21; James Meek, *Private Island: Why Britain Now Belongs to Someone Else* (London: Verso, 2014). For the export of PFI, see Chris Holden, 'Exporting Public–Private Partnerships in Healthcare: Export Strategy and Policy Transfer', *Policy Studies* 30, no. 3 (2009): 313–32.
87. 'Building Anxiety', *Health Service Journal* 109, no. 5644 (1999): 13–14, 16, quote on 13.
88. The King's Fund, *An Independent Audit of the NHS Under Labour (1997–2005)* (London: King's Fund, 2005), 66.
89. Andrew Walsh, 'A Legal Perspective on Risk Management in Public–Private Partnership', in Akintola Akintoye, Matthias Beck and Cliff Hardcastle (eds), *Public–Private Partnerships: Managing Risks and Opportunities* (Oxford: Blackwell Science, 2004), 158–9.
90. HMSO, *Health and Medicines Act* (London: HMSO, 1988), 5–8.
91. House of Commons Health Committee, *NHS Charges: Third Report of Session 2005–06* (London: HMSO, 2006), 35–7.
92. Adam Kay, *This Is Going To Hurt: Secret Diaries of a Junior Doctor* (London: Picador, 2018), 81.
93. NHS Estates, *Design Guide: The Design of Hospital Main Entrances* (London: HMSO, 1993), 41.
94. This paragraph draws from Ian Martin, 'Postcards from an Accidental Inpatient', *Building Design*, 20 October 2006, 12–13.
95. The remainder of this paragraph's comments on PFI draws from HM Treasury, 'Private Finance Initiative and Private Finance 2 Projects: 2015 Summary Data', 2016; 'Death Knell Sounded for PFI Contracts', *Financial Times*, 30 October 2018, 8; John Appleby, 'Making Sense of PFI', Nuffield Trust, 2017, https://www.nuffieldtrust.org.uk/resource/making-sense-of-pfi.
96. 'Flagship PFI Hospital "Technically Bankrupt"', *Guardian*, 16 December 2005, https://www.theguardian.com/uk/2005/dec/16/publicservices.topstories3. See also Jane Lethbridge, 'Public Enterprises in the Healthcare Sector – A Case Study of Queen Elizabeth Hospital, Greenwich, England', *Journal of Economic Policy Reform* 17, no. 3 (2014): 224–35.
97. Allyson Pollock and David Price, 'PFI and the National Health Service in England' (2013), https://www.allysonpollock.com/wp-content/uploads/2013/09/AP_2013_Pollock_PFILewisham.pdf, statistic on 9.
98. Gordon Brown, *A Modern Agenda for Prosperity and Social Reform* (London: Social Market Foundation, 2004), 27–8. The National Audit Office's criticism of the costs of PFI led to its abandonment; see National Audit Office, 'PFI and PFI2', 2018.

99. For PFI design as a typology, see Owen Hatherley, 'The Death and Life of PFI Urbanism: Vagaries of Style and Politics in British Cities, 2009–Present' in Juliet Odgers, Mhairi McVicar and Stephen Kite (eds), *Economy and Architecture* (Abingdon: Routledge, 2015), 191–203.
100. Architects complained about the apathy of the Royal Institute of British Architects (RIBA) towards PFI design; see 'RIBA Must Take On PFI Right Now', *Building Design*, 11 October 2002, 6.
101. Prince Charles's involvement provoked consternation among architects; see 'Charles: Prognosis on NHS "Tsar"', *Architects' Journal* 214 (2001), 4; For *The Times* quote, see 'Bad Health', *The Times*, 15 October 2001, 19.
102. 'Doubts Over PFI Hospitals', *Building Design*, 22 September 2000, 5.
103. MRC, 11/2/9/3/1-6, UNISON, *The PFI Experience: Voices from the Frontline* (London: UNISON, 2003), 10–12.
104. 'Doubts Over PFI Hospitals', *Building Design*.
105. For problems with Wonford Hospital and other NHS buildings, see 'Falling-Down Sickness', *The Economist*, 12 September 1987, 28, 31–2.
106. By the end of the Labour government, public sector procurement broadly delivered projects on time and under budget to the same extent as the private sector; see Paul Hare, 'PPP and PFI: The Political Economy of Building Public Infrastructure and Delivering Services', *Oxford Review of Economic Policy* 29, no. 1 (2013): 95–112, especially 108.
107. Matthew G. Dunnigan and Allyson M. Pollock, 'Downsizing of Acute Inpatient Beds Associated with Private Finance Initiative: Scotland's Case Study', *British Medical Journal* 326, no. 7395 (2003): 905; 'PFI Doubts as Hospital Runs Out of Beds', *Building Design*, 20 July 2001, 4.
108. Office of Health Economics, *OHE Guide to UK Health and Health Care Statistics*, 102.
109. The King's Fund, 'NHS Hospital Bed Numbers: Past, Present, Future', 2021, https://www.kingsfund.org.uk/publications/nhs-hospital-bed-numbers.
110. The following comments on the Cumberland Infirmary's lack of space are drawn from 'Inspectors Slam PFI Hospital in Report', *Guardian*, 27 February 2003, 11.
111. MRC, 11/2/9/3/1-6, John Lister, *PFI in the NHS: A Dossier* (2001).
112. MRC, 854/1/2/17, 'Oxford TUC stickers', 2005.
113. This paragraph's comments on the Royal Liverpool University Hospital draw from 'Remembering Sam Semoff', *Open Democracy*, 2018, https://www.opendemocracy.net/en/ournhs/remembering-sam-semoff-american-in-exile-fighting-to-defend-nhs/; 'Royal Liverpool Hospital Plan Wins High Court Battle but Faces New Challenge', *Liverpool Echo*, 17 November 2010, https://www.liverpoolecho.co.uk/news/liverpool-news/royal-liverpool-hospital-plan-wins-3390675.
114. On Carillion, see National Audit Office, *Investigation into the Government's Handling of the Collapse of Carillion* (London: National Audit Office, 2018).
115. Klein, *New Politics of the NHS*, 305.
116. 'Inside Fermanagh's State of the Art Hospital', BBC News, 15 June 2012, https://www.bbc.co.uk/news/uk-northern-ireland-18443335.
117. 'Trust Unveils What Single Bedrooms Will Look Like in the New Royal', *Building Better Healthcare*, 18 April 2016, https://www.buildingbetterhealthcare.com/news/article_page/Trust_unveils_what_single_bedrooms_will_look_like_in_the_new_Royal/117440.
118. Youseff El-Gingihy, *How to Dismantle the NHS in 10 Easy Steps* (Winchester: Zero Books, 2015), 17–18.
119. For the debate about single rooms in the NHS, see NHS Estates, *Exploring the Patient Environment* (London: HMSO, 2004), especially 4–5 for Ulrich's views.

120. Sam Nahas et al, 'Patient Experience in Single Rooms Compared with the Open Ward for Elective Orthopaedic Admissions', *Musculoskeletal Care* 14, no. 1 (2016): 57–61, especially 57.
121. This paragraph draws from NHS Estates, *The Architectural Healthcare Environment and Its Effects on Patient Health Outcomes* (London: HMSO, 2003), especially 13–14.
122. For further debate, see Hugh Pennington and Chris Isles, 'Should Hospitals Provide All Patients with Single Rooms?', *British Medical Journal* 347, no. 7927 (2013): 18–19.
123. For LIFT, see 'Long-Term Cure', *Building Design*, 10 September 2004, 18–21.
124. The remainder of this paragraph draws on Amion Consulting, 'The Impact of the Local Improvement Finance Trust Programme' (London: Community Health Partnerships, 2014), 3–4, 7. For the Wilberforce Centre, see HLM Architects, 'Case Study: Wilberforce', https://hlmarchitects.com/projects/wilberforce/.
125. HMSO, *Health and Social Care Act* (London: HMSO, 2012).
126. Colin Leys and Stewart Player, *The Plot Against the NHS* (London: Merlin Press, 2011); Jacky Davis and Raymond Tallis (eds), *NHS SOS: How the NHS Was Betrayed – And How We Can Save It* (London: Oneworld, 2013); Alyson Pollock, *The End of the NHS* (London: Verso, 2019).
127. The figures on private sector involvement in the rest of this paragraph draw from Helen Buckingham and Mark Dayan, 'Privatisation in the English NHS: Fact or Fiction?', The Nuffield Trust, 2019, https://www.nuffieldtrust.org.uk/news-item/privatisation-in-the-englishnhs-fact-or-fiction.
128. Kate Bayliss, 'Can England's National Health System Reforms Overcome the Neoliberal Legacy?', *International Journal of Health Services* 52, no. 4 (2022): 480–91, quote on 481.
129. Nick Krachler and Ian Greer, 'When Does Marketisation Lead to Privatisation? Profit-making in English Health Services After the 2012 Health and Social Care Act', *Social Science & Medicine* 124 (2015): 215–23.
130. Katey Logan, 'Customers Who Don't Buy Anything! The Introduction of Free Dispensing at Boots the Chemists', in Crane and Hand (eds), *Posters, Protests, and Prescriptions*, 150–74, quote on 150.
131. John Appleby and Sally Gainsbury, 'The Past, Present and Future of Government Spending on the NHS', The Nuffield Trust, 2022, https://www.nuffieldtrust.org.uk/news-item/the-past-present-and-future-of-government-spending-on-the-nhs.
132. 'NHS Commissioners Are Ignoring Guidelines by Rationing Cataract Surgery', *British Medical Journal*, 2019, https://www.bmj.com/company/newsroom/nhs-commissioners-are-ignoring-guidelines-by-rationing-cataract-surgery/.

CHAPTER 8 BIRTHDAYS AND THE ENDURANCE OF SOCIAL DEMOCRACY

1. The comments on the Ellesmere protest draw from the BBC documentary programme *Can You Afford the Doctor? Life Before the NHS* (1988), found in WC, 1463V. For the politics of hospital closures, see Ellen Stewart, Kathy Dodworth and Angelo Ercia, 'The Everyday Work of Hospital Campaigns: Public Knowledge and Activism in the UK's National Health Services', in Crane and Hand (eds), *Posters, Protests, and Prescriptions*, 103–24.
2. The wider meanings of NHS anniversaries are understudied, but they have been used as a device to demonstrate policy changes over time; see Martin Powell, 'Exploring 70 Years of the British National Health Service through Anniversary Documents', *International Journal of Health Policy Management* 7, no. 7 (2018): 574–80.
3. An 'invented tradition' is a set of practices which inculcate values and behaviour through repetition, which implies continuity with the past; Eric Hobsbawm,

'Inventing Traditions', in Eric Hobsbawm and Terence Ranger (eds), *The Invention of Tradition* (Cambridge: Cambridge University Press, 2012), 1–14.

4. Local variety continued: the government's involvement did not amount to a rigid 'state-sponsored history'. For discussion of the term, see Berber Bevernage and Nico Wouters, 'State-Sponsored History after 1945: An Introduction', in Berber Bevernage and Nico Wouters (eds), *The Palgrave Handbook of State-Sponsored History after 1945* (London: Palgrave Macmillan, 2017), 1–36.
5. Peter Burke, 'Co-memorations. Performing the Past', in Karin Tilmans, Frank van Vree and Jay M. Winter (eds), *Performing the Past: Memory, History, and Identity in Modern Europe* (Amsterdam: Amsterdam University Press, 2010), 105–18.
6. Raphael Samuel, *Theatres of Memory. Volume 1: Past and Present in Contemporary Culture* (London: Verso, 1994), quote on 25. See also Peter Mandler, *History and National Life* (London: Profile, 2002), 93–142; Laura Carter, *Histories of Everyday Life: The Making of Popular Social History in Britain, 1918–1979* (Oxford: Oxford University Press, 2021).
7. Jon Lawrence notes the continued existence of a 'vernacular social democracy' in the twenty-first century; see 'Vernacular Social Democracy and the Politics of Labour', *Renewal* 28, no. 3 (2020): 38–42.
8. NA, MH 55/2205, 'Tenth Anniversary of National Health Service', 1958.
9. NA, MH 55/2205, 'Minister of Health's Message', 1958.
10. Comments on the 1968 conference are drawn from NA, MH 77/243, 20th Anniversary, Minutes of Proceedings, First Day. For Jennie Lee, see Jennie Lee, *My Life with Nye* (London: Cape, 1980).
11. Local and national newspapers did often mark notable NHS anniversaries; see, for instance, 'Health Service 'Birthday'', *Skegness Standard*, 9 July 1958, 1.
12. 'Birthday Lunch for the NHS', *Daily Telegraph*, 1 June 1978, 11.
13. 'Callaghan Appeals for End to Strikes in Health Service', *Daily Telegraph*, 6 July 1978, 6.
14. NA, BN 10/137, 'Cardiac Arrest Team', 'Geriatric Care', 'Blood Grouping in Laboratory', 'Child Nursing'.
15. MRC, 1179/4/3/22, Fightback, 'Special: NHS 30th Anniversary Flyer', 1978.
16. MRC, MSS.292D/847.01/1, TUC, 'NHS Day Press Conference – July 5', 28 June 1984.
17. MRC, MSS.292D/847.01/1, NUPE Press Release, 2 July 1984.
18. MRC, MSS.292D/847.01/1, N.H.S. Day Gala Evening Flyer, 1984.
19. MRC, MSS.292D/847.01/1, TUC, 'NHS Campaign', 25 October 1984.
20. This paragraph draws from MRC, MSS.292D/847.01/1, Minutes of the TUC Health Services Committee, 11 December 1984.
21. See MRC, MSS.292D/847.01/1, P.S. Armitage to Martin Jacques, 28 February 1985.
22. This paragraph draws from MRC, MSS.292D/847.01/2, Minutes of the TUC Health Services Committee, 24 October 1985 and 26 June 1986.
23. MRC, MSS.292D/847.01/2, NHS Day '86 Flyer (1986).
24. Kevin Hickson (ed.), *Neil Kinnock: Saving the Labour Party?* (London: Routledge, 2022).
25. CCA, KNNK 11/1/1, 'Speech to Socialist Health Association', 5 November 1983; 'Statement on Health', 4 June 1987.
26. CCA, KNNK 11/1/16, 'Programme Sunday 3 July', 1988.
27. This paragraph's comments on the imagery of the event are drawn from MRC, 864/185, 'NHS 40th Birthday Slides', 1988.
28. CCA, KNNK 11/1/1, 'Speech by the Rt Hon Neil Kinnock MP at the Alexandra Palace' (3 July 1988).
29. House of Commons, 'NHS (40th Anniversary)', 13 July 1988, vol. 137, 282–3.

30. Office of Health Economics, *People as Patients and Patients as People* (London: OHE, 1988), 30–2.
31. '40th Anniversary Celebrations', *Gwent Gazette,* 14 July 1988, 3.
32. 'Birthday Support for Crisis-Hit NHS', *Reading Evening Post,* 16 June 1988, 7.
33. MRC, 864/185, 'NHS 40th Birthday Slides', 1988.
34. NA, JA53/885, 'NHS50 National Liaison Steering Group Members', 1998.
35. See, for example, NA, JA53/955, Richard Chew to Peter Addison-Child, 18 January 1998.
36. NA, JA53/893, 'The Vision Thing', 1998.
37. NA, JA53/893, 'Communicating the New NHS', 1998.
38. WC, Med.pam O/S WA500 1998N57n, NHS 50th Anniversary Logo: Application Guidelines', 1998.
39. NA, JA53/954, 'Branding Kit', 17 March 1998.
40. NA, JA53/959, 'Delivering Better Public Services – Fast Primary Care: Branding Issues, Discussion Paper' (March 1999).
41. For further discussion of the NHS logo, see Steve Mathieson, 'Brand Designs', *Health Service Journal* 114, no. 5893 (2004): 36–7; 'NHS Blue: The Colour of Universal Healthcare', Wellcome Collection, https://wellcomecollection.org/articles/WyjcSigAACsALDg1 (2018).
42. Sally Sheard, 'Epilogue: 'I'm afraid[,] there's no NHS', in Crane and Hand (eds), *Posters, Protests, and Prescriptions*, 323–31, quote on 324.
43. This paragraph draws on NA, JA53/955, 'Summary of National Activities June and July 1998'; NA, JA53/885, Minutes of National Liaison Steering Group Meeting, 21 July 1998.
44. 'The Big Picture', *NHS Magazine,* no. 13 (Summer 1998), 19–33.
45. The association of the NHS with hands began at its foundation, through assertions of its caring qualities. These themes were extended in the postwar years through cultural productions such as the long-running BBC television documentary about surgery, *Your Life in Their Hands* (which began in 1958).
46. WC, Med.pam O/S WA500 1998N57n, 'NHS 50th Anniversary: 50 Ways to Celebrate', 1998.
47. For a spread of the activities, see 'Here's Looking at You', *Nursing Times,* 15–21 July 1998, 12–13.
48. WC, Med.pam O/S WA500 1998N57n, 'Dear Colleague Letter', 1998.
49. NA, JA53/885, Minutes of National Liaison Steering Group Meeting, 21 July 1998.
50. BFI, BFI Identifier: 506685. Sarah Manwaring-White. *The Prescription (One of Three).* Directed by Jon Woods. Manchester: Granada Television, 1998.
51. 'NHS: Celebration for Bureaucrats', *Daily Mail,* 5 July 1988, 34.
52. Patrick Wright, *On Living in an Old Country: The National Past in Contemporary Britain* (London: Verso, 1985). Raphael Samuel disagreed with this interpretation in *Theatres of Memory*, 263–71.
53. For Labour and history, see Nathan Yeowell (ed.), *Rethinking Labour's Past* (London: I.B. Tauris, 2022).
54. NA, BN 10/136, Brian Abel-Smith, *National Health Service: The First Thirty Years* (London: HMSO, 1978).
55. NA, BN 10/136, Brian Abel-Smith, *National Health Service*, 7.
56. Quotes in this paragraph draw on TUC East Midlands Region, *Life Before the National Health Service* (Matlock: TUC East Midlands Region – Health Services Committee, 1988), 5, 20, 24.
57. CCA, KNNK 11/1/1, 'Speech to the Gwent Medical Society', 5 July 1985.
58. BFI, BFI Identifier: 505194. Twenty Twenty Television. *Pennies from Bevan.* Directed by John Brownlow. London: Twenty Twenty Television, 14 June 1998.

59. '20 Questions', *Nursing Times*, 1–7 July 1998, 28.
60. James E. Cronin, *New Labour's Pasts: The Labour Party and Its Discontents* (London: Routledge, 2004), 4. Its supporters made similar claims; see Philip Gould, *The Unfinished Revolution: How the Modernisers Saved the Labour Party* (London: Abacus, 1999).
61. Emily Robinson, *History, Heritage and Tradition in Contemporary British Politics: Past Politics and Present Histories* (Manchester: Manchester University Press, 2012), 122–47; Steven Fielding, 'New Labour and the Past', in Duncan Tanner, Pat Thane and Nick Tiratsoo (eds), *Labour's First Century* (Cambridge: Cambridge University Press, 2000), 367–92.
62. BOD, 'Speech by the Prime Minister the Rt Hon Tony Blair MP', 2 July 1998.
63. Gordon Brown, *My Life, Our Times* (London: Vintage, 2018), 10, 162.
64. WC, Med.pam O/S WA500 1998N57n, 'Fact Sheet No. 1 Trends 1948 – Present', 1998.
65. 'Times Change for the Better', *Liverpool Echo,* 4 July 1998, 5. Shortly after this event, doctors at Alder Hey were accused of removing hundreds of body parts from children without their parents' consent.
66. David G. Green, *Working-Class Patients and the Medical Establishment: Self-Help in Britain from the Mid-Nineteenth Century to 1948* (Aldershot: Gower, 1985), quotes in this paragraph on 4, 200. See also David G. Green, *Challenge to the NHS: A Study of Competition in American Health Care and the Lessons for Britain* (London: IEA, 1986).
67. CCA, KNNK 11/1/1, 'Speech by the Rt Hon Neil Kinnock MP at the Alexandra Palace'.
68. Directed by Geoffrey Sax. 'Friends of St. James', *The New Statesman*. Series 1, Episode 5. Yorkshire Television, 1987.
69. Paul Heaton, Ian Peter Cullimore, Anthony Key. 'Flag Day'. Universal Music, 1986.
70. WC, Med.pam O/S WA500 1998N57n, 'NHS 50th Anniversary: 50 Ways to Celebrate'.
71. Comments about the Lewisham pamphlet are drawn from WC, Lewisham Hospital NHS Trust, *A Rich Past . . . An Exciting Future: The Lewisham Hospital NHS Trust Celebrates 50 Years* (1998).
72. WC, Ruskin College Agewell Group, *From Cradle to Grave: 50 Years of the NHS. Memories of Before and After 1948* (1998).
73. Eve Worth argues that critical memories of pre-1948 health care were passed down through generations: see *The Welfare State Generation*, 18–22.
74. Oral historians have long examined the gaps between personal testimony and dominant historical accounts; see Luisa Passerini, *Memory and Totalitarianism* (Oxford: Oxford University Press, 1992).
75. TUC East Midlands Region, *Life Before the National Health Service*, 19.
76. For nostalgia, see Hannah Rose Woods, *Rule Nostalgia: A Backwards History of Britain* (London: Penguin, 2022); Hatherley, *Ministry of Nostalgia*; Agnes Arnold-Forster, 'Nostalgia', The Emotions Lab, https://emotionslab.org/emotion/nostalgia/.
77. WC, BBC, 'NHS At 50: The Ethical Age' (London: BBC Radio 4, 1998).
78. NA, JA53/893, 'The Vision Thing'.
79. 'Health Workers Talk about the Old Times', *Middlesex Chronicle*, 16 July 1998, 14.
80. Comments about the Bury St Edmunds events are drawn from 'Hospital Faces Welcome Cut on Red Ribbon Day', *Bury Free Press*, 10 July 1998, 27.
81. This paragraph draws on Baker, 'Beyond the Island Story?', especially 413–21; 'Was London Olympics Opening Ceremony A "Socialist" Spectacle?, *Forbes*, 30 July 2012, https://www.forbes.com/sites/parmyolson/2012/07/30/was-london-olympics-opening-ceremony-a-socialist-spectacle/?sh=7900ef227d9c.

82. 'In Full: Cameron on the NHS at 60', BBC News, 2008, http://news.bbc.co.uk/1/hi/uk_politics/7168355.stm.
83. For NHS funding and waiting lists in the 2010s, see John Appleby, 'Squeezed as Never Before', The King's Fund, 2015, https://www.kingsfund.org.uk/blog/2015/10/nhs-spending-squeezed-never; 'NHS Pressures in England: Waiting Times, Demand, and Capacity', House of Commons Library, 2019, https://commonslibrary.parliament.uk/nhs-pressures-in-england-waiting-times-demand-and-capacity/.
84. '2016 Vote Leave Video Is Compared to Current State of Brexit Britain', *London Economic*, 2022, https://www.thelondoneconomic.com/news/watch-2016-vote-leave-video-is-compared-to-current-state-of-brexit-britain-327338/. For the unreliability of the £350 million statistic mentioned later in this paragraph, see UK Statistics Authority (2016), https://uksa.statisticsauthority.gov.uk/news/uk-statistics-authority-statement-on-the-use-of-official-statistics-on-contributions-to-the-european-union/.
85. 'Nigel Farage's Anti-Immigrant Poster Reported to Police', *Guardian*, 16 June 2016, https://www.theguardian.com/politics/2016/jun/16/nigel-farage-defends-ukip-breaking-point-poster-queue-of-migrants.

CONCLUSION

1. Author's conversation with June Rosen, 5 September 2022; 'Girl Who Served Bevan Breakfast Marks Anniversary at First NHS Hospital', *Express & Star*, 5 July 2018, https://www.expressandstar.com/news/uk-news/2018/07/05/girl-who-served-bevan-breakfast-marks-anniversary-at-first-nhs-hospital/.
2. Westminster Abbey, *A Service to Celebrate the 70th Anniversary of the National Health Service* (London: Barnard & Westwood, 2018).
3. 'Hostile Environment: Anatomy of a Policy Disaster', *Guardian*, 27 August 2018, https://www.theguardian.com/uk-news/2018/aug/27/hostile-environment-anatomy-of-a-policy-disaster.
4. Polly Morland, *A Fortunate Woman: The Story of a Country Doctor* (London: Picador, 2022), quote on 141.
5. Data on COVID-19 is drawn from 'Mortality Analyses', Coronavirus Resource Center, Johns Hopkins University & Medicine, September 2022, https://coronavirus.jhu.edu/data/mortality; Veena Raleigh, 'Deaths from Covid-19 (Coronavirus): How Are They Counted and What Do They Show?', King's Fund, August 2022, https://www.kingsfund.org.uk/publications/deaths-covid-19.
6. Siva Anandaciva, 'Was Building the NHS Nightingale Hospitals Worth the Money?', King's Fund, May 2021, https://www.kingsfund.org.uk/blog/2021/04/nhs-nightingale-hospitals-worth-money.
7. 'Covid-19: Government's Use of VIP Lane for Awarding PPE Contracts Was Unlawful, Says Judge', *British Medical Journal*, 13 January 2022, https://www.bmj.com/content/376/bmj.o96.
8. Jacqui Wise, 'Covid-19: Ten Conservative MPs and Peers Referred Companies to "VIP Lane" That Won £1.6 billion of PPE Contracts', *British Medical Journal* 375, no. 816 (2021): 2825.
9. Owen Jones, 'While the UK's Key Workers Lack PPE, Ministers Clapping for Them Is an Insult', *Guardian*, 23 April 2020, https://www.theguardian.com/commentisfree/2020/apr/23/uk-key-workers-ppe-ministers-clapping-protect-nhs.
10. Anita Charlesworth, 'Years of Underinvestment Made the UK's Death Toll So Much Higher Than It Need Have Been', The Health Foundation, 19 February 2021, https://www.health.org.uk/news-and-comment/blogs/years-of-underinvestment-made-the-uks-death-toll-so-much-higher.

11. Centre for Cities, 'Cities Outlook: 2019', 2019, https://www.centreforcities.org/reader/cities-outlook-2019/a-decade-of-austerity; Mia Gray and Anna Barford, 'The Depth of the Cuts: The Uneven Geography of Local Government Austerity', *Cambridge Journal of Regions, Economy and Society* 11, no. 3 (2018): 541–63.
12. Michael Marmot et al, *Health Equity in England: The Marmot Review 10 Years On* (London: Institute of Health Equity, 2020).
13. Adam Tinson, 'What Geographic Inequalities in Covid-19 Mortality Rates and Health Can Tell Us about Levelling Up', The Health Foundation, July 2021, https://www.health.org.uk/news-and-comment/charts-and-infographics/what-geographic-inequalities-in-covid-19-mortality-rates-can-tell-us-about-levelling-up.
14. Grace Redhead and Jesse Olszynko-Gryn, 'Radical Object: The Black Report', *History Workshop Online*, 25 August 2020, https://www.historyworkshop.org.uk/radical-object-the-black-report/.
15. The Black Report gained notoriety as a Pelican paperback: Sir Douglas Black, Peter Townsend and Nick Davidson, *Inequalities in Health: The Black Report* (Harmondsworth: Penguin, 1982), quotes from 15–16.
16. Michael Marmot and Richard Wilkinson (eds), *Social Determinants of Health* (Oxford: Oxford University Press, 1999).
17. Institute of Fiscal Studies, 'The Health Impacts of Sure Start', 2021, https://ifs.org.uk/publications/health-impacts-sure-start.
18. See, for instance, Daniel Waterfield, 'To Save the NHS, Let's Stop Worshipping It Like a God', *Guardian*, 12 March 2015, https://www.theguardian.com/commentisfree/2015/mar/12/save-nhs-health-service; Theodore Dalrymple, 'It's Time We Stopped Treating the NHS Like a Religion', *Sun*, 5 July 2018, https://www.thesun.co.uk/news/6700162/its-time-we-stopped-treating-the-nhs-like-a-religion/.
19. Melissa Benn, *Life Lessons: The Case for a National Education Service* (London: Verso, 2018).
20. Tim Knox, 'How to Fix the NHS', *Spectator*, 26 July 2022, https://www.spectator.co.uk/article/how-to-fix-the-nhs/.
21. The Commonwealth Fund, *Mirror, Mirror on the Wall: How the U.S. Health Care System Compares Internationally* (New York: The Commonwealth Fund, 2010).
22. 'Three in Five Globally Say Their Healthcare System is Overstretched', Ipsos, 2022, https://www.ipsos.com/en/three-five-globally-say-their-healthcare-system-overstretched.
23. 'Decade of Neglect Means NHS Unable to Tackle Care Backlog, Report Says', *Guardian*, 12 December 2022, https://www.theguardian.com/society/2022/dec/12/decade-of-neglect-means-nhs-unable-to-tackle-care-backlog-report-says.
24. The rest of this paragraph's discussion of public opinion draws from Dan Wellings, 'Has the Public Fallen Out of Love With the NHS?', King's Fund, October 2022, https://www.kingsfund.org.uk/blog/2022/10/has-public-fallen-out-love-nhs.

SELECT BIBLIOGRAPHY

For a full bibliography, visit https://www.yalebooks.co.uk/page/detail/?k=9780300268270

ARCHIVES

APS	American Philosophical Society Archives, Philadelphia, PA, US
BA	Bristol Archives, Bristol, UK
BBCWAC	BBC Written Archives Centre, Reading, UK
BCA	Black Cultural Archives, London, UK
BFI	British Film Institute Archives, London, UK
BL	The British Library, London, UK
BOD	Bodleian Library Archives and Manuscripts, Oxford, UK
BUA	Bristol University Archives, Bristol, UK
CCA	Churchill College Archives, Cambridge, UK
CPA	Conservative Party Archive, Oxford, UK
DHC	Devon Heritage Centre, Exeter, UK
ERO	Essex Records Office, Chelmsford, UK
FDRL	Franklin D. Roosevelt Presidential Library, Hyde Park, NY, US
GA	Glamorgan Archives, Cardiff , UK
HHC	Hull History Centre, Hull, UK
LA	Lambeth Archives, London, UK
LMA	London Metropolitan Archives, London, UK
LRO	Liverpool Record Office, Liverpool, UK
LSE	London School of Economics Library Archives, London, UK
MOA	Mass Observation Archives, The Keep, Sussex, UK
MRC	Modern Records Centre, University of Warwick, Coventry, UK
NA	National Archives, Kew, London, UK
NARC	North Auckland Research Centre, Auckland, NZ
NUAA	Norwich Union/Aviva Archive, Norwich, UK
NVHK	New Victoria Hospital Records, Kingston, London, UK
NYAM	New York Academy of Medicine Archives, New York, NY, US
PHM	Labour Party Archive, People's History Museum, Manchester, UK
RAC	Rockefeller Archive Center, Sleepy Hollow, NY, US
RCP	Royal College of Physicians Archives, London, UK
TL	The Tamiment Library and Robert F. Wagner Archives, New York, NY, US
UCB	University of California Berkeley Archives, Berkeley, CA, US
UCSC	University of California Santa Cruz Special Collections, Santa Cruz, CA, US

ULA University of Liverpool Special Collections and Archives, Liverpool, UK
UMA University of Manchester Archives, Manchester, UK
WC Wellcome Collection, London, UK

CONVERSATIONS UNDERTAKEN BY THE AUTHOR

Fernando, Ossie. 4 May 2022.
Pizzey, Jack. 20 November 2017.
Rosen, June. 5 September 2022.
Vanson, Yvette. 25 October 2017.

PUBLISHED PRIMARY SOURCES

Abel-Smith, Brian. *The Hospitals, 1800–1948: A Study in Social Administration in England and Wales.* London: Heinemann, 1964.

Abel-Smith, Brian and Kathleen Gales. *British Doctors at Home and Abroad.* London: Codicote Press, 1964.

Abel-Smith, Brian and Peter Townsend. *The Poor and the Poorest.* London: G. Bell & Sons, 1965.

Arrow, Kenneth. 'Uncertainty and the Welfare Economics of Medical Care', *American Economic Review* 53, no. 5 (1963): 941–73.

Ascher, Kate. *The Politics of Privatisation: Contracting Out Public Services.* Basingstoke: Macmillan, 1987.

Auld, Philip. *Honour a Physician.* London: Hollis & Carter, 1959.

Balint, Michael. *The Doctor, His Patient and the Illness.* New York: International Universities Press, 1957.

Berger, John. *A Fortunate Man: The Story of a Country Doctor.* New York: Pantheon Books, 1967.

Bevan, Aneurin. *In Place of Fear.* London: Heinemann, 1952.

Black, Sir Douglas, Peter Townsend and Nick Davidson. *Inequalities in Health: The Black Report.* Harmondsworth: Penguin, 1982.

Blair, Tony. *A Journey.* London: Arrow, 2011.

Bowlby, John. *Maternal Care and Mental Health.* Geneva, Switzerland: World Health Organization, 1951.

Brown, Gordon. *My Life, Our Times.* London: Vintage, 2018.

Bryant, Arthur. *BUPA, 1947–1968: A History of the British United Provident Association.* London: BUPA, 1968.

Calnan, Michael, Sarah Cant and Jonathan Gabe. *Going Private: Why People Pay for Their Health Care.* Buckingham: Open University Press, 1993.

Campion, Sarah. *National Baby.* London: Ernest Benn, 1950.

Cartwright, Ann. *Human Relations and Hospital Care.* London: Routledge & Kegan Paul, 1964.

— *Patients and Their Doctors: A Study of General Practice.* New York: Atherton Press, 1967.

Castle, Barbara. *The Castle Diaries 1974–76.* London: Weidenfeld & Nicolson, 1980.

Clarke, Ken. *Kind of Blue: A Political Memoir.* London: Macmillan, 2016.

Coyle, Angela. *Dirty Business: Women's Work and Trade Union Organisation in Contract Cleaning.* Birmingham: West Midlands Low Pay Unit, 1986.

Cronin, A.J. *The Citadel.* London: Victor Gollancz, 1937.

Doll, Richard and Austin Bradford Hill. 'Smoking and Carcinoma of the Lung', *British Medical Journal* 2, no. 4682 (1950): 739–48.

Drabble, Margaret. *The Millstone.* London: Weidenfeld & Nicolson, 1965.

Eckstein, Harry. *The English Health Service: Its Origins, Structure, and Achievements.* Cambridge, MA: Harvard University Press, 1958.

Emecheta, Buchi. *Second-Class Citizen.* London: Allison & Busby, 1974.

Fellowship for Freedom in Medicine. *The Supply of Doctors and the Future of the British Medical Profession.* London: FFM, 1962.

Gemmill, Paul F. *Britain's Search for Health: The First Decade of the National Health Service.* Philadelphia: University of Pennsylvania Press, 1960.
Giddens, Anthony. *The Third Way: The Renewal of Social Democracy.* Cambridge: Polity Press, 1998.
Green, David G. *Working-Class Patients and the Medical Establishment: Self-Help in Britain from the Mid-Nineteenth Century to 1948.* Aldershot: Gower, 1985.
Halsey, A.H. and Josephine Webb (eds). *Twentieth-Century British Social Trends.* New York: St Martin's Press, 2000.
Hinks, M. Dorothy. *'The Most Cruel Absence of Care'.* London: King's Fund, 1974.
HMSO. *Health Centres: A Design Guide.* London: HMSO, 1970.
— *Health and Medicines Act.* London: HMSO, 1988.
— *Health and Social Care Act.* London: HMSO, 2012.
— *A Hospital Plan for England and Wales.* London: HMSO, 1962.
— *An Interim Report to the Consultative Council on Medical and Allied Services.* London: HMSO, 1920.
— *Mental Health Act.* London: HMSO, 1959.
— *National Health Service Act.* London: HMSO, 1946.
— *The National Health Service and Community Care Act.* London: HMSO, 1990.
— *National Health Service Reorganisation Act.* London: HMSO, 1973.
— *The National Insurance Act.* London: HMSO, 1911.
— *Report of the Committee to Consider the Future Numbers of Medical Practitioners and the Appropriate Intake of Medical Students.* HMSO: London, 1957.
— *Social Insurance and Allied Services.* London: HMSO, 1942.
Hollingsworth, Mark. *MPs for Hire: The Secret World of Political Lobbying.* London: Bloomsbury, 1991.
Institute of Economic Affairs. *Monopoly or Choice in Health Services?: A Symposium of Contrasting Approaches.* London: IEA, 1964.
James, Paul and William Tatton-Brown. *Hospitals: Design and Development.* London: Architectural Press, 1986.
Jefferys, Margot and Hessie Sachs. *Rethinking General Practice: Dilemmas in Primary Medical Care.* London: Tavistock Publications, 1983.
Jewkes, John and Sylvia Jewkes. *The Genesis of the British National Health Service.* Oxford: Blackwell, 1961.
Johnson, Donald McIntosh. *The British National Health Service: Friend or Frankenstein?.* London: Christopher Johnson, 1962.
Kay, Adam. *This Is Going to Hurt: Secret Diaries of a Junior Doctor.* London: Picador, 2018.
King Edward's Hospital Fund for London. *An Independent Audit of the NHS under Labour (1997–2005).* London: King's Fund, 2005.
— *Noise Control in Hospitals.* London: King's Fund, 1958.
Lee, Jennie. *My Life with Nye.* London: Cape, 1980.
Lees, D.S. *Health through Choice: An Economic Study of the British National Health Service.* London: IEA, 1961.
Lindsey, Almont. *Socialized Medicine in England and Wales: The National Health Service, 1948–1961.* Chapel Hill, NC: University of North Carolina Press, 1962.
Lister, John (ed.). *Cutting the Lifeline: The Fight for the NHS.* London: Journeyman, 1988.
Marmot, Michael, Jessica Allen, Tammy Boyce, Peter Goldblatt and Joana Morrison. *Health Equity in England: The Marmot Review 10 Years On.* London: Institute of Health Equity, 2020.
Marmot, Michael and Richard Wilkinson. *Social Determinants of Health.* Oxford: Oxford University Press, 1999.
Mass Observation. *Meet Yourself at the Doctor's.* London: Faber and Faber, 2009.
Moore, Benjamin. *The Dawn of the Health Age.* Edinburgh: Ballantyne Press, 1911.
Morland, Polly. *A Fortunate Woman: The Story of a Country Doctor.* London: Picador, 2022.

Murray, David Stark. *Health for All.* London: Victor Gollancz, 1942.
Nightingale, Florence. *Notes on Hospitals.* London: Longman, Green, Longman, Roberts, and Green, 1863.
Office of Health Economics. *OHE Guide to UK Health and Health Care Statistics.* London: OHE, 2013.
Owen, David. *In Sickness and in Health: The Politics of Medicine.* London: Quartet Books, 1976.
Pinker, Robert. *English Hospital Statistics, 1861–1938.* London: Heinemann, 1966.
Political and Economic Planning. *Report on the British Health Services: A Survey of the Existing Health Services in Great Britain with Proposals for Future Development.* London: PEP, 1937.
Powell, John Enoch. *A New Look at Medicine and Politics.* London: Pitman Medical, 1966.
Raphael, Winifred. *Patients and Their Hospitals.* London: King's Fund, 1969.
Reynolds, Z. Nia. *When I Came to England: An Oral History of Life in 1950s and 1960s Britain.* London: Black Stock, 2014.
Robb, Barbara. *Sans Everything: A Case to Answer.* London: Nelson, 1967.
Robb, Douglas. *BUPA 1968–1983: A Continuing History.* London: BUPA, 1984.
Roberts, Ffrangcon. *The Cost of Health.* London: Turnstile Press, 1952.
Seldon, Arthur. *After the N.H.S.* London: IEA, 1968.
Shute, Nevil. *The Far Country.* London: Heinemann, 1952.
Summerskill, Edith. *Wanted – Babies: A Trenchant Examination of a Grave National Problem.* London: Hutchinson, 1943.
Taylor, Stephen. *Good General Practice.* Oxford: Oxford University Press, 1955.
Thatcher, Margaret. *The Downing Street Years.* New York: HarperCollins, 1993.
Titmuss, Richard. *Commitment to Welfare.* London: Allen & Unwin, 1968.
— *Problems of Social Policy.* London: HMSO, 1950.
Titmuss, Richard and Brian Abel-Smith. *The Cost of the National Health Service in England and Wales.* Cambridge: Cambridge University Press, 1956.
TUC East Midlands Region. *Life Before the National Health Service.* Matlock: TUC East Midlands Region – Health Services Committee, 1988.
Tudor Hart, Julian. 'The Inverse Care Law', *The Lancet* 297, no. 7696 (1971): 405–12.
Webb, Sidney and Beatrice Webb. *The Break-up of the Poor Law: Being Part One of the Minority Report of the Poor Law Commission.* London: Longman, Green & Co., 1909.
Westminster Abbey. *A Service to Celebrate the 70th Anniversary of the National Health Service.* London: Barnard & Westwood, 2018.

SECONDARY SOURCES

Addison, Paul. *The Road to 1945: British Politics and the Second World War.* London: Quartet Books, 1977.
Arnold-Forster, Agnes. 'Racing Pulses: Gender, Professionalism and Health Care in Medical Romance Fiction', *History Workshop Journal* 91, no. 1 (2021): 157–81.
Babikian, Catherine. ' "Partnership not Prejudice": British Nurses, Colonial Students, and the National Health Service, 1948–1962', *Journal of British Studies* 60, no. 1 (2021): 140–68.
Bailkin, Jordanna. *The Afterlife of Empire.* Berkeley: University of California Press, 2012.
Baker, Catherine. 'Beyond the Island Story?: The Opening Ceremony of the London 2012 Olympic Games as Public History', *Rethinking History* 19, no. 3 (2015): 409–28.
Baldwin, Peter. *The Politics of Social Solidarity: Class Bases of the European Welfare State, 1875–1975.* Cambridge: Cambridge University Press, 1990.
Bar-Haim, Shaul. ' "The Drug Doctor": Michael Balint and the Revival of General Practice in Postwar Britain', *History Workshop Journal* 86, no. 1 (2018): 114–32.
Bartel, Fritz. *The Triumph of Broken Promises: The End of the Cold War and the Rise of Neoliberalism.* Cambridge, MA: Harvard University Press, 2022.

SELECT BIBLIOGRAPHY

Bates, Victoria. '"Humanizing" Healthcare Environments: Architecture, Art and Design in Modern Hospitals', *Design for Health* 2, no. 1 (2018): 5–19.

Beaumont, Caitríona. *Housewives and Citizens: Domesticity and the Women's Movement in England, 1928–64.* Manchester: Manchester University Press, 2013.

Beers, Laura. 'Labour's Britain, Fight for it Now!', *Historical Journal*, vol. 52, no. 3 (2009): 667–95.

Begley, Philip and Sally Sheard. 'McKinsey and the "Tripartite Monster": The Role of Management Consultants in the 1974 NHS Reorganisation', *Medical History* 63, no. 4 (2019): 390–410.

Berridge, Virginia. *Marketing Health: Smoking and the Discourse of Public Health in Britain 1945–2000.* Oxford: Oxford University Press, 2007.

Bevir, Mark. *New Labour: A Critique.* London: Routledge, 2005.

Birn, Anne-Emanuelle, Laura Nervi and Eduardo Siqueira. 'Neoliberalism Redux: The Global Health Policy of Cooptation in Latin America and Beyond', *Development and Change* 47, no. 4 (2016): 734–59.

Bivins, Roberta. *Contagious Communities: Medicine, Migration, and the NHS in Post-War Britain.* Oxford: Oxford University Press, 2015.

— 'Picturing Race in the British National Health Service, 1949–1988', *Twentieth Century British History* 28, no. 1 (2017): 83–109.

Black, Lawrence and Hugh Pemberton (eds). *An Affluent Society?: Britain's Post-War 'Golden Age' Revisited.* Aldershot: Ashgate, 2004.

Black, Lawrence, Hugh Pemberton and Pat Thane (eds). *Reassessing 1970s Britain.* Manchester: Manchester University Press, 2013.

Boughton, John. *Municipal Dreams: The Rise and Fall of Council Housing.* London: Verso, 2018.

Bowman, Andrew, Ismail Ertürk, Peter Folkman, Julie Froud, Colin Haslam, Sukhdev Johal, Adam Leaver, Mick Moran, Nick Tsitsianis and Karel Williams. *What a Waste: Outsourcing and How It Goes Wrong.* Manchester: Manchester University Press, 2015.

Brotherton, P. Sean. *Revolutionary Medicine: Health and the Body in Post-Soviet Cuba.* Durham, NC: Duke University Press, 2012.

Brown, Wendy. *Undoing the Demos: Neoliberalism's Stealth Revolution.* Cambridge, MA: MIT Press, 2015.

Calder, Angus. *The People's War: Britain, 1939–1945.* New York: Pantheon Books, 1969.

Carr, Richard. *March of the Moderates: Bill Clinton, Tony Blair, and the Rebirth of Progressive Politics.* London: I.B. Tauris, 2019.

Carter, Laura. *Histories of Everyday Life: The Making of Popular Social History in Britain, 1918–1979.* Oxford: Oxford University Press, 2021.

Chettiar, Teri. '"More than a Contract": The Emergence of a State-Supported Marriage Welfare Service and the Politics of Emotional Life in Post-1945 Britain', *Journal of British Studies* 55, no. 3 (2016): 566–91.

Chorev, Nitsan. *The World Health Organization between North and South.* Ithaca, NY: Cornell University Press, 2012.

Clark, Peder. '"Problems of Today and Tomorrow": Prevention and the National Health Service in the 1970s', *Social History of Medicine* 33, no. 3 (2020): 981–1000.

Cockett, Richard. *Thinking the Unthinkable: Think-Tanks and the Economic Counter-Revolution, 1931–1983.* London: HarperCollins, 1995.

Cohen, Deborah. *Family Secrets: Shame and Privacy in Modern Britain.* Oxford: Oxford University Press, 2013.

Cooper, Melinda. *Family Values: Between Neoliberalism and the New Social Conservatism.* New York: Zone Books, 2017.

Cowan, David. 'The "Progress of a Slogan": Youth, Culture, and the Shaping of Everyday Political Languages in Late 1940s Britain', *Twentieth Century British History* 29, no. 3 (2018): 435–58.

Crane, Jennifer. '"Save Our NHS": Activism, Information-Based Expertise and the "New Times" of the 1980s', *Contemporary British History* 33, no. 1 (2019): 52–74.
Crane, Jennifer and Jane Hand (eds). *Posters, Protests, and Prescriptions: Cultural Histories of the National Health Service in Britain.* Manchester: Manchester University Press, 2022.
Cronin, James E. *New Labour's Pasts: The Labour Party and Its Discontents.* London: Routledge, 2004.
Cueto, Marcos, Theodore M. Brown and Elizabeth Fee. *The World Health Organization: A History.* Cambridge: Cambridge University Press, 2019.
Cutler, Tony. 'Dangerous Yardstick? Early Cost Estimates and the Politics of Financial Management in the First Decade of the National Health Service', *Medical History* 47, no. 2 (2003): 217–38.
— 'Economic Liberal or Arch Planner? Enoch Powell and the Political Economy of the Hospital Plan', *Contemporary British History* 25, no. 4 (2011): 469–89.
Davies, Aled. *The City of London and Social Democracy: The Political Economy of Finance in Britain, 1959–1979.* Oxford: Oxford University Press, 2017.
Davies, Aled, Ben Jackson and Florence Sutcliffe-Braithwaite. *The Neoliberal Age?: Britain since the 1970s.* London: UCL Press, 2021.
Davies, William. *The Limits of Neoliberalism: Authority, Sovereignty and the Logic of Competition.* London: SAGE, 2014.
Davis, Angela. *Modern Motherhood: Women and Family in England, 1945–2000.* Manchester: Manchester University Press, 2012.
Davis, Jacky and Raymond Tallis (eds). *NHS SOS: How the NHS Was Betrayed – and How We Can Save It.* London: Oneworld, 2013.
DeVane, Ed. 'Pilgrim's Progress: The Landscape of the NHS Hospital, 1948–70', *Twentieth Century British History* 32, no. 4 (2021): 534–52.
Digby, Anne. *The Evolution of British General Practice 1850–1948.* Oxford: Oxford University Press, 1999.
Doyle, Barry M. *The Politics of Hospital Provision in Early Twentieth-Century Britain.* London: Pickering & Chatto, 2014.
Edgerton, David. *The Rise and Fall of the British Nation: A Twentieth-Century History.* London: Allen Lane, 2018.
— *Science, Technology and British Industrial 'Decline'.* Cambridge: Cambridge University Press, 1996.
Edwards, Amy. '"Financial Consumerism": Citizenship, Consumerism and Capital Ownership in the 1980s', *Contemporary British History* 31, no. 2 (2017): 210–29.
Eley, Geoff. *Forging Democracy: The History of the Left in Europe, 1850–2000.* Oxford: Oxford University Press, 2002.
Esping-Andersen, Gøsta. *The Three Worlds of Welfare Capitalism.* Princeton, NJ: Princeton University Press, 1990.
Fair, Alistair. '"Modernization of Our Hospital System": The National Health Service, the Hospital Plan, and the "Harness" Programme, 1962–77', *Twentieth Century British History* 29, no. 4 (2018): 547–75.
Fielding, Steven, Peter Thompson and Nick Tiratsoo. *"England Arise!": The Labour Party and Popular Politics in 1940s Britain.* Manchester: Manchester University Press, 1995.
Finlayson, Geoffrey B. A. M. *Citizen, State, and Social Welfare in Britain 1830–1990.* Oxford: Oxford University Press, 1994.
Fontaine, Philippe. 'Blood, Politics, and Social Science: Richard Titmuss and the Institute of Economic Affairs, 1957–1973', *Isis* 93, no. 3 (2002): 401–34.
Fox, Daniel M. *Health Policies, Health Politics: The British and American Experience, 1911–1965.* Princeton, NJ: Princeton University Press, 1986.
Francis, Martin. 'The Labour Party: Modernisation and the Politics of Restraint', in Becky Conekin, Frank Mort and Chris Waters (eds), *Moments of Modernity: Reconstructing Britain, 1945–1964*, 152–70. New York: New York University Press, 1999.

Francis, Matthew. '"A Crusade to Enfranchise the Many": Thatcherism and the "Property-Owning Democracy"', *Twentieth Century British History* 23, no. 2 (2012): 275–97.
Fraser, Derek. *The Evolution of the British Welfare State: A History of Social Policy since the Industrial Revolution.* London: Palgrave, 2017.
Freeden, Michael. *Ideologies and Political Theory: A Conceptual Approach.* Oxford: Clarendon Press, 1996.
Garland, David. 'The Emergence of the Idea of the "Welfare State" in British Political Discourse', *History of the Human Sciences* 35, no. 1 (2022): 132–57.
Gilroy, Paul. *There Ain't No Black in the Union Jack: The Cultural Politics of Race and Nation.* London: Routledge, 2002.
Gingrich, Jane. *Making Markets in the Welfare State: The Politics of Varying Market Reforms.* Cambridge: Cambridge University Press, 2011.
Gorsky, Martin. 'The National Health Service 1948–2008: A Review of the Historiography', *Social History of Medicine* 21, no. 3 (2008): 437–60.
— 'The Political Economy of Health Care', in Mark Jackson (ed.), *The Oxford Handbook of the History of Medicine*, 429–49. Oxford: Oxford University Press, 2011.
Gorsky, Martin, John Mohan and Tim Willis. *Mutualism and Health Care: British Hospital Contributory Schemes in the Twentieth Century.* Manchester: Manchester University Press, 2006.
Gosling, George Campbell. *Payment and Philanthropy in British Healthcare, 1918–48.* Manchester: Manchester University Press, 2017.
Grandy, Christine. 'Cultural History's Absent Audience', *Cultural and Social History* 16, no. 5 (2019): 643–63.
Griffith, Ben, Steve Iliffe and Geof Rayner. *Banking on Sickness: Commercial Medicine in Britain and the USA.* London: Lawrence and Wishart, 1987.
Hall, Stuart. 'New Labour's Double-Shuffle', *Soundings* 2003, no. 24 (2004): 10–24.
— 'Racism and Reaction', in Stuart Hall, Sally Davidson, David Featherstone, Michael Rustin and Bill Schwartz (eds), *Selected Political Writings: The Great Moving Right Show and Other Essays*, 142–57. Durham, NC: Duke University Press, 2017.
Hardy, Anne. *Health and Medicine in Britain since 1860.* Basingstoke: Palgrave, 2001.
Harris, Jose. *William Beveridge: A Biography.* Oxford: Clarendon, 1997.
Harvey, David. *A Brief History of Neoliberalism.* Oxford: Oxford University Press, 2005.
Hatherley, Owen. *The Ministry of Nostalgia.* London: Verso, 2016.
Hayes, Nick. 'Did We Really Want a National Health Service? Hospitals, Patients and Public Opinions before 1948', *English Historical Review* 127, no. 526 (2012): 625–61.
Hayes, Nick and Barry M. Doyle. 'Eggs, Rags and Whist Drives: Popular Munificence and the Development of Provincial Medical Voluntarism between the Wars', *Historical Research* 86, no. 234 (2013): 712–40.
Haynes, Douglas M. *Fit to Practice: Empire, Race, Gender, and the Making of British Medicine, 1850–1980.* Rochester NY: University of Rochester Press, 2017.
Higgins, Joan. *The Business of Medicine: Private Health Care in Britain.* Basingstoke: Macmillan, 1988.
Hilton, Matthew. *Consumerism in Twentieth-Century Britain: The Search for a Historical Movement.* Cambridge: Cambridge University Press, 2003.
Hilton, Matthew, Chris Moores and Florence Sutcliffe-Braithwaite. 'New Times Revisited: Britain in the 1980s', *Contemporary British History* 31, no. 2 (2017): 145–65.
Hinton, James. *The Mass Observers: A History, 1937–1949.* Oxford: Oxford University Press, 2013.
Hobsbawm, Eric. *Age of Extremes: The Short Twentieth Century, 1914–1991.* London: Michael Joseph, 1994.
— 'Inventing Traditions', in Eric Hobsbawm and Terence Ranger (eds), *The Invention of Tradition*, 1–14. Cambridge: Cambridge University Press, 2012.
Hoffman, Beatrix. *Health Care for Some: Rights and Rationing in the United States since 1930.* Chicago: University of Chicago Press, 2012.

Hogg, Christine. *Patients, Power and Politics: From Patients to Citizens.* London: SAGE, 1999.
Holland, Patricia, Hugh Chignell and Sherryl Wilson. *Broadcasting and the NHS in the Thatcherite 1980s: The Challenge to Public Service.* London: Palgrave Macmillan, 2013.
Jackson, Ben. 'Richard Titmuss versus the IEA: The Transition from Idealism to Neo-Liberalism in British Social Policy', in Lawrence Goldman (ed.), *Welfare and Social Policy in Britain since 1870: Essays in Honour of Jose Harris*, 147–61. Oxford: Oxford University Press, 2019.
— 'Social Democracy', in Michael Freeden, Lyman Tower Sargent and Marc Stears (eds), *The Oxford Handbook of Political Ideologies*, 348–63. Oxford: Oxford University Press, 2013.
Jackson, Ben and Robert Saunders (eds). *Making Thatcher's Britain.* Cambridge: Cambridge University Press, 2012.
Jacobs, Lawrence R. *The Health of Nations: Public Opinion and the Making of American and British Health Policy.* Ithaca, NY: Cornell University Press, 1993.
Jarausch, Konrad H. *Out of Ashes: A New History of Europe in the Twentieth Century.* Princeton, NJ: Princeton University Press, 2015.
Johnson, Jennifer. *The Battle for Algeria: Sovereignty, Health Care, and Humanitarianism.* Philadelphia: University of Pennsylvania Press, 2016.
Jones, Harriet and Michael Kandiah. *The Myth of Consensus: New Views on British History, 1945–64.* Basingstoke: Macmillan, 1996.
Judt, Tony. *Ill Fares the Land.* New York: Penguin Books, 2010.
— *Postwar: A History of Europe since 1945.* London: Heinemann, 2005.
Kavanagh, Dennis and Peter Morris. *Consensus Politics from Attlee to Thatcher.* Oxford: Blackwell, 1989.
Kefford, Alistair. 'Housing the Citizen-Consumer in Post-war Britain: The Parker Morris Report and the Even Briefer Life of Social Democracy', *Twentieth Century British History* 29, no. 2 (2018): 225–58.
Kettunen, Pauli, Saara Pellander and Miika Tervonen (eds). *Nationalism and Democracy in the Welfare State.* Cheltenham: Edward Elgar Publishing, 2022.
King, Laura. *Family Men: Fatherhood and Masculinity in Britain, c. 1914–1960.* Oxford: Oxford University Press, 2015.
Kisacky, Jeanne. *Rise of the Modern Hospital: An Architectural History of Health and Healing, 1870–1940.* Pittsburgh, PA: University of Pittsburgh Press, 2017.
Klein, Rudolf. *The New Politics of the NHS: From Creation to Reinvention*, 7th edn. Boca Raton, FL: CRC Press, 2013.
Kyiakides, Christopher and Satnam Virdee. 'Migrant Labour, Racism and the British National Health Service', *Ethnicity & Health* 8, no. 4 (2003): 283–305.
Kynaston, David. *Family Britain, 1951–57.* London: Bloomsbury, 2009.
Lawrence, Jon. *Me, Me, Me? The Search for Community in Post-War England.* Oxford: Oxford University Press, 2019.
Levene, Alysa, Martin A. Powell, John Stewart and Becky Taylor. *Cradle to Grave: Municipal Medicine in Interwar England and Wales.* Oxford: Peter Lang, 2011.
Lewis, Jane. *What Price Community Medicine?: The Philosophy, Practice and Politics of Public Health Since 1919.* Brighton: Wheatsheaf Books, 1986.
Leys, Colin and Stewart Player. *The Plot against the NHS.* London: Merlin Press, 2011.
Livingston, Julie. *Improvising Medicine: An African Oncology Ward in an Emerging Cancer Epidemic.* Durham, NC: Duke University Press, 2012.
Longpré, Nicole. '"An Issue That Could Tear Us Apart": Race, Empire, and Economy in the British (Welfare) State, 1968', *Canadian Journal of History* 46, no. 1 (2011): 63–95.
Lowe, Rodney. *The Welfare State in Britain since 1945.* Basingstoke: Macmillan, 2005.
Lyons, John F. *America in the British Imagination: 1945 to the Present.* New York: Palgrave Macmillan, 2013.

MacKillop, Eleanor, Sally Sheard, Philip Begley and Michael Lambert (eds). *The NHS Internal Market*. Liverpool: Department of Public Health and Policy, University of Liverpool, 2018.
Maier, Charles S. *In Search of Stability: Explorations in Historical Political Economy.* Cambridge: Cambridge University Press, 1987.
Mandler, Peter. *The Crisis of the Meritocracy: Britain's Transition to Mass Education since the Second World War.* Oxford: Oxford University Press, 2020.
— *History and National Life*. London: Profile, 2002.
McKibbin, Ross. *Class and Cultures: England, 1918–1951*. Oxford: Oxford University Press, 1998.
Meek, James. *Private Island: Why Britain Now Belongs to Someone Else.* London: Verso, 2014.
Mencher, Samuel. *Private Practice in Britain: The Relationship of Private Medical Care to the National Health Service*. London: G. Bell & Sons, 1967.
Millward, Gareth. *Sick Note: A History of the British Welfare State.* Oxford: Oxford University Press, 2022.
Mirowski, Philip and Dieter Plehwe (eds). *The Road from Mont Pèlerin: The Making of the Neoliberal Thought Collective.* Cambridge, MA: Harvard University Press, 2009.
Mohan, John. *A National Health Service? The Restructuring of Health Care in Britain since 1979.* Basingstoke: Macmillan, 1995.
Mold, Alex. *Making the Patient-Consumer: Patient Organisations and Health Consumerism in Britain.* Manchester: Manchester University Press, 2015.
— 'Repositioning the Patient: Patient Organizations, Consumerism, and Autonomy in Britain during the 1960s and 1970s', *Bulletin of the History of Medicine* 87, no. 2 (2013): 225–49.
Monnais-Rousselot, Laurence and David Wright, eds. *Doctors Beyond Borders: The Transnational Migration of Physicians in the Twentieth Century.* Toronto: University of Toronto Press, 2016.
Moore, Martin D. 'Waiting for the Doctor: Managing Time and Emotion in the British National Health Service, 1948–80', *Twentieth Century British History* 33, no. 2 (2022): 203–29.
Moran, Michael. *Governing the Health Care State: A Comparative Study of the United Kingdom, the United States and Germany*. Manchester: Manchester University Press, 1999.
Mort, Frank. 'The Permissive Society Revisited', *Twentieth Century British History* 22, no. 2 (2011): 269–98.
Moyn, Samuel. *The Last Utopia: Human Rights in History.* Cambridge, MA: Harvard University Press, 2010.
Mudge, Stephanie L. *Leftism Reinvented: Western Parties from Socialism to Neoliberalism.* Cambridge, MA: Harvard University Press, 2018.
Murphy, Colm. *Futures of Socialism: 'Modernisation', the Labour Party and the British Left, 1973–1997.* Cambridge: Cambridge University Press, 2023.
Nuttall, Jeremy and Hans Schattle (eds). *Making Social Democrats: Citizens, Mindsets, Realities: Essays for David Marquand.* Manchester: Manchester University Press, 2018.
Offer, Avner. 'The Market Turn: From Social Democracy to Market Liberalism', *Economic History Review* 70, no. 4 (2017): 1051–71.
O'Hara, Glen. *From Dreams to Disillusionment: Economic and Social Planning in 1960s Britain.* Basingstoke: Palgrave Macmillan, 2007.
Olszynko-Gryn, Jesse. 'The Feminist Appropriation of Pregnancy Testing in 1970s Britain', *Women's History Review* 28, no. 6 (2019): 869–94.
Omran, Abdel R. 'The Epidemiologic Transition: A Theory of the Epidemiology of Population Change', *The Milbank Quarterly* 83, no. 4 (2005): 731–57.
Ortolano, Guy. *Thatcher's Progress: From Social Democracy to Market Liberalism through an English New Town.* Cambridge: Cambridge University Press, 2019.

— *The Two Cultures Controversy: Science, Literature and Cultural Politics in Postwar Britain.* Cambridge: Cambridge University Press, 2009.

Owens, Deirdre Benia Cooper. *Medical Bondage: Race, Gender, and the Origins of American Gynecology.* Athens, GA: University of Georgia Press, 2017.

Packard, Randall. *A History of Global Health: Interventions into the Lives of Other Peoples.* Baltimore, MD: Johns Hopkins University Press, 2016.

Pedersen, Susan. *Family, Dependence, and the Origins of the Welfare State: Britain and France, 1914–1945.* Cambridge: Cambridge University Press, 1993.

Pelling, Henry. 'The Working Class and the Welfare State', in Henry Pelling (ed.), *Popular Politics and Society in Late Victorian Britain*, 1–18. London: Palgrave Macmillan, 1979.

Perry, Kennetta Hammond. *London Is the Place for Me: Black Britons, Citizenship, and the Politics of Race.* Oxford: Oxford University Press, 2015.

Phillips-Fein, Kim. *Invisible Hands: The Making of the Conservative Movement from the New Deal to Reagan.* New York: W.W. Norton, 2009.

Pickstone, John V. *Medicine and Industrial Society: A History of Hospital Development in Manchester and Its Region.* Manchester: Manchester University Press, 1985.

Pierson, Paul. *Dismantling the Welfare State?: Reagan, Thatcher, and the Politics of Retrenchment.* Cambridge: Cambridge University Press, 1994.

Polanyi, Karl. *The Great Transformation: The Political and Economic Origins of Our Time.* Boston, MA: Beacon Press, 1944.

Pollock, Allyson. *NHS PLC: The Privatisation of Our Health Care.* London: Verso, 2004.

Porter, Dorothy. *Health, Civilization, and the State: A History of Public Health from Ancient to Modern Times.* London: Routledge, 1999.

Porter, Roy. 'The Patient's View: Doing Medical History from Below', *Theory and Society* 14, no. 2 (1985): 175–98.

Quinton, Laura. 'Britain's Royal Ballet in Apartheid South Africa, 1960', *Historical Journal* 64, no. 3 (2021): 750–73.

Redhead, Grace. '"A British Problem Affecting British People": Sickle Cell Anaemia, Medical Activism and Race in the National Health Service, 1975–1993', *Twentieth Century British History* 32, no. 2 (1 June 2021): 189–211.

Renwick, Chris. *Bread for All: The Origins of the Welfare State.* London: Allen Lane, 2017.

Rieger, Bernhard. 'Making Britain Work Again: Unemployment and the Remaking of British Social Policy in the Eighties', *English Historical Review* 133, no. 562 (2018): 634–66.

Rivett, Geoffrey. *From Cradle to Grave: Fifty Years of the NHS.* London: King's Fund, 1998.

Robinson, Emily. *History, Heritage, and Tradition in Contemporary British Politics: Past Politics and Present Histories.* Manchester: Manchester University Press, 2012.

Robinson, Emily, Camilla Schofield, Florence Sutcliffe-Braithwaite and Natalie Tomlinson. 'Telling Stories about Post-war Britain: Popular Individualism and the "Crisis" of the 1970s', *Twentieth Century British History* 28, no. 2 (2017): 268–304.

Rodgers, Daniel T. *Age of Fracture.* Cambridge, MA: Belknap Press, 2011.

— *Atlantic Crossings: Social Politics in a Progressive Age.* Cambridge, MA: Harvard University Press, 1998.

Roemer, Milton. *National Health Systems of the World, Vol. 1, The Countries.* Oxford: Oxford University Press, 1991.

Rose, Sonya O. *Which People's War?: National Identity and Citizenship in Wartime Britain, 1939–1945.* Oxford: Oxford University Press, 2003.

Rosenberg, Charles E. *The Care of Strangers: The Rise of America's Hospital System.* New York: Basic Books, 1987.

Samuel, Raphael. *Theatres of Memory. Volume 1: Past and Present in Contemporary Culture.* London: Verso, 1994.

Sassoon, Donald. *One Hundred Years of Socialism: The West European Left in the Twentieth Century.* London: I.B. Tauris, 1996.

Saunders, Jack. 'Emotions, Social Practices and the Changing Composition of Class, Race and Gender in the National Health Service, 1970–79: "Lively Discussion Ensued"', *History Workshop Journal* 88, no. 1 (2019): 204–28.
Saunders, Robert. 'Crisis? What Crisis? Thatcherism and the Seventies', in Ben Jackson and Robert Saunders (eds), *Making Thatcher's Britain*, 25–42. Cambridge: Cambridge University Press, 2012.
Schofield, Camilla. *Enoch Powell and the Making of Postcolonial Britain.* Cambridge: Cambridge University Press, 2013.
Seaton, Andrew. '"Against the Sacred Cow": NHS Opposition and the Fellowship for Freedom in Medicine, 1948–72', *Twentieth Century British History* 26, no. 3 (2015): 424–49.
— 'The Gospel of Wealth and the National Health: The Rockefeller Foundation and Social Medicine in Britain's NHS, 1945–60', *Bulletin of the History of Medicine* 94, no. 1 (2020): 91–124.
Shapira, Michal. *The War Inside: Psychoanalysis, Total War, and the Making of the Democratic Self in Postwar Britain.* Cambridge: Cambridge University Press, 2013.
Sheard, Sally. 'A Creature of Its Time: The Critical History of the Creation of the British NHS', *Michael Quarterly* 8, no. 4 (2011): 428–41.
— *The Passionate Economist: How Brian Abel-Smith Shaped Global Health and Social Welfare.* Bristol: Policy Press, 2013.
Shepherd, John. *Crisis? What Crisis?: The Callaghan Government and the British 'Winter of Discontent'.* Manchester: Manchester University Press, 2013.
Shilliam, Robbie. *Race and the Undeserving Poor: From Abolition to Brexit.* Newcastle upon Tyne: Agenda Publishing, 2018.
Simpson, Julian. M. *Migrant Architects of the NHS: South Asian Doctors and the Reinvention of British General Practice (1940s–1980s).* Manchester: Manchester University Press, 2018.
Slobodian, Quinn. *Globalists: The End of Empire and the Birth of Neoliberalism.* Cambridge, MA: Harvard University Press, 2018.
Snow, Stephanie J. and Angela F. Whitecross. 'Making History Together: The UK's National Health Service and the Story of Our Lives since 1948', *Contemporary British History* 36, no. 3 (2022): 403–29.
Stedman Jones, Daniel. *Masters of the Universe: Hayek, Friedman, and the Birth of Neoliberal Politics.* Princeton, NJ: Princeton University Press, 2012.
Stevens, Rosemary. *Medical Practice in Modern England: The Impact of Specialization and State Medicine.* New Brunswick, NJ: Transaction, 2003.
Stewart, John. *The Battle for Health: A Political History of the Socialist Medical Association, 1930–51.* Aldershot: Ashgate, 1999.
— 'Ideology and Process in the Creation of the British National Health Service', *Journal of Policy History* 14, no. 2 (2002): 113–34.
Subramanian, Divya. 'The Townscape Movement and the Politics of Post-War Urbanism', *Twentieth Century British History* 32, no. 3 (2021): 392–415.
Sutcliffe-Braithwaite, Florence. *Class, Politics, and the Decline of Deference in England, 1968–2000.* Oxford: Oxford University Press, 2018.
— 'Neo-Liberalism and Morality in the Making of Thatcherite Social Policy', *Historical Journal* 55, no. 2 (2012): 497–520.
Tanner, Duncan. *Political Change and the Labour Party, 1900–1918.* Cambridge: Cambridge University Press, 1990.
Thane, Pat. *Foundations of the Welfare State.* London: Longman, 1996.
Thomas-Symonds, Nicklaus. *Nye: The Political Life of Aneurin Bevan.* London: I.B. Tauris, 2014.
Thomson, Mathew. *Lost Freedom: The Landscape of the Child and the British Post-War Settlement.* Oxford: Oxford University Press, 2013.
Timmins, Nicholas. *The Five Giants: A Biography of the Welfare State.* London: HarperCollins, 2001.

Tomes, Nancy. *Remaking the American Patient: How Madison Avenue and Modern Medicine Turned Patients into Consumers.* Chapel Hill, NC: University of North Carolina Press, 2016.
Tomlinson, Jim. 'Inventing "Decline": The Falling Behind of the British Economy in the Postwar Years', *Economic History Review* 49, no. 4 (1996): 731–57.
— 'Managing the Economy, Managing the People: Britain c.1931–70', *Economic History Review* 58, no. 3 (2005): 555–85.
— 'Tale of a Death Exaggerated: How Keynesian Policies Survived the 1970s', *Contemporary British History* 21, no. 4 (2007): 429–48.
Tooze, Adam. *The Deluge: The Great War and the Remaking of Global Order, 1916–1931.* London: Penguin, 2015.
Toye, Richard. *The Labour Party and the Planned Economy, 1931–1951.* Cambridge: Cambridge University Press, 2003.
Vargha, Dóra. *Polio across the Iron Curtain: Hungary's Cold War with an Epidemic.* Cambridge: Cambridge University Press, 2018.
Vernon, James. 'The Local, the Imperial and the Global: Repositioning Twentieth-Century Britain and the Brief Life of Its Social Democracy', *Twentieth Century British History* 21, no. 2 (2010): 404–18.
— *Modern Britain: 1750 to the Present.* Cambridge: Cambridge University Press, 2017.
Vinen, Richard. *Thatcher's Britain: The Politics and Social Upheaval of the Thatcher Era.* London: Simon & Schuster, 2009.
Waddington, Keir. 'Problems of Progress: Modernity and Writing the Social History of Medicine', *Social History of Medicine* 34, no. 4 (2021): 1053–67.
Wailoo, Keith. *Dying in the City of the Blues: Sickle Cell Anemia and the Politics of Race and Health.* Chapel Hill, NC: University of North Carolina Press, 2001.
Waters, Chris. '"Dark Strangers in Our Midst": Discourses of Race and Nation in Britain, 1947–1963', *Journal of British Studies* 36, no. 2 (1997): 207–38.
Webster, Charles (ed.). *Aneurin Bevan on the National Health Service.* Oxford: Wellcome Unit for the History of Medicine, 1991.
— *The Health Services since the War. Volume I. Problems of Health Care: The National Health Service before 1957.* London: HMSO, 1988.
— *The Health Services since the War. Volume II. Government and Health Care: The National Health Service 1958–1979.* London: HMSO, 1996.
— *The National Health Service: A Political History.* Oxford: Oxford University Press, 2002.
Webster, Wendy. *Englishness and Empire, 1939–1965.* Oxford: Oxford University Press, 2005.
Weisz, George. *Chronic Disease in the Twentieth Century: A History.* Baltimore, MD: Johns Hopkins University Press, 2014.
Wetherell, Sam. *Foundations: How the Built Environment Made Twentieth-Century Britain.* Princeton, NJ: Princeton University Press, 2020.
Whipple, Amy. 'Revisiting the "Rivers of Blood" Controversy: Letters to Enoch Powell', *Journal of British Studies* 48, no. 3 (2009): 717–35.
White, Alan. *Who Really Runs Britain?: The Private Companies Taking Control of Benefits, Prisons, Asylum, Deportation, Security, Social Care and the NHS*, updated edn. London: Oneworld, 2017.
Williams, Stephen and R.H. Fryer. *Leadership and Democracy: the History of The National Union of Public Employees. Volume 2, 1928–1993.* London: Lawrence & Wishart, 2011.
Williamson, Charlotte. *Towards the Emancipation of Patients: Patients' Experience and the Patient Movement.* Bristol: Policy Press, 2010.
Williamson, Clifford. 'The Quiet Time? Pay-beds and Private Practice in the National Health Service: 1948–1970', *Social History of Medicine* 28, no. 3 (2015): 576–95.
Willis, Julie, Philip Goad and Cameron Logan. *Architecture and the Modern Hospital, Nosokomeion to Hygeia.* Abingdon: Routledge, 2019.
Wills, Clair. *Lovers and Strangers: An Immigrant History of Post-War Britain.* London: Allen Lane, 2017.

Wilson, Dolly Smith. 'A New Look at the Affluent Worker: The Good Working Mother in Post-War Britain', *Twentieth Century British History* 17, no. 2 (2006), 206–29.
Wood, Bruce. *Patient Power?: The Politics of Patients' Associations in Britain and America.* Buckingham: Open University Press, 2000.
Woods, Hannah Rose. *Rule Nostalgia: A Backwards History of Britain.* London: Penguin, 2022.
Worth, Eve. *The Welfare State Generation: Women, Agency and Class in Britain since 1945.* London: Bloomsbury, 2022.
Wright, David, Nathan Flis and Mona Gupta. 'The "Brain Drain" of Physicians: Historical Antecedents to an Ethical Debate, c. 1960–79', *Philosophy, Ethics, and Humanities in Medicine* 24, no. 3 (2008): 1–8.
Wright, David, Sasha Mullally and Mary Colleen Cordukes. ' "Worse than Being Married": The Exodus of British Doctors from the National Health Service to Canada, c.1955–75', *Journal of the History of Medicine and Allied Sciences* 65, no. 4 (2010): 546–75.
Wright, Patrick. *On Living in an Old Country: The National Past in Contemporary Britain.* London: Verso, 1985.
Yeowell, Nathan (ed.). *Rethinking Labour's Past.* London: I.B. Tauris, 2022.
Zweiniger-Bargielowska, Ina. *Austerity in Britain: Rationing, Controls, and Consumption, 1939–1955.* Oxford: Oxford University Press, 2000.

INDEX

INDEX

INDEX